NURSING IN TODAY'S WORLD

Challenges, Issues, and Trends

Janice Rider Ellis, R.N., Ph.D.
Professor of Nursing
Shoreline Community College
Seattle, Washington

Celia Love Hartley, R.N., M.N.
Professor and Director of Nursing Education
Shoreline Community College
Seattle, Washington

with illustrations by
Kari Berger, B.A.
Bainbridge Island, Washington

NURSING IN TODAY'S WORLD

Challenges, Issues, and Trends

Fourth Edition

J.B. Lippincott Company
Philadelphia

New York   London   Hagerstown

Sponsoring Editor: David Carroll
Coordinating Editorial Assistant: Amy Stonehouse
Project Editor: Melissa McGrath
Indexer: Betty Herr Hallinger
Design Coordinator: Christopher Laird
Cover Designer: Lou Fuiano
Production Manager: Helen Ewan
Production Coordinator: Kathryn Rule
Compositor: Tapsco, Incorporated
Printer/Binder: R. R. Donnelley & Sons Company
Cover Printer: R. R. Donnelley & Sons Company

Fourth Edition

6 5 4 3 2

Library of Congress Cataloging in Publications Data

Ellis, Janice Rider.
    Nursing in today's world : challenges, issues, and trends / Janice Rider Ellis, Celia Love Hartley : with illustrations by Kari Berger.
    —4th ed.
        p.   cm.
    Includes bibliographical references and index.
    ISBN 0-397-54916-4
    1. Nursing. 2. Nursing—Practice. I. Hartley, Celia Love.
II. Title.
    [DNLM: 1. Nursing—United States. WY 16 E47n]
RT82.E45   1992
610.73—dc20
DNLM/DLC
for Library of Congress   91-29909
                                                                CIP

Preface

The fourth edition of *Nursing in Today's World: Challenges, Issues, and Trends,* like the previous editions, represents an effort on our part to present content essential to nursing practice that is often viewed by students as secondary or less important than the courses with a clinical component. Certainly, the largest segment of the educational preparation of any student pursuing a nursing career is spent developing a theoretical foundation for and applying the clinical aspects of care. The rapidly increasing body of nursing knowledge and the new technologies that have reshaped nursing practice demand that the new graduate have a sound understanding of nursing theory that will guide the performance of the many psychomotor skills that comprise the art and science of nursing. Likewise, it is important that nurses who will fill the role demanded of today's professional possess an understanding of the development, heritage, and history of nursing as a profession; the many studies that have helped us to know more about ourselves and our profession, its struggles, controversies, and victories; and the battles that are yet to be waged and won. It is also important for the student to be aware of the many issues to which there are no ready solutions and the questions that are likely to remain unanswered, or that can be answered only on an individual basis. It is for this aspect of nursing that *Nursing in Today's World* is written. Our challenge has been to present this content in a format that will keep students' interest and provide incentive to explore these issues in greater depth.

Students need to know how nursing relates to society as a whole. What impact does nursing have on society and, conversely, what impact does society have on the practice of nursing? What are the effects of legal, ethical, bioethical, legislative, and political concerns? What type of image does the public hold of nurses and nursing? How should this image be changed?

Students can benefit additionally from information that will help them into the nursing profession. This includes knowledge of opportunities in nursing as well as the specifics of applying and interviewing for positions, understanding the hospital environment and how it is structured, anticipating conflicts that may occur in their professional roles, and understanding the organizations that represent nursing. Students with this preparation will be in a better position to practice nursing as it exists today and influence the development of future nursing practice.

We have written this book as an introduction to that task. It is our hope that it will assist you with your course in "Issues," "Trends," or "Professional Adjustments," or with such material integrated into other courses. Each chapter is preceded by a list of general objectives designed to guide you to an understanding of the information that follows. Additional bibliographical references at the end of each chapter lend direction to each of you seeking a more in-depth exploration of a given topic.

We recognize that many of the topics presented in the context of this book have enough subject matter to fill an entire textbook or, in cases such as bioethical issues, an entire encyclopedia. Our purpose is to provide you with an overview of basic information necessary to move into the nursing role, while at the same time stimulating a desire for further reading. Changes in our society occur so rapidly that many of our most heavily and heatedly debated issues are history by the time they can be placed in a textbook. While time adds perspective, day-to-day reading of newspapers and periodicals is vital to remain informed; thus, we encourage students using this book to read additional materials to be completely up to date.

With each edition we have tried to make this book more responsive to your needs. Nursing education, as it responds to the changing world of work, is a dynamic process. Today some leaders in nursing curriculum development and teaching are encouraging the art of story-telling as a valuable teaching technique. As you examine *Nursing in Today's World,* we hope you will value the stories used to illustrate our points of emphasis—stories of real people and their problems, stories of legal challenges, and stories of some of the individuals who have helped to paint the kaleidoscope of nursing history. Through the cartoon-like illustrations, we hope you will gain a varied visual introduction to nursing issues that will provide some humor, as well as gratification, to your commitment to nursing.

In accomplishing our task, many thanks are in order, and we hesitate for fear of omitting anyone. Certainly we need to acknowledge the support of our colleagues at Shoreline Community College who continue to bring new issues to our attention. One colleague in particular deserves special mention: Karine (Kasey) Gvard, who completed a degree in jurisprudence while teaching full time, reviewed our legal chapter for accuracy and content. We are deeply appreciative of her help and comments. As we worked at perfecting the content of the fourth edition, we have also appreciated the comments of fellow educators throughout the

United States who have used our text and offered enthusiastic support and constructive criticism of the content. Your continued suggestions and recommendations will be valued. We also need to thank our students, who provide one of the best audits of our ability to set forth this content clearly and interestingly. Certainly our list of acknowledgments would be incomplete if we did not express our heart-felt thanks for the emotional support provided by our respective husbands, Ivan and Gordon, and our families, who have allowed us to put the book first when necessary. And last, but not least, we thank the editors of the J.B. Lippincott Company for their help with this text.

Janice Rider Ellis, PhD, RN
Celia Love Hartley, MN, RN

Contents

12   Understanding the Traditional Health Care Settings   *429*

13   Organizations for and About Nursing   *461*

Appendix A: State Boards of Nursing   *487*

Appendix B: Nursing-Related Organizations   *493*

NURSING IN TODAY'S WORLD

Challenges, Issues, and Trends

Unit I

Understanding the Development of Nursing as a Profession

As you seek a career in nursing you can best appreciate the role and responsibilities you are being prepared to assume if you have an understanding of the history and development of the profession. Nursing is considered a relatively young profession by many people. Others challenge that it has yet to achieve professional status. The educational processes by which we prepare nurses continue to experience change and modification. Are you interested in how this might affect you and your career in nursing? In this unit we present a history of nursing as it grew from an apprentice-type training to a profession that encompasses doctoral degrees. We also discuss the various educational routes by which you can prepare for a role as a nurse and conclude with a discussion of the future of nursing education.

1

Nursing as a Developing Profession

Objectives

After completing this chapter, you should be able to

1. *Identify reasons the profession has had difficulty defining nursing.*

2. *Give a definition of nursing and identify the theorist who defines nursing similarly.*

3. *Using the formal characteristics provided, determine whether you believe nursing is a profession.*

4. *Describe the health care practices in the early civilizations.*

5. *Discuss the three major historical images of the nurse.*

6. *Describe how each of these historical images has influenced the development of nursing as a profession.*

7. *Explain the significance of the "Dark Ages of Nursing" to the development of the nursing profession.*

8. *Discuss the contribution of Florence Nightingale to the development of nursing as a profession.*

9. *Identify some early hospitals established in the Americas.*

> *10. Describe the early development of nursing schools in the United States.*
> *11. Discuss factors that have affected the image of nursing today.*
> *12. List at least three studies about nursing and explain their significance.*

What is nursing? Is nursing an art or a science? If both, which should receive the primary emphasis? How should or can "hunches" and "gut feelings" exist in a world surrounded by scientific rationale? Should nursing be considered a profession or an occupation? What factors have affected its emergence as a profession? Does it possess a unique body of knowledge? Is the nurse a professional? If so, what education is required for professional standing? Should the educational preparation for nursing occur in a variety of settings that award differing degrees? How will the skills of graduates from various programs be differentiated in practice? Do differing levels of competence exist in the practice of clinical nursing? What is the position of the nurse in relation to other members of the health care team? What is the exclusive role of the nurse? What forces have had a hand in the development of that role? What is the future of that role? What should we remember from our past that will assist with the development of nursing for the future? These are only some of the questions being asked by nurses about nurses and nursing today. Not all the questions have acceptable answers. Some of the answers that are given provide the basis for debate and dialogue among nurses, health care providers, and the public as health care consumers. As a novice, joining the ranks of those who have preceded you, it is important that you have a grasp of the issues that have challenged, and in some instances plagued, nursing over the years. As the nurse of the 21st century, you may have a direct impact on some of the answers to these questions. Some of the issues that surround nursing today are presented in this chapter.

NURSING DEFINED

Defining nursing is difficult. Nurses themselves cannot agree on a single definition. This is due in part to nursing's historical background. Very little is known other than by inference about the work of the nurse in prehistory. Yet Donahue (1985, p 2) writes, "From the dawn of civilization, evidence prevails to support the premise that *nurturing* has been essential to the preservation of life. Survival of the human race, therefore, is inextricably intertwined with the development of nursing."

Distinguishing Nursing From Medicine

Clear and concise definitions of nursing are also impeded by the lack of separation or an obvious distinction from medicine. For example, it is not unusual to hear a prospective nursing student say, "I've always been interested in the medical field, so I decided to go into nursing." Something of an interdependence exists between the two professions, medicine and nursing, and they have somewhat paralleled one another in historical development. However, anyone who has been involved in the profession of nursing for any period of time will be quick to assure you that differences exist. Primarily these are focused on the major goal of each profession. In general, medicine is concerned with the diagnosis and treatment (cure when possible) of disease. Nursing is concerned with caring for the person in a variety of health-related situations. Thus we think of medicine being involved in the cure of the patient and nursing with the care of that patient.

With the advancing technology in the health care fields, the varying areas of specialization, the different routes to educational preparation, and the variety of practice settings and roles occupied by the nurse, it is critical that nurses provide clear information for themselves as well as for the public. To state that you are a registered nurse says little about what you do. It conveys nothing about where you are employed or about your educational background. The words "nurse" and "nursing" have been applied to a wide variety of health care activities in many different settings performed by many variously educated people. The old adage "A nurse, is a nurse, is a nurse" is out of place in our highly technical health care delivery system that struggles to keep "high touch" and "high tech" compatible.

The Effect of Technology on the Definition of Nursing

Technological advances have significantly affected the definition of nursing and the role of the nurse. This is reflected in the comments made by a colleague after looking in a late-1950s medical-surgical nursing textbook to see how nurses managed the care of a patient with an aortic aneurysm in 1960. She found that nurses did not usually manage such patients because these patients seldom lived long enough to require any nursing care. Today such patients are in intensive care units making a good, although cautious, recovery after careful diagnosis that perhaps requires angiography, sonography, or tomography; delicate surgery to excise and repair the distention of the artery; and specialized critical care nursing. "A nurse is a nurse is a nurse" would certainly not reflect with any specificity the role of the person who would provide care to this patient, the skills needed to fulfill the expected behaviors, or the diversity that exists within the profession.

Nurses in many positions have been required to assume ever greater levels of responsibility. Paradoxically, they have not always been given the official authority, autonomy, or recognition that would be expected to accompany those responsibilities. Fortunately, in recent years there has been more appreciation of the role nurses are filling in the health care delivery system.

Early Definitions of Nursing

Beginning with the simplest definition, a nurse is a person who nourishes, fosters, and protects—a person who is prepared to care for the sick, injured, and aged. In this sense "nurse" is used as a noun and is derived from the Latin *nutrix*, which means "nursing mother." Another early use of the word "nurse" was associated with the meaning of a woman who suckled a child, usually not her own—a wet nurse. Dictionary definitions of nurse also include such words as "suckles or nourishes,"

Figure 1–1. In recent years there has been more appreciation of the role nurses are filling.

"to take care of a child or children," "to bring up; rear." In this way "nurse" is used as a verb, deriving from the Latin *nutrire,* which means "to suckle and nourish." With such an origin it is understandable that people generally have associated nursing with women.

References to "the nurse" can be found in the Talmud and in the Old Testament, although the role of this person is not clearly stated. It was probably more similar to that of the wet nurse than to that of someone who tended the sick. Slowly, over the centuries, the word "nurse" has evolved to refer to a person who cares for or tends to the needs of the sick. Florence Nightingale, in her *Notes on Nursing: What It Is, and What It Is Not,* described the nurse's role as one that would "put the patient in the best condition for nature to act upon him" (Nightingale, 1954, p 133).

It is more than just a coincidence that the development of nursing as a profession has been inextricably tied to the role that women occupied in a society at that given time and to the forces that were impacting that society. People who functioned in the capacity of nurses were undoubtedly more concerned about carrying out the responsibilities of the role than about defining the role. Throughout the years we have seen the concepts of nurse and nursing grow and evolve from one of the nurse as mother, nourishing and nurturing children, to one of nurse without sexual connotation and encompassing ever-expanding and challenging services to people needing health care.

Definitions of Nurse Theorists

As nursing has grown as a profession, various nursing theorists have developed definitions of nursing that are consistent with their conceptual frameworks. Table 1-1 presents the definitions of some of the theorists.

In 1958, Virginia Henderson was asked by the nursing service committee of the International Council of Nurses to describe her concept of basic nursing. Hers is one of the most widely accepted definitions of nursing:

> The unique function of the nurse is to assist the individual, sick or well, in the performance of those activities contributing to health or its recovery (or to peaceful death) that he would perform unaided if he had the necessary strength, will or knowledge. And to do this in such a way as to help him gain independence as rapidly as possible (Henderson, 1966, p 15).

Nursing as Defined by Organizations

In 1965, the American Nurses Association (ANA) published the "First Paper on Education for Nursing." Within that paper were iden-

Table 1–1. Definitions of Nursing Developed by Major Theorists

Florence Nightingale (1859)	The goal of nursing is to put the patient in the best condition for nature to act upon him, primarily by altering the environment.
Hildegard Peplau (1952)	Nursing is viewed as an interpersonal process involving interaction between two or more individuals that has as its common goal assisting the individual who is sick or in need of health care.
Virginia Henderson (1955)	Nursing's role is to assist the individual (sick or well) to carry out those activities . . . he would perform unaided if he had the necessary strength, will, or knowledge.
Faye Abdellah (1960)	Nursing is a service to individuals, families, and society based on an art and science that molds the attitudes, intellectual competencies, and technical skills of the individual nurse into the desire and ability to help people cope with their health care needs, and is focused around twenty-one nursing problems.
Ernestine Wiedenbach (1969)	Nursing is a helping, nurturing, and caring service rendered with compassion, skill, and understanding in which sensitivity is key to assisting the nurse to identify the problem.
Ida Jean Orlando (1972)	Nursing's unique and independent role concerns itself with an individual's need for help in an immediate situation for the purpose of avoiding, relieving, diminishing, or curing that individual's sense of helplessness.
Dorothea Orem (1980)	Nursing is concerned with the individual's need for self-care action, which is the practice of activities that individuals initiate and perform on their own behalf in maintaining life, health, and well-being.
Dorothy E. Johnson (1980)	Nursing is an external regulatory force that acts to preserve the organization and integration of the patient's behavior at an optimal level under those conditions in which the behavior constitutes a threat to physical or social health, or in which illness is found.
Imogene M. King (1981)	The focus of nursing is the care of human beings resulting in the health of individuals

(continued)

Table 1–1. **Definitions of Nursing Developed by Major**
            Theorists *(continued)*

	and health care for groups who are viewed as open systems in constant interaction with their environment.
Betty Neuman (1982)	Nursing responds to individuals, groups, and communities who are in constant interaction with environmental stressors that create disequilibrium. A critical element is the client's ability to react to stress and factors that assist with reconstitution or adaptation.
Sister Callista Roy (1984)	The goal of nursing is the promotion of adaptive responses (those things that positively influence health) that are affected by the person's ability to respond to stimuli. Nursing involves manipulating stimuli to promote adaptive responses.
Martha E. Rogers (1984)	Nursing is an art and science that is humanistic and humanitarian and directed toward the unitary human and is concerned with the nature and direction of human development.

tified significant aspects of nursing. It stated "essential components of professional nursing practice include care, cure, and coordination" (American Nurses' Association, 1965, p 107). Others would concur that it is both an art and a science: an art in the sense that it is composed of skills that require expertness and proficiency for their execution and a science in the sense that it requires systematized knowledge derived from observation, study, and research carried on in such a way that they will determine the principles for what is being studied.

Again in 1980, the ANA, through their Social Policy Statement, provided yet another definition of nursing: "Nursing is the diagnosis and treatment of human responses to actual or potential health problems" (American Nurses' Association, 1980, p 9). That definition had widespread effect and was realized in the language used in some of the nursing diagnoses we use today.

In 1982, the National Council of State Boards of Nursing (NCSBN) developed a Model Nurse Practice Act. The single most important part of any nurse practice act is the legal definition of nursing practice. This is necessary because it provides the foundation for education, licensure, scope of practice of the profession, and when necessary, the basis for corrective actions against the nurse who violates the practice act. The committee that developed the act had difficulty arriving at a precise and succinct definition. It found a lack of consensus within the literature and the profession. The committee was looking for a definition that would clearly differentiate nursing from the practice of any other health care discipline. It was looking for terms that would describe the essential elements unique to nursing but that would be broad enough to include all levels of nurses who should be licensed to practice. In reaching for these goals the committee found that the term *nursing* was not differentiating or limiting and therefore did not use it in the definition. As a working alternative the National Council incorporated currently accepted concepts of the nursing process and proposed that the practice of nursing be defined around these concepts (Pavelka, 1982).

As the profession grows and responsibilities change, undoubtedly we will continue to redefine and refine our definition of nursing. In being responsive to changes, nursing becomes even more closely aligned with professions such as law, theology, and education in which changing practices have required greater precision and refinement of definitions of the profession.

CHARACTERISTICS OF A PROFESSION

Since the 1950s some nursing leaders have been primarily concerned about providing an explicit definition of nursing, whereas others have examined, challenged, and defended nursing's standing as a profession. Certainly at the time nursing and nursing education were evolving in the United States no one asked if nursing qualified as a profession. As a matter of fact, there is evidence that from an early date the word "profession" was associated with nursing. Strauss (1966) gives as an example a magazine article entitled "A New Profession for Women" that appeared in 1882. The article described nursing reform and carried with it a picture of Isabel Hampton. Strauss (1966) also refers to writings of Lizabeth Price, published in 1892, in which nursing was discussed as a profession.

From a period of time lasting approximately from the 1950s through the 1970s or mid 1980s nursing periodically was reviewed against the characteristics of a profession. The activities for which nurses were responsible, the legal ramifications of practice, and particularly the education of future nurses were subjected to the scrutiny of sociologists and nursing leaders who found it challenging to examine nursing against established standards. The stated characteristics of a profession (Flexner, 1915; Bixler and Bixler, 1945: Pavalko, 1971) generally include the following:

- Possesses a well-defined and well-organized body of knowledge that is on an intellectual level and can be applied to the activities of the group.
- Enlarges that systematic body of knowledge and improves education and service through use of the scientific method.
- Educates its practitioners in institutions of higher education.
- Functions autonomously in the formulation of professional policy and in the control of professional activity.
- Has developed within the group a code of ethics.
- Attracts to the profession individuals who recognize this occupation as their life work and who desire to contribute to the good of society through service to others.
- Strives to compensate its practitioners by providing autonomy, continuous professional development, and economic security.

Some critics challenge that nursing falls short of meeting these criteria. Some of nursing's leaders would also claim that nursing falls short of fulfilling a professional role (Schlotfeldt, 1987; Newman, 1990). In light of that challenge it might be helpful to explore each of the above criteria as it might be applied to nursing.

A Body of Specialized Knowledge

A major criticism often levied at nursing is that nursing has no "body of specialized knowledge" that belongs uniquely to nursing. Critics state that nursing borrows from biological sciences, social sciences, and medical science, and then combines the various skills and concepts to call it "nursing." Nursing leaders and theorists disagree as to whether nursing is a unique profession or one borrowed from other disciplines. In fact, this amalgamation and synthesis of some areas with application to another may be one of the unique qualities of nursing. Nursing researchers are also working to develop an organized body of knowledge that is unique to nursing. Even simple tasks, such as the length of time required to get an accurate reading on a rectal thermometer, are being researched and recorded. Other nurses are working to advance the standing of nursing through the development of a code of ethics, standards of practice, and

Figure 1–2. Some continue to question whether nursing truly can support the title of "profession."

peer review. Nursing theorists are challenging the work of one another in efforts to identify and describe the general principles that govern nursing practice. (See Chapter 3 for more information on nursing theories.) As the result of these efforts become realized, fewer challenges regarding nursing's specialized body of knowledge occur.

Use of the Scientific Method to Enlarge the Body of Knowledge

Critical to any profession is its ability to grow and change as the world changes. Equally important is the method by which those changes occur. They cannot take place in a haphazard, random, or hit-or-miss fashion. In other words, they must be well thought out. Data must be systematically gathered and carefully analyzed, the problem(s) must be correctly identified, alternative solutions must be sought, the best approach selected and implemented, and the results thoroughly evaluated. As a student of nursing you already recognize that this has been applied to nursing practice through the nursing process. It is also being applied to nursing research. Through research and practice we add to the established body of nursing knowledge. Tangible proof of this growth can be monitored in the quick turnover in nursing textbooks. One seldom finds a clinical text in use in a quality program that has a publication date that is in excess of 4 years old. Accreditation criteria set down for nursing programs by the national accrediting agencies require that libraries be stocked with texts and periodicals that are up to date. All of this is a reflection of the growth of the body of knowledge we call nursing.

Education Within Institutions of Higher Education

Perhaps no issue in nursing has been any more controversial than the education of its practitioners. Nursing's heritage, like that of medicine, was one of an appreticeship beginning. Students were assigned to experienced practitioners who taught the skills with which they were knowledgeable. Once those skills were acquired the student moved into the world of employment. Our earliest programs of education were located in hospitals rather than universities. (See Chapter 2 for more information on the history of nursing education.) Over time the setting in which nurses are educated has changed. Today by far the majority of nursing programs preparing registered nurses are located in collegiate settings, either the community college or the senior college or university. However, some controversy still exists with regard to 2-year versus 4-year nursing education and to the "technical" aspects of patient care. All these issues will be discussed at length later in this book as we continue to study the profession of nursing.

Control of Professional Policy and Professional Activity

Most critics reviewing professions against standards for professions place emphasis on the ability of any group to develop its own policy and to function fairly autonomously. To some extent, this has always been a problem for nursing and is likely to continue to be so for some time to come. Traditionally the nurse works under the orders of the patient's private physician, often in a hospital setting. The physician gives the orders that are to be implemented by the nurse, and the agency or hospital sets the policies under which that care is delivered. Only in the last half-century has nursing made significant inroads in defining the unique role of the nurse in "care" as opposed to "cure" of the patient. Today nurses have achieved autonomy with regard to the nursing care of patients and are also accountable for the care provided. The practice acts in some states may even provide for an expanded role of the nurse that gives prescriptive authority to nurses who have completed the necessary educational preparation to be so licensed. Nursing diagnosis, once challenged as an inappropriate responsibility for nurses, has come to be expected. In some practice settings, nurses are eligible for third-party payment; that is, they can be reimbursed by insurance companies for the care they have provided. While nurses continue to carry out the medical regimen outlined by physicians, in many areas a more collaborative relationship is beginning to occur and the contribution of the nurse is receiving more recognition.

A Code of Ethics

Although the challenge of some of the criteria of a profession may leave some question when applied to nursing, that is not the case with regard to developing and implementing a code of ethics. The general standard for professional behavior of nurses in the United States is the ANA Code for Nurses. This document was developed by the ANA and is periodically revised to address current issues in practice. The International Council of Nurses, housed in Geneva, Switzerland, has also developed a code for nurses that reiterates many of the behaviors outlined in the ANA Code for Nurses. The international code sets the standards for ethical practice by nurses throughout the world. Copies of both of these codes and more discussion of the ethical conduct of nurses are found in Chapter 6.

Nursing as a Lifetime Commitment

Bixler and Bixler (1945) emphasized in their listing of criteria for professions that a profession should attract people of intellectual and personal qualities who exalt service above personal gain and who recognize their chosen occupation as a lifework. Pavalko (1971) also identified as a significant criteria the sense of commitment the members have toward work as a lifetime or at least a long-term pursuit rather than as a stepping-stone to another profession. Studies of nursing indicate that most individuals gaining educational preparation for nursing remain within the profession, although concern has been voiced regarding the "burnout" that occurs from stress (see Chapter 11). Most individuals who have been nurses continue to identify themselves as such long after they have retired. Of even greater emphasis today is the tendency of individuals to enter the profession of nursing at one educational level and to continue to advance in practice and education by pursuing additional degrees and experience. The concept of "articulation" between variously positioned degree granting institutions is very much in the forefront of nursing today. More discussion of articulation in nursing education is found in Chapter 2.

Service to the Public

Various theorists list criteria for professions that discuss concepts of altruism, service to the public, and dedication. Some suggest that altruism, or the desire to provide for the good of society, must be the worker's motivating force. Nurses have long struggled with the ambiguity that can result from this concept. Possessing a history with a strong religious heritage, the giving of oneself at all costs helped frame the image of nursing and nurses. As nursing has come of age as a profession, some of our thinking is changing to recognize that "giving away" one's services should not be considered professional. Because nurses expect appropriate remuneration for services rendered does not suggest that they are less than dedicated to the patients for whom they are caring and the care that is being given. Providing service to the public should not be thought of as requiring the sacrifice of one's financial security. One can list medicine, law, dentistry, and engineering as some examples of other professions in which the practitioners are amply rewarded financially for the services provided. Greater discussion of nurses and collective bargaining is included in Chapter 9.

DIFFERENTIATING BETWEEN THE TERMS *PROFESSION* AND *PROFESSIONAL*

The practice of nursing involves many activities that may be performed by many caregivers. These people include nurse aides or assistants, orderlies, practical nurses, and registered nurses prepared for entry into nursing through any of several educational avenues (see Chapter 2). Each of these caregivers is contributing to nursing as a profession. To meet the nursing needs of the public, it is essential that caregivers function at various levels of practice. This had led to confusion about the use of the terms *profession* and *professional*. Is there is a difference in looking at the practice of nursing in its totality and at the practice of professional nursing?

A popular view of a profession involves the approach a person has to an occupation. Most professionals are seriously concerned about their occupation, strive for excellence in performance, and demonstrate a sense of ethics and responsibility in relationship to their occupation. As mentioned previously, such people consider their work a lifelong endeavor rather than a stepping-stone to another field of employment. They place a positive value on being termed professional and perceive being termed nonprofessional or technical as an adverse reflection on their status, position, and motivation.

Others consider the attributes of professionalism to have a great deal to do with attitude, dress, conduct, and deportment. Often built into this concept of the professional are the personal values and stereotypes held by the person doing the evaluating. For example, some would perceive the "truly professional" nurse as the person who is dressed in a starched white uniform and cap, whose hair is off her collar, and whose shoes are freshly polished. Others may perceive the "professional nurse" as the one who is open and kind in interpersonal relationships, who focuses on the needs of others, and who is tactful and skillful in interview techniques.

In at least one instance, federal legislation has helped to establish a list of characteristics of a professional. Public Law 93-360 (1974), which governs collective bargaining activities, defines the professional employee as follows:

> (a) any employee engaged in work (i) predominantly intellectual and varied in character as opposed to routine mental, manual, mechanical, or physical work; (ii) involving the consistent exercise of discretion and judgment in its performance; (iii) of such a character that the output produced or the result accomplished cannot be standardized in relation to a given period of time; (iv) requiring knowledge of an advanced type in a field of science or learning customarily acquired by a prolonged course of specialized intellectual instruction and study in an institution of higher learning or a hospital, as distinguished from a general academic education or from an apprenticeship or from training in the performance of routine mental, manual, or physical processes; or
>
> (b) any employee, who (i) has completed the courses of specialized intellectual instruction and study described in clause (iv) of paragraph (a), and

(ii) is performing related work under the supervision of a professional person to qualify himself to become a professional employee as defined in paragraph (a).

As you can see, the sociological and legal definitions are much more restrictive than the popular view of the term *professional*. One of the difficulties is the communication block that results from people using the term in different ways. When one person is using a restrictive, sociological definition and the other person responds from a standpoint of personal belief and feeling, agreement is almost impossible.

Debate over the use of the terms *profession* and *professional* in nursing is widespread. One can better understand the debate if one knows something about the historical development of the field of nursing.

HEALTH CARE IN ANCIENT CULTURES

The life of the primitive societies was necessarily a nomadic one. People wandered in search of food, warmth, and an environment compatible with life. It is believed that these primitive groups moved from the interior parts of Europe and Asia to the warmer climate found around the Mediterranean Sea, in India, and in China. The Mediterranean Sea was thought to occupy the center of the earth with all areas to its east known as "eastern" and those to the west known as "western" (Donahue, 1985). Located in the Near East were the countries of Egypt, Persia (Iran), Babylonia (Iraq), Assyria, and Palestine. The sophistication of health care practices varied considerably from one culture to another.

Egypt

The oldest medical records so far discovered and deciphered are those from Egypt, dating back as far as 3000 BC. Early records were carved on stone or were written on papyrus. Ancient Egyptians, who settled along the Nile (while other cultures were settling along the Indus, Euphrates, and Tigris rivers), developed community planning that helped to avoid public health problems, especially those related to disease transmitted through water sources. Egypt is credited with being one of the healthiest of ancient countries, perhaps because of the progress it made in the fields of hygiene and sanitation. Strict rules were developed around such things as cleanliness, food, drink, exercise, and sexual relations. The Egyptians also established a "house of death," which was located at a site away from civilization. People in this early culture classified more than 700 drugs and developed the art of embalming. Their skill in bandaging was carried over for history to observe in mummies. It is also believed that they were skilled in dentistry, often filling teeth with gold. The oldest known medical books come from this society. The books outline surgical techniques and methods of birth control, describe disease processes, and suggest remedies. Out of this culture came the first physician known to history, Imhotep (2900–2800 BC). He was recognized as a surgeon, an architect, a temple priest, a scribe, and a magician. Although women in ancient Egypt received more respect than in some other Eastern countries, it is not clear whether nurses existed as such. Most likely they served as "wet nurses" and as midwives.

Persia (Iran)

One of the most extensive empires of the Near East was that of the Persians. Their warlike nature resulted in their conquering much of the fertile land in that area. By religion they professed the power of Zoroaster, a prophet who wrote the sacred books of Persia. His writing introduced the world to the concept of two creators—one good, one evil—and sacred elements of fire, earth, and water. The Persian society adopted the culture of the land they conquered, which included much of the medical and surgical practices of Egypt. They established early schools to prepare priest-physicians, from which evolved three types of physicians—those who healed by the knife, those who healed with herbs, and those who healed through exorcism.

Babylonia (Iraq)

Babylonia, like Egypt, was located in an area known as the Fertile Crescent and the Cradle of Civilization. The area was so named because of its well-watered soil and warm climate, a combination that was favorable to the establishment of civilizations. The life-style of the Babylonians was entirely different from that of the Egyptians. Each city was a complete community in itself, governed by a divine ruler and a priest-king. It was believed that illness was the punishment for sinning and for displeasing the gods. A cure was brought about by purifying the body, usually by incantations and the use of herbs. Temples, in which the purification occurred, became centers of medical care.

The Babylonians were skilled mathematicians and astronomers. It is not surprising, therefore, that many of their beliefs were based on nature study and the potency of numbers and on observations of the movement of stars and planets. Horoscopes were cast in terms of a person's birth and the position of the planets on that occasion. The Babylonians were fond of the number seven, which still holds a high place in the superstitions of various cultures. From this culture developed the famous Code of Hammurabi (Hammurabi was then the king of Babylonia) in 1900 BC. (The principal source of this code is a stone monument found in 1901 and preserved today in the Louvre in Paris.) This code may represent the first sliding scale for fee payment by dividing the public into three classes. Those classified as "gentlemen" might expect to pay their surgeons in silver coins rather than in goods or services. A surgeon who bungled an operation on a "gentleman" carried heavy obligations, since the surgeon might have his hands cut off if the surgery went poorly. This makes the malpractice rates absorbed by physicians today seem more palatable.

Assyria

The Babylonians were succeeded by the Assyrians, a warlike tribe. Their laws were severe, with the death penalty frequently being invoked. They supported the belief that illness was punishment for sin and that a person's body could be occupied by evil spirits. Thus, the practice of medicine was developed around superstitious beliefs.

Palestine

The Hebrews made their home in the area called Palestine, adjacent to Egypt. Primarily an agricultural society, the country was ruled by kings. The Hebrews are credited with more democratic sharing of knowledge than any of the other ancient civilizations. Through the leadership of Moses, the adopted son of the Egyptian pharaoh's daughter, the Hebrews developed the Mosaic Code, which represented an organized method of disease prevention. The code emphasized isolation of persons with communicable diseases and differentiated clean from unclean. Bible scriptures such as Leviticus 7:16–19 and 19:5–8, which forbade that meat be eaten past the third day after the animal was slaughtered, were no doubt written because of the warm climate and the lack of refrigeration. The Hebrew culture recognized one god who had power over life and death. From this belief evolved the role of the priest as supervisor of medical practices relating to cleansing and purification. Priest-physicians took on the function of health inspectors.

India

Located in the southern part of the Far East, India was essentially isolated by mountains from other parts of the world. Excavations indicate that the first civilizations (2500–1500 BC) were highly developed with systems of sanitation, bathrooms and public baths, and other amenities. The Vedic age began in 1500 BC and the people worshiped the eternal spirit Brahma. Brahmanism (also known as Hinduism) was to become a major religion of the country. Sources of information about health practices come from the Vedas, a sacred book of Brahmanism dating back as far as 1600 BC. Medicine, as described in these books, apparently included major and minor surgery, children's diseases, and diseases of the nervous and urinary systems. Their surgery may have been the most highly developed of any ancient culture. Also developing out of this early religion was stratification of the society into four different castes. Later Buddhism was to emerge as the major religion of early India. During the Buddhist period, India is credited with an advanced understanding of disease prevention, hygiene and sanitation, medicine, and surgery. The importance of prenatal care to both mother and infant seemed well understood and practiced. In disregarding the caste system of the earlier religion, Buddhism made education and the right to peace possible for everyone. Public hospitals were constructed during this time, and some vital statistics were collected. The early hospitals were staffed with nurses whose qualifications were similar to those expected of today's practical nurse, except that the Indian nurses were all men. When Buddhism fell, the hospitals were abolished (Donahue, 1985).

China

The ancient Chinese followed the teachings of Confucius, who sought to relieve the country's oppression by reviving ancient customs. Patriarchal rule dominated, and emphasis was placed on the value of the family as a unit. Ancestor worship attained great importance. Woman's role was seen as being vastly inferior to man's, her major value being determined by the number of sons she could produce. Early Chinese established the philosophy of the yang and the yin. The yang represented the active, positive, masculine force of the universe, and the yin represented the passive, negative, feminine force. These two forces were always contrasted to and complementary with each other. Health practices focused on prevention and good health resulted from a balance between the yang and the yin.

The Chinese also developed acupuncture skills that are still being practiced today. No faith was placed in the patient's history as a diagnostic tool, and diagnosis was made on the basis of a complicated pulse theory. The Chinese had elaborate materia medica, and many of the drugs they used, such as ephedrine, are used in modern medicine.

Greece

This culture occupied a peninsula that jutted out into the Mediterranean Sea from the southeastern part of Europe. The ancient Greek culture is remembered in part for its worship of gods and goddesses and for the emphasis that was placed on healthy bodies. (Remember that the Greeks started the Olympic games.) In Greek mythology, Asklepios (sometimes spelled Aesculapius or Asclepius), son of Apollo, was the chief healer. He is usually represented as carrying a staff, to show that he traveled from place to place, around which is entwined a serpent, representing wisdom and immortality. (Some persons believe that when the army medical services fashioned the caduceus, the symbol of the medical profession, the staff and serpent that were incorporated into the symbol came from this legend.)

Exquisite temples, located on beautiful sites, were built as shrines to Asklepios and became social and intellectual centers as well as places to obtain cures. The curative process usually began with animal sacrifice and continued through various purifying processes. In addition to these shrines, two other institutions offered care to the sick in ancient Greece. The xenodochium was an institution that first offered care to travelers and later cared for people who were sick and injured. This may have been the forerunner of the city or country hospital as we know it today. The iatrion was a facility offering ambulatory care and would correspond to our outpatient clinics.

It is rather surprising that from this Greek society, so heavily steeped in mythology, animal sacrifice, and faith in the power of the gods, was to come the Father of Medicine. Hippocrates was born about 400 BC on the island of Cos. He stressed a natural cause for disease, treated the whole patient in a patient-centered approach to care, and introduced the scientific method of solving patient problems. He also taught the necessity of accurate observations and careful record keeping. Hippocrates did not attribute ill health to an infliction by the gods but rather believed that health depended on equilibrium existing between the mind and body and the environment. From this evolved the humoral theory of disease, which has lasted for centuries.

Many early physicians were also from Greece, although they often practiced their skills in Rome after Greece was conquered by the Roman Empire. Galen, Aesclepiades, and Pedanim Dioscorides were all Greek physicians who worked in Rome.

Rome

The medical advancements of the ancient Romans fell short of those of the Greeks. Medical practices were often borrowed from the countries the Romans conquered, and the physicians from those countries were made slaves who provided medical services to the Romans. The Romans clung to gods, superstition, and herbs when faced with disease, although hygiene and sanitation were fairly well established. Many homes were equipped with baths, and cleanliness was valued. The role of women was considerably different from that in other ancient cultures. Women were allowed to hold property, appear in public, and campaign publicly for causes they believed should be advanced, and they could entertain guests and sit with them at the table.

The Americas

No definite date can be assumed for the historical recording of civilization of the area that was to be known as the Americas. It is thought that early inhabitants probably came from Central Asia, gaining access across a land bridge in the Bering Strait into Alaska. Like other early tribes they were nomadic, seeking food and shelter. Several groups including the Incas and the Aztecs developed a high level of civilization. Medicine men were responsible for curing ills of both the body and the mind, and disease was believed to result from displeasing gods. The sun god was particularly important to these cultures. Rites, ceremonies, herbal treatment, charms, and, in some instances, human sacrifice contributed to healing practices. Little is known about the role of the nurse in these early civilizations, although the status enjoyed by women was good.

As you can see from the previous discussion, the writing about early health care makes almost no mention of nursing or nurses. Health practices varied depending on level of development of the society. Ritualistic ceremonies and worship of gods was common and the role of healer was assumed by various individuals within the culture. Each primitive society had its own curative agents, taboos, and practices, some more advanced than others. Absent from most cultures was a sound theory of disease.

HISTORICAL PERSPECTIVES OF NURSING

Although the ancient cultures developed medicine as a science and profession, they showed little evidence of establishing a foundation for nursing. With the possible exceptions of the male attendants of the early Buddhist culture in India and the midwives, who had an established role in several cultures, nursing, as we think of it, did not exist. It was not until the early Christian period that nursing was to take root.

Muriel Uprichard identifies three heritages from the past that tend to inhibit the progress of nursing. They are "the folk image of the nurse brought forward from primitive times, the religious image of the nurse inherited from the medieval period, and the servant image of the nurse created by the Protestant-capitalist ethic of the 16th to 19th century" (Uprichard, 1973, p 24). Whether they impeded progress, certainly these concepts of the nurse have had an impact.

The Folk Image of the Nurse

Since the time of the first mother, women have carried the major responsibility for the nourishing and the nurturing of children and for caring for elderly and aging members of the family. It is difficult, however, when examining the pages of history, to pinpoint a particular time or place for the beginnings of nursing as we know it. It is reasonable to assume that early tribes and civilizations had needs for health care. It is also reasonable to assume that within those tribes and civilizations, there would come forth people who demonstrated adeptness and special interests in meeting the needs of the sick, the injured, and women bearing children. The education of these people was largely by trial and error, advancing those methods that appeared successful, and by the sharing of information with one another. Superstition and magic played a significant role in the treatment rendered; folklore abounded, and a close relationship existed between religion and the healing arts.

Nursing skills primarily evolved from intuition. For example, during the process of planning a diet for the family, the wise woman noticed that eating certain foods resulted in episodes of diarrhea and vomiting, whereas eating other herbs, roots, and leaves had a soothing effect on the body. Families developed recipes that were handed down from generation to generation.

The Religious Image of the Nurse

The first continuity in the history of nursing began with Christianity. Christ's teachings admonished people to love and care for their neighbors. With the establishment of churches in the Christian era, groups were organized as orders whose primary concern was to care for the sick, the poor, orphans, widows, the aged, slaves, and prisoners, all done in the name of charity and Christian love. Christ's precepts placed women and men on a parity, and the early church made both men and women deacons, with equal rank. Unmarried women had opportunities for service that were never imagined earlier. While these opportunities represented positive changes, as nursing developed an image closely tied to religion and religious orders, strict discipline was expected. Absolute attendance to the orders of persons in higher rank (priest or physicians) was demanded. This type of thinking was to follow nursing for many years.

Of particular significance in the history of nursing are the deaconesses in the Eastern churches. These women, who were required to be unmarried or widowed, were often widows or daughters of Roman officials, and thus had breeding, culture, wealth, and position. These dedicated young women practiced "works of mercy" that included feeding the hungry, clothing the naked, visiting the imprisoned, sheltering the homeless, caring for the sick, and burying the dead. The deaconesses were the early counterparts to the community health nurses of today. When they entered homes to distribute food and medicine they carried a basket, which would later become the visiting nurse bag of today. No discussion of nursing history would be complete without mentioning Phoebe, who is often referred to as the first deaconess and the first visiting nurse. She carried Paul's letters and cared for him and many others. In the Epistle to the Romans, dated about AD 58, reference is made to Phoebe and to her work.

Not clearly distinguished from the deaconesses were the widows and the virgins. The members of the *Order of Widows* had not necessarily been married. It seems that the title was used to designate respect for age. If married, a member was required to be widowed only once, and vows were taken never to remarry. The *Order of Virgins* emphasized virginity as essential to purity of life, and virgins ranked equal to the clergy. These three groups—deaconesses, widows, and virgins—shared many common characteristics and carried out similar responsibilities. Because these women often visited the sick in their homes, they are sometimes recognized as the earliest organized group of public health nurses. The movement peaked in Constantinople about AD 400, when a staff of 40 deaconesses lived and worked under the direction of Olympia, a powerful and deeply religious deaconess. The influence of the deaconess order diminished in the fifth and sixth centuries, when church decrees removed clerical duties and rank from the deaconess.

Although the position of deaconess originated in the Eastern Church, it spread west to Gaul and Ireland. In Rome, women who served in comparable positions were known as *matrons*. Active during the fourth and fifth centuries, these women held independent positions and had great wealth, which they contributed to charity and to nursing. Among these Christian converts were three women who contributed significantly to nursing.

St. Marcella

St. Marcella established the first monastery for women in her own beautiful and palatial home, which became a center for Christian study and teaching. It was here that St. Jerome worked on translation of the Bible while teaching Christian principles. Marcella herself was regarded as an authority on difficult scriptural passages. Her home was later invaded by warriors who expected to find valuables stored there. When they found little more than a bare building, they whipped Marcella, hoping that she would reveal the hiding places of riches. After the assault she is said to have fled to a nearby church where she died.

Fabiola

Fabiola is said to have studied at Marcella's home. She was reputably a beautiful woman from a great and wealthy Roman family; however, she was unhappy in her first marriage and so divorced her husband and remarried. She converted to Christianity and, after the death of her second husband, began her career of charity. On becoming a Christian, Fabiola realized that her new beliefs made marriage after divorce a sin. She publicly acknowledged this, committed her life to charitable work, and in AD 380 built the first public hospital in Rome described as a *nosocomium*. Here she cared for the sick and poor whom she gathered from the streets and highways, personally washing and treating wounds and sores that repulsed others. St. Jerome tells of some of her work and her attributes in his writings. She died about 399, and scores of Romans are said to have attended her funeral to show their respect for her.

St. Paula

St. Paula was also a scholar of Marcella. Widowed, learned, and wealthy, she is said to have assisted St. Jerome in the translation of the writings of the prophets. St. Paula traveled to Palestine and devoted a fortune to the establishment of hospitals and inns for pilgrims traveling to Jerusalem. In Bethlehem she organized a monastery, built hospitals for the sick, and developed hospices for pilgrims, where tired travelers and the ill were cared for. Some credit her with being the first to teach nursing as an art rather than as a service.

The Role of the Monastic Orders

Also developing during this time were the monastic orders. Through them young men and women were able to follow careers of their choice while living a Christian life. One of the earliest organizations for men in nursing, the Parabolani brotherhood, was established at this time. Responding to needs created by the Black Plague, this group reportedly organized a hospital and traveled throughout Rome caring for the sick.

The order of Benedictines, which still exists, was founded during this period. Such famous monastic nurses as St. Brigid, St. Scholastica (a twin sister of St. Benedict), and St. Hilda were founding schools, tending to the sick, and giving to the poor. The monasteries played a large role in the preservation of culture and learning as well as in offering refuge to the persecuted, care to the sick, and education to the uneducated. The learning of the classical period would have been lost when the empire fell were it not for the monks and monasteries. During this period (approximately AD 50 to 800) the first hospitals also were established. These hospitals, located outside the monastery walls, are still standing. There were more than 700 hospitals in England by the middle of the 16th century. The Hotel Dieu in Lyons was established in 542 and the Hotel Dieu in Paris, around 650. The Hotel Dieu in Paris was staffed by the first order specifically devoted to nursing, the Augustinian Sisters. The Santo Spirito Hospital in Rome, the largest medieval hospital, was established by papal order in 717.

The Crusades, which swept northern Europe, were to last for almost 200 years (1096–1291). The deaconess movement, suppressed by the Western churches, became all but extinct. Military nursing orders evolved as a result of the Crusades. The Knights Hospitallers of St. John was one such order. It was organized to staff two hospitals that were located in Jerusalem. The Knights, organized as a nursing order, at times were required to defend the hospital and its patients. For this reason they wore a suit of armor under their habits. On the habit was the Maltese cross. The same cross was to be used later on a badge designed for the Nightingale School. The badge became the forerunner of the nursing pin as we know it today. The symbolism of the pin dates back to the 16th century, when the privilege of wearing a coat of arms was limited to noblemen who served their kings with distinction. As centuries passed the privilege was extended to schools and to craft guilds, and the symbols of wisdom, strength, courage, and faith appeared on buttons, badges, and shields. The pins of many schools of nursing are fashioned after a cross of some kind. In Germany a similar order of Knights Hospitallers was formed called the Teutonic Knights. They functioned much as did the group in Rome and were identified by their black habit worn over a white cloak with a black cross embroidered in gold on the shoulder (Donahue, 1985). Orders of lay sisters called *consorores* developed to assist with the hospital work but were not granted the status of the Knights.

Secular orders of nurses also came into existence at this time in history. Operating much like the monastic orders, members of this group could terminate their vocations at any time and were not bound to the vows of monastic life. Examples of the secular orders include the Order of Antonines (1095); the Beguines of Flanders, Belgium (1184); the Misericordia (1244); and the Alexian Brothers, founded during the bubonic plague epidemic of 1348. The only nursing education offered to these dedicated people was in the form of an apprenticeship; a newcomer to the organization would be assigned to a more experienced person and would learn from that person.

The inquiring student is encouraged to seek greater depth of knowledge about the orders, their purposes and goals, and the lives of those who devoted their energies to the care of the sick and the poor by consulting the nursing references given at the end of this chapter.

The Servant Image of the Nurse

The Middle Ages were followed by the Renaissance (occurring from the 14th through the 16th centuries) and the Reformation. During the Renaissance, also known as the Age of Discovery, a new impetus was given to education, but not to medical education, which was still caught up in the humoral theory of disease, or to nursing education, which was all but nonexistent.

The Reformation, a religious movement that started with the work of Martin Luther, began in Germany in 1517. It resulted in a revolt against the supremacy of the pope and the formation of Protestant churches across Europe. Monasteries were closed, religious orders were dissolved, and the work of women in these orders became almost extinct.

Also associated with the Reformation was a change in the role of women. The Protestant Church, which stood for freedom of religion and thought, did not allow much freedom for women. Once revered by the church and encouraged toward charitable activities, women of the Reformation were deemed subordinate to men. Their role was within the confines of the home; their duties were those of bearing children and caring for the home. Work in hospitals no longer appealed to women of high birth. Hospital care was relegated to "uncommon" women, a group comprising prisoners, prostitutes, and drunks.

Women faced with earning their own living were forced to work as domestic servants; and although nursing was considered a domestic service, it was not a desirable one. Pay was poor; the hours were long; the work was strenuous. The nurse was considered the most menial of servants. Thus developed what may be called the "Dark Ages of Nursing."

The image of nurses and nursing during this time was described by Charles Dickens through the characters of Sairey Gamp and Betsy Prig in his book *Martin Chuzzlewit:*

Figure 1-3. From the Middle Ages to the 19th century, nursing was often left to "uncommon women."

She was a fat old woman, this Mrs. Gamp, with a husky voice and a moist eye, which she had a remarkable power of turning up, and only showing the white of it. Having very little neck, it cost her some trouble to look over herself, if one may say so, at those to whom she talked. She wore a very rusty black gown, rather the worse for snuff, and a shawl and bonnet to correspond. . . . The face of Mrs. Gamp—the nose in particular—was somewhat red and swollen, and it was difficult to enjoy her society without becoming conscious of a smell of spirits. Like most persons who have attained to great eminence in their profession, she took to hers very kindly; insomuch, that setting aside her natural predilections as a woman, she went to a lying-in or a lying-out with equal zest and relish (Dickens, 1936, p 318).

Mrs. Prig was of the Gamp build, but not so fat; and her voice was deeper and more like a man's. She had also a beard (Dickens, 1936, p 417).

The 16th and 17th centuries found Europe devastated by famine, plague, filth, and horror. In England, for example, King Henry VIII had effectively eliminated organized monastic relief provided to orphans and other displaced persons. Throughout Europe vagrancy and begging abounded, and those caught begging were often severely punished by being branded, beaten, or chained in galleys where they served as oarsmen. Knowledge of hygiene was insufficient; the poor suffered the most. Social reform was inevitable. Several nursing groups were organized. These groups gave money, time, and service to the sick and the poor, visiting them in their homes and ministering to their needs. Such groups include the Order of the Visitation of Mary, St. Vincent de Paul, and in 1633, the Sisters of Charity. The last group became an outstanding secular nursing order. They developed an educational program for the intelligent young women they recruited that included experience in a hospital as well as visiting in the homes. Receiving help, counsel, and encouragement from St. Vincent de Paul, the Sisters expanded their services to include caring for abandoned children. In 1640, St. Vincent established the Hospital for Foundlings in Paris.

The Beginning of Change

Countries remaining Catholic escaped some of the disorganization caused by the Reformation. During the 1500s the Spanish and the Portuguese began traveling to the New World. In 1521, Cortes conquered the capital of the Aztec civilization in Mexico and renamed that capital Mexico City. Early colonists to the area included members of Catholic religious orders, who became the doctors, nurses, and teachers of the new land. In 1524 the first hospital on the American continent, the Hospital of Immaculate Conception, was built in Mexico City. Mission colleges were founded. The first medical school in America was founded in 1578 at the University of Mexico.

Farther north, Jacques Cartier sailed up the St. Lawrence River in 1535 and established French settlements in Nova Scotia. In 1639, three Augustinian nuns arrived in Quebec to staff the Hotel Dieu. Jeanne Mance, who had been educated at an Ursuline Convent, arrived in Montreal in 1641 to care for the Iroquois Indians and the colonists. The Ursuline Sisters of Quebec are credited with attempting to organize the first training for nurses on this continent. They taught the Indian women of the area to care for their sick.

The first hospital founded in what was to become the United States was started in Philadelphia, at the urging of Benjamin Franklin, in 1751.

Franklin believed that the public had a duty to provide care to the poor, friendless, sick, and insane. A bill was passed that year authorizing the establishment of the Pennsylvania Hospital (Kalisch and Kalisch, 1986).

In Europe, outstanding men of medicine began to make vital and valuable contributions to medical knowledge. William Harvey (1578–1657), who became known as the father of modern medicine, theorized first about circulation of the blood. Anton van Leeuwenhoek (1632–1723) used a microscope to delineate bacteria and protozoa. Later, Rene Laennec (1781–1826) described the pathology of tuberculosis; Ignatz Semmelweis (1818–1865) explained the relationship between hand-washing, or the lack of it, and puerperal fever; Louis Pasteur (1822–1895) discovered anaerobic bacteria and the process of pasteurization; and Joseph Lister (1827–1912) developed aseptic technique. In the United States Oliver Wendell Holmes (1809–1894) wrote the classic *The Contagiousness of Puerperal Fever*, published 5 years before the medical community became aware of the work of Semmelweis.

Among lay persons influencing social change during this time was a young minister in Kaiserwerth, Germany, Theodore Fliedner (1800–1864). With the assistance of his first wife, Friederike, Fliedner revived the deaconess movement by establishing a training institute for deaconesses at Kaiserwerth in 1836. During a fund-raising tour through Holland and England, Pastor Fliedner met Elizabeth Fry of England, who had brought about reform at Newgate Prison in England. Greatly impressed with Mrs. Fry's accomplishments, the Fliedners followed her example and first worked with women prisoners in Kaiserwerth. Later they opened a small hospital for the sick, and Gertrude Reichardt, the daughter of a physician, was recruited as their first deaconess. The endeavors at Kaiserwerth included care of the sick, visitations and parochial work, and teaching. A course in nursing was developed that included lectures by physicians. No small part was played by Friederike, who helped bring Theodore's visionary plans to fruition and who was herself much dedicated to the deaconess movement. While away from home promoting deaconess activities, she learned that one of her children had died. A second child died shortly after her return, and she herself died in 1842, after the birth of a premature infant. Pastor Fliedner was also assisted in his work by his second wife, Caroline Bertheau, who had some nursing experience before her marriage. In 1849 Pastor Fliedner journeyed to the United States, where he helped to establish the first Motherhouse of Kaiserwerth Deaconesses in Pittsburgh, Pennsylvania.

In England, at about the same time, Elizabeth Fry (1780–1845) organized the Institute of Nursing Sisters, often called the Fry Sisters, a secular group. To follow were the Sisters of Mercy, a Roman Catholic group formed by Catherine McAuley (1787–1841), and another Catholic group called the Irish Sisters of Charity, formed by Mary Aikenhead (1787–1858).

THE NIGHTINGALE INFLUENCE

The three images discussed (the folk image, the servant image, and the religious image) all influenced the development of nursing, but in the latter half of the 18th century one woman changed the form and direction of nursing and succeeded in establishing it as a respected field of endeavor. This outstanding woman was Florence Nightingale.

Born May 12, 1820, the second daughter of a wealthy family, she was named after the city in which she was born, Florence, Italy. Because of her family's high social and economic standing, she was cultured, well traveled, and educated. At the age of 17 she had mastered several languages and mathematics and was extremely well read. Through the influential people she met, she was expected to select a desirable mate, marry, and take her place in society. Florence Nightingale had other ideas. She wanted to become a nurse. To her family this was unthinkable. She continued to travel with her family and their friends. In her travels she met Mr. and Mrs. Sidney Herbert, who were becoming interested in hospital reform. Miss Nightingale began collecting information on public health and hospitals and soon became recognized as an important authority on the subject.

Through friends she learned about Pastor Fliedner's institute at Kaiserwerth. Because it was a religious institution under the auspices of the church, she could go there, although she could not go to English hospitals. In 1851 she spent 3 months studying at Kaiserwerth.

In 1853, she started working with a committee that supervised an "Establishment for Gentlewomen During Illness." She eventually was appointed superintendent of the establishment. As her knowledge of hospitals and nursing reform grew, she was consulted by both reformers and physicians who were beginning to see the need for "trained" nurses. Still her family objected to her activities.

When the Crimean War broke out, war correspondents wrote about the abominable manner in which the sick and wounded soldiers were cared for by the British Army. Florence Nightingale, by then a recognized authority on hospital care, wrote to her friend Sir Sidney Herbert, who was then secretary of war, and offered to take a group of 38 nurses to the Crimea. At the same time he had written a letter requesting her assistance in resolving this national crisis. Their letters crossed in the mail. Her achievements in the Crimea were so outstanding, although they seriously affected her own health, that she was later recognized in 1907 by the Queen of England, who awarded her the Order of Merit.

In 1856 she returned to England, her health broken. Much has been written of her "illness," many suggesting it was, to a large degree, a neurosis. She retreated to her bedroom, and for the next 43 years conducted her business from her secluded apartment.

Throughout her lifetime Florence Nightingale wrote extensively about hospitals, sanitation, health and health statistics, and especially about nursing and nursing education. She crusaded for and brought about great reform in nursing education.

In 1860 she devoted her efforts to the creation of a school of nursing at Saint Thomas' Hospital in London, financed by the Nightingale Fund. Among the basic principles on which Miss Nightingale established her school were the following:

The nurses should be trained in teaching hospitals associated with medical schools and organized for that purpose.

The nurses would be carefully selected and should reside in nurses' houses that would be fit to form discipline and character.

The school matron would have final authority over the curriculum, living, and all other aspects of the school.

The curriculum would include both theoretical material and practical experience.

Teachers would be paid for their instruction.

Records would be kept on the students, who would be required to attend lectures, take quizzes, write papers, and keep diaries.

In many other ways Florence Nightingale advanced nursing as a profession. She believed that nurses should spend their time caring for patients, not cleaning; that nurses must continue learning throughout their lifetime and not become "stagnant"; that nurses should be intelligent and should use that intelligence to improve conditions for the patient; and that nursing leaders should have social standing. She had a vision of what nursing could and should be.

Florence Nightingale died in her sleep at the age of 90. The week during which she was born is now honored as National Hospital Week. The enthusiastic student is encouraged to learn more about this fascinating woman in Cecil Woodham-Smith's book *Florence Nightingale*.

EARLY SCHOOLS IN THE UNITED STATES

After the establishment of the Nightingale School in England, nursing programs flourished, and the Nightingale system spread to other countries, including the United States. It was extended to America in 1849 when Pastor Fliedner arrived in Pittsburgh with four deaconesses. They assumed responsibility for the Pittsburgh Infirmary, which was the first Protestant hospital in the United States. The hospital is now called Passavant Hospital. Since that time, nursing education has grown in the United States.

The Civil War broke out in the United States in 1861. Although social reform was on its way, nursing was still in an embryonic, unorganized stage. Responding to the nursing needs created by the war, women volunteered to help, and after a brief training course, they performed nursing duties. Dorothea Dix, already well known for her concern for the mentally ill, was appointed superintendent of women nurses for the Union Army. Clara Barton, who served as a volunteer with the Sixth Massachusetts Regiment, was instrumental in founding the American Red Cross in 1882. Clara Barton's birthplace in Boston, Massachusetts, is maintained as a museum by the Unitarian Universalist Women's Federation, who also operate the Clara Barton Camp for Girls with diabetes, as a living memorial to this dedicated humanitarian.

African-American nurses, such as Harriet Tubman and Susie Taylor, carried out nursing duties for the Union army while supporting anti-slavery activities for the blacks. Mary Ann (Mother) Bickerdyke challenged the work of lazy, corrupt medical officers. Jane Stuart Woolsey and her sisters Georgeanna and Abby championed for standards of selection and training for nurses of the Union nurse corps. The Woolseys continued their efforts to establish sound nurse training schools after the Civil War. Students who want to learn more about the nurses of the Civil War should explore the writings of Walt Whitman, who was a nurse during this time, and Louisa May Alcott. Both wrote poignantly about nursing and war conditions of this period.

The conditions exposed during the civil war coupled with the popularity of Florence Nightingale in England provided the impetus necessary to heighten the interest in nursing education in the United States. In 1869 the American Medical Association established a committee to study the issue. The New England Hospital for Women and Children established a 1-year program to train nurses in 1872, and by 1873 three additional schools were opened: the Bellevue Training School in New York City, the Connecticut Training School, and the Boston Training

School. The evolution of nursing education in the United States is fully discussed in Chapter 2.

THE IMAGE OF NURSING TODAY

During the late 1970s and early 1980s a great deal of time and energy was invested in studying the image of nursing. Much of this work was done by Beatrice and Phillip Kalisch, who have written prolifically about the topic. Much of their writing deals with segments of an overall study of the image of the nurse in various forms of the mass media, including radio, movies, television, newspapers, magazines, and novels. Kalisch and Kalisch believe that popular attitudes and assumptions about nurses and what nurses contribute to the patient's welfare can influence the future of nursing to a large extent. It is their contention that since the 1970s, the popular image of the nurse has not only failed to reflect changing professional conditions but also assumed derogatory traits that have undermined public confidence in and respect for the professional nurse. Nurses should be concerned about negative or incorrect images because such images can influence the attitudes of patients, policymakers, and politicians. Negative attitudes about nursing may also turn away many capable prospective nurses, who will choose another career that offers greater appeal in stature, status, and salary.

In studying nurses on television (the single most important source of information in the country), Kalisch and Kalisch found that nurses often had no substantive role in the television stories. Often the nurse was part of the hospital background scenery for the physician characters, whose careers were viewed as more important and who scored high on such attributes as ambition, intelligence, rationality, aggression, self-confidence, and altruism. When nurses were singled out, most of the attention was directed toward solving the nurse's personal problems, as opposed to portraying her role as a nurse. The nurse frequently was portrayed as the "handmaiden" to the physician and scored high on such attributes as obedience, permissiveness, conformity, flexibility, and serenity. It is interesting to note that nurses ranked lower than physicians on such items as humanism, self-sacrifice, duty, and family concern, all of which are values traditionally ascribed to nurses (Kalisch and Kalisch, 1982a).

Kalisch and Kalisch found a rise and fall in the image of nurses in motion pictures, with the high point occurring during the war years of the 1940s and the low point occurring in the 1970s, when the nursing profession was denigrated and satirized in many films. This latter fact will have an impact on the attitudes of prospective nurses because the largest proportion of moviegoers each year are adolescents. The earlier, positive images of nurses usually came from films that were biographies of outstanding nurses such as Sister Kenny, who worked with polio patients, or Edith Cavell, a World War I heroine who was shot by the Germans for helping Allied soldiers escape from occupied Belgium. For a time the nurse-detective was a popular theme in films; such nurses were portrayed as being intelligent, perceptive, confident, sophisticated, composed, tough, and assertive. During the 1970s, however, nurses in films often were portrayed as being malevolent and sadistic (e.g., the roles of Nurse Ratched in *One Flew Over the Cuckoo's Nest* and Nurse Diesel in *High Anxiety*). This was the lowest point in the history of films for the nurse figure with regard to such values as duty, self-sacrifice, achievement, integrity, virtue, intelligence, rationality, and kindness. Few films centered on the individual achievement or personal autonomy of the nurse. When compared with the physician's role, nursing was seen as less important (Kalisch and Kalisch, 1982c).

In studying the image of nursing in novels, Kalisch and Kalisch analyzed 207 books. As was true of the review of films and television, they found that the nurse in the novel was almost always female, usually single, childless, white, and younger than the age of 35.

Because nurses almost always have been depicted in novels as women, emphasis has also been on traditional female roles (i.e., wife, mistress, mother). Three nurse stereotypes have resulted: (1) the nurse as man's companion, (2) the nurse as man's destroyer, and (3) the nurse as man's mother or the mother of his children. The man of the novel was often a physician. Novelists of the 1970s and 1980s have, as was seen in movies, often maligned their nurse characters, ignoring the nurses' professional motivations and health care perspectives (Kalisch and Kalisch, 1982b).

Muff (1982) has analyzed feminine myths and stereotypes and has elaborated on nursing stereotypes. In looking at books about nurses written for school-aged children (e.g., *Cherry Ames, Sue Barton, Kathy Martin,* and *Penny Scott*) she has made the following conclusions. Nursing is described as glamorous; medicine and nursing are imbued with a sense of mystery and elitism; nursing is simplistic; nurses move from job to job; and nurses are subservient and deferential, following orders, running errands, and idolizing the physicians for whom they work. All of the nurses in these books were educated in hospital-based diploma programs in which the hard-earned "R.N." was finally won after hours of hospital service, although the Martin and Scott series were both written in the 1960s.

Muff (1982) has also examined the role of the nurse as it is captured

Figure 1–4. Nurses should be concerned about negative or incorrect images because these are sure to influence the attitudes of patients, policy-makers, and politicians.

in the romance novel. In many instances appearances (e.g., color and condition of the hair) were most important, and the nurse was portrayed as a "pure" girl, dressed in white, whose main aim was to get a man, usually the doctor. Those women who were not looking for husbands were in nursing for altruistic reasons, and duty and self-sacrifice were glamorized. Muff also found that the image of the nurse as found in the novel generally could be classified into one of the following categories: ministering angels, handmaidens, battle-axes, fools, and whores. She also stated that the stereotypes of nursing presented by television and films usually would fit one of these categories. When reviewing the nurse image on get-well cards, she had to add a new category, that of "token torturer."

Only newspapers and news magazines tended toward realism rather than fantasy. News articles tended to cover information about the nursing shortage, including some reasons for it, for example, working conditions, salaries, benefits, and hardships. Articles also provided information about new nursing roles, or special features, such as nurses in Viet Nam (Muff, 1982). With the outbreak of war in the Middle East in 1991, nurses received positive recognition by the various media. Nurses serving in reserve status with branches of the military were among the first called up when the conflict began. Although some might argue that nursing has better things to do than worry about how the nurse is revealed in the media, a consistently misrepresented image can negatively affect the way the public thinks about nurses. Misrepresentation of nursing may be responsible, to some degree, for the nationwide decline of applicants to nursing programs during the late 1970s and early 1980s. This decline will have an effect on the nation's health care industry, and therefore nurses have begun measures to help correct their image in the public's eye. In 1981 the National League for Nursing (NLN) prepared a videotape, entitled *Nursing: A Career for All Reasons,* that attempted to attract and recruit ambitious and intelligent men and women into nursing. The NLN also formed the Task Force on Nursing's Public Image in 1982. Nurses are organizing as groups to make their force felt politically. Individual nurses are responding to television advertisements or programs that portray nurses and nursing in a negative light with letters and telephone calls. In instances in which a product was involved, a boycott on the purchase of that item has proved to be a fairly effective way to bring about a change. Actions such as these were responsible for the discontinuance of a television show title "The Nightingales" that cast nursing in an inaccurate and demeaning image.

   In response to serious concerns about the nursing shortage, the National Commission on Nursing Implementation Project organized a campaign sponsored by the Advertising Council designed to combat the nation's acute nursing shortage by enhancing the image of nursing as a career that is prestigious, desirable, and respected. The theme of the campaign was "If caring were enough, anyone could be a nurse." The Council supplied television stations across the country with attractive, fast-moving public service announcements depicting nurses managing life-threatening situations. Radio stations ran announcements targeted to students in high school and to individuals who might change careers asking "Do you care about people? Are you smart enough to study biology and anatomy? Do you have the guts for a challenging career?" Newspapers and magazines carried advertisements that read, "After 4 years of college, you look for a job. . . . After nursing school, a job's looking for you." Job satisfaction was emphasized in other ads. The costs of running the advertisements came from donations received from a long list of interested organizations and agencies concerned about health care. Some of the air time and magazine and poster space in newspapers and magazines was donated by the media.

Another recruitment campaign was initiated by the Texas Hospital Association that focused on the positive image of nursing depicted in the television program "China Beach." The "McMurphy Nursing Project," which took its name from the character Colleen McMurphy featured in the program, made video tapes available at no cost to every junior, middle, and senior high school in the nation. They believed that Collen McMurphy presented a positive role model while at the same time affording a realistic picture of nursing as a career.

STUDIES FOR AND ABOUT NURSING

As schools of nursing grew in number, the quality of many of the schools and their graduates often suffered, and many of Florence Nightingale's admonitions regarding nursing education were forgotten. Nurses, doctors, friends, and critics of nursing became concerned about the inadequate preparation being offered. Before the problem could be corrected, it was necessary to learn more about the programs, how nurses were being used in the employment market, and the problems that resulted. To accomplish this, studies about nursing and nurses were initiated.

We recognize that many students in nursing are not excited by studies, especially those conducted years ago. However, the development of nursing as a profession has been affected by them, and it seems important that the significant studies be discussed. We think you will recognize some reoccurring themes that remain current today.

Although the first studies were not begun until the early 1900s, the number of studies since the 1950s is voluminous. It is impossible to pick up any professional publication and not find mention of some new study in progress. In an effort to classify and catalog references to these studies, Virginia Henderson has prepared *A Nursing Studies Index*. In 1952 a group of nurses, under the sponsorship of the Association of Collegiate Schools of Nursing, launched a new journal called *Nursing Research,* which was designed to disseminate information about nursing research.

Early Studies

One of the earliest studies was carried out under the guidance of M. Adelaide Nutting in 1912. Published by the U.S. Bureau of Education, it was entitled *The Educational Status of Nursing*. The study investigated what and how students were being taught at the time and under what conditions students were living. Although it did not receive the attention it probably deserved, it began to establish nursing as a profession and led the way to later studies.

The Winslow-Goldmark Report, sometimes simply called the Goldmark Report, followed in 1923. This was also referred to as *The Study of Nursing and Nursing Education in the United States* (Winslow-Goldmark Report, 1923). The report focused on the preparation of public health nurses, teachers, administrators, clinical learning experiences of students, and the financing of schools. Subsequently, the Yale University School of Nursing was established.

A three-part study, sponsored by the Committee on the Grading of Nursing Schools, was conducted in the years 1928 to 1934. The first part, which was socioeconomic in nature and entitled "Nurses, Patients, and Pocketbooks," attempted to determine if there was a shortage of nurses in the United States; the second part, an "Activity Analysis of Nursing," looked at nurses' activities that could be used as a basis for improving the curricula in nursing schools; part three, "Nursing Schools Today and Tomorrow," described the schools of the period and made recommendations for professional schools.

The last of the early studies that we mention was not really a study but often is referred to as one because of its far-reaching effects. *A Curriculum Guide for Schools of Nursing*, published in 1937, was a revised version of earlier publications. It outlined the curricula for a 3-year course, emphasizing sound educational teaching procedures. It was read and followed by many schools that were operating programs at that time.

Midcentury Studies

By the 1950s studies about nurses and nursing were numerous and dealt with many aspects of the profession. Only a few of those studies are mentioned here.

Of particular significance was a study published in 1948 entitled *Nursing for the Future*. Conducted by Esther Lucille Brown, the study is also known as the Brown report. Funded by the Carnegie Foundation, the study was done to determine society's need for nursing, and recommendations were made for higher education for nurses. It prompted serious examination of professional education and pointed out weaknesses in the existing educational programs. The investigators recommended that basic schools of nursing be placed in universities and colleges and encouraged the recruitment of large numbers of men and members of minority groups into nursing schools. This report set the stage for studies of nursing education that followed in the 1950s and 1960s and for recommendations that were to continue into the 1990s.

The Ginzberg report was published the same year. This study reviewed problems centering around the current and prospective shortage of nurses. The conclusions and recommendations were published in the book entitled *A Program for the Nursing Profession.* The study recommended that nursing teams consisting of 4-year professional nurses, 2-year registered nurses, and 1-year practical nurses be developed. Some of these conclusions are not far from where we are now.

In 1958, a study entitled *Twenty Thousand Nurses Tell Their Story* was published. It was part of a 5-year research project that was conceived by the ANA and financially supported by nurses throughout the country. The report was prepared by Everett C. Hughes, a professor of sociology at the University of Chicago. The study looked at nurses, what they were doing, their attitudes toward their jobs, and their job satisfaction. As a result, nurses learned a great deal about themselves.

Another significant study was initiated by Mildred Montag in 1952. This study on *Community College Education for Nursing* resulted in the creation of associate degree nursing education (see Chapter 2).

Significant Studies of the 1960s and 1970s

In 1961 the Surgeon General of the U.S. Public Health Service appointed a 25-member panel called the Consultant Group of Nursing. This group was to advise him on nursing needs and identify the role of the federal government in assessing nursing services to the nation. In 1963 this group presented a report entitled "Toward Quality in Nursing," which recommended a national investigation of nursing education that would place emphasis on the criteria for high-quality patient care. After publication of this report, the ANA and the NLN appropriated funds and established a joint committee to study ways to conduct and finance such a national inquiry. It was decided that the study would expand to consider probable requirements in professional nursing to occur over several decades to come as well as examine changing practice and educational patterns of the present time. W. Allen Wallis, president of the University of Rochester, headed the study. Financing was obtained from the American Nurses Foundation, the Kellogg Foundation, the Avalon Foundation, and an anonymous benefactor. The National Commission for the Study of Nursing and Nursing Education was set up as an independent agency and functioned as a self-directing group. The commissioners, 12 in all, were chosen for their broad knowledge of nursing, for their skills in related disciplines, or for their competencies in relevant fields, with no commissioner representing a particular interest group or position. In August 1967, at the first meeting of the commission, Jerome P. Lysaught was appointed director to conduct the planning and operation of the inquiry.

The study focused on the supply and demand for nurses, nursing roles and functions, nursing education, and nursing as a career. The commission found it necessary not only to examine these key concerns but also to relate these issues to the social system that provides care to the public.

The final report of the commission, entitled *An Abstract for Action*, was published in 1970. It included 58 specific recommendations and concluded with four central recommendations. It also listed three basic priorities: (1) increased research in both the practice and education of nurses, (2) enhanced educational systems and curricula based on research, and (3) increased financial support for nurses and for nursing.

The four general recommendations were as follows:

1. That the Federal Division of Nursing, the National Center for Health Services Research and Development, other governmental agencies, and private foundations appropriate grant funds or research contracts to investigate the impact of nursing practice on the quality, effectiveness, and economy of health care

2. That the same agencies and foundations appropriate research funds and research contracts for basic and applied research into the nursing curriculum, articulation of educational systems, instructional methodologies, and facilities design so that the most functional, effective, and economic approaches are taken in the education and development of future nurses

3. That each state have, or create, a master planning committee that will take nursing education under its purview, with such committees to include representatives of nursing, education, other health care professions, and the public, to recommend specific guidelines, means for implementation, and deadlines to ensure that nursing education is positioned in the mainstream of American educational patterns

4. That federal, regional, state, and local governments adopt measures for the increased support of nursing research and education. Priority should be given to construction grants, institutional grants, advanced traineeships, and research grants and contracts. It was further recommended that private funds and foundations support nursing research and educational innovations where such

activities are not publicly aided. It was recommended that funds come from the federal government, and public and private agencies (National Commission for the Study of Nursing and Nursing Education, 1970).

In 1973 a progress report from the National Commission for the Study of Nursing and Nursing Education concerning the status of the implementation of the recommendations of the original report was published under the title *From Abstract into Action*. The commission believed that it was imperative that nursing achieve the goals established in the recommendations so that nursing could emerge as a full profession and in the interest of optimal health care for this country.

Studies of the 1980s and Early 1990s

One of the major studies of nursing conducted in the 1980s was that of the National Commission on Nursing. This group was composed of a forum of thirty commissioners from disciplines such as nursing, hospital management, business, government, education, and medicine, all of whom were concerned about the current nursing-related problems in the health care system, especially the apparent shortage of nurses. The commission was sponsored by the American Hospital Association, Hospital Research and Educational Trust, and the American Hospital Supply Corporation. Its chairman was H. Robert Cathcart. The group began its work in September 1980 and had seven charges, which were as follows (National Commission on Nursing, 1981, p 1):

1. Analyze the internal and external forces that influence the environment of nurses at work.

2. Identify the effects of professional nursing issues on nursing practice in health care agencies.

3. Assess the professional characteristics of nurses in relation to the organizational structure of health care agencies.

4. Explore the motivation and incentives for nursing education and nursing practice.

5. Analyze the relationship among education, nursing practice, and professional interaction in the health care agency.

6. Develop a platform of issues to be dealt with in the commission activities.

7. Plan methods to enhance the professional status and top management role of the nurse through research to define status and role, publication of information to describe or explain status and

role in relation to health care, and demonstration projects to provide models for problem resolution, development, and reshaping of relationships and structures in health care agencies.

Moving from these charges, the commission began systematically to examine and evaluate data sources. Journal articles, state studies, and policy documents were reviewed. A series of public hearings held in six major cities across the nation provided the opportunity for input about nursing issues from each region of the country. Two open forums also were held. After the hearings the commission conducted an Inventory of Innovative Programs and Projects.

The highlights of these findings, along with the commission's recommendations and future action plans, were published in the initial report of the group in September 1981. The final recommendations were published in 1983. Although the findings and recommendations are too lengthy to be included in this chapter in their entirety, it is important to mention the five major categories of issues identified by the study (National Commission on Nursing, 1981, p 5):

1. The status and image of nursing, which includes changes in the nursing role

2. The interface of nursing education and practice, including models for education to prepare for practice

3. The effective management of the nursing resource, including such factors as job satisfaction, recruitment, and retention

4. The relationship among nursing, medical staff, and hospital administration, including nursing's participation in decision making

5. The maturing of nursing as a self-determining profession, including defining and determining the nature and scope of practice, the role of nursing leadership, increasing decision making in nursing practice, and the need for unity in the nursing profession.

A series of publications that explore the work of the National Commission on Nursing is available from the Hospital Research and Educational Trust, 840 North Lake Drive, Chicago, Illinois. The publication *New Directions in Nursing* deals with nursing practice, credentialing, licensure, accreditation, and education.

Many of these issues are discussed in other sections of this book. A number of the issues are not new to nursing; most of them will not be completely resolved in the next decade. Thus you as a new graduate will have the opportunity to influence the outcome.

Many of the commission's findings were no surprise to people who are involved with nursing. Included was information that indicated that physicians and health care administrators often did not understand the role of nurses in patient care and that traditional and outdated images of nurses (including Victorian stereotypes and traditional male-female relationships) impeded acceptance of current roles. Some physicians and administrators perceived nurses as being overeducated, and they did not support an increase in the nurse's authority to make decisions concerning health care.

The findings that individuals and nursing groups are not unified in defining fundamental, professional goals for nursing, and that nursing, as a profession, lacks cohesiveness and a clear understanding of its role and direction were no revelations to many seasoned nurses. These same people were also not astonished to learn of the numerous and diverse associations that represent nursing but lack any arrangement to determine common goals for nursing education, practice, and credentialing. The disagreement and confusion about educational preparation for nurses and the controversy about entry into practice were identified as further blocks to the advancement of the profession. Clearly there is a need for a system of nursing education that promotes realistic expectations, provides appropriate support for practice and advancement, and includes educational mobility in nursing.

Following in the footsteps of the National Commission of Nursing was the National Commission on Nursing Implementation Project, which began in 1985. Funded by the W. K. Kellogg Foundation for 3 years, the project was co-sponsored by the NLN, the ANA, the American Organization of Nurse Executives, and the American Association of Colleges of Nursing. Administered by the American Nurses' Foundation, it had as its purpose to provide leadership in seeking consensus about the appropriate education and credentialing for basic nursing practice, effective models for the delivery of nursing care, and the means for developing and testing nursing knowledge. The focus of this project was to lay the groundwork and take action wherever possible to support effective, high-quality nursing care delivery in the immediate and long-range future.

The results of another study of nursing were released in January 1983. This 2-year study, mandated under the 1979 Nurse Training Amendments, was conducted by the Institute of Medicine Committee on Nursing and Nursing Education and was funded by the Department of Health and Human Services at a cost of $1.6 million. The objectives of the study included providing advice regarding federal support for nursing education, to gain more information about nurses such as why they do not seek employment in medically underserved areas and why they leave the profession, and to make recommendations regarding measures to improve the supply and use of nursing resources (Institute of Medicine Study, 1983).

The Institute of Medicine study made 21 specific recommendations to Congress. The study found that the shortage of nurses of the 1960s and 1970s had largely disappeared and that federal support of nursing education should focus on graduate study. The first recommendation of the study was that the federal government discontinue efforts to increase the supply of "generalist nurses."

The fallacies in these findings were soon realized. Across the nation nursing enrollments plummeted in the late 1980s. When combined with the expanded roles being assumed by nurses and the increased need for nurses in the delivery of health care throughout the nation, this soon resulted in a serious national shortage of nurses. These shortages are of a critical nature in specific areas such as certain geographic areas and in services to certain groups such as geriatric and economically disadvantaged patients.

Responding to the increasing need for nurses, many of the studies of the early 1990s focused on the roles of nurses in the delivery of health care and on educational patterns that would encourage capable individuals to choose nursing as a career and programs that would facilitate educational mobility. Issues related to nurses' image and the nursing shortage merged. A new Commission on the National Nursing Shortage replaced the Federal Commission on Nursing, and $275,000 was budgeted to assist in its function. This commission had as its role developing strategies to decrease the nursing shortage, which included areas related to recruitment, retention, restructuring of nursing services for most effective utilization of nursing personnel, and gathering data about nursing and the information systems used in nursing.

CONCLUSION

There are two major trends that will shape the direction of nursing. Education for nursing has moved progressively into the mainstream of education in postsecondary settings and away from vocational apprenticeship-type preparation. There has been a move toward more research in nursing as a theoretical foundation for nursing education and practice.

Discussions that focus on nursing's relative status as a profession and the appropriate educational requirements have paled in the national concern about the nursing shortage. While theorists may continue to debate such issues, more action is being devoted to recruitment.

Nurses have been delivering health care for many years in the best way they are able without waiting for definitive answers to questions about nursing. Perhaps part of the strength of nursing is that whatever our personal philosophical concerns, we continue to see the patient, or client, as the appropriate focus for our major efforts.

REFERENCES

Abdellah FG: Patient-Centered Approaches to Nursing. New York, Macmillian, 1960

American Nurses' Association: Nursing: A Social Policy Statement. Kansas City, MO, American Journal of Nursing Co, 1980

American Nurses' Association: First Position on Education for Nursing. Am J Nurs 65(12):106–111, 1965

Bixler GK, Bixler RW: The professional status of nursing. Am J Nurs 45(9):730, 1945

Dickens C: Martin Chuzzlewit. *In* The Works of Charles Dickens, Vol II. New York, Books Inc, 1936

Donahue MP: Nursing: The Finest Art. St Louis, CV Mosby, 1985

Flexner A: *In* Bernard LA, Walsh M: Leadership: The Key to the Professionalization of Nursing. New York, John Wiley & Sons, 1981

Henderson V: The Nature of a Science of Nursing. New York, Macmillan, 1966

I.O.M. study sees need for funds in graduate, specialty areas. Am J Nurs 83(3): 343, 344, 454, 1983.

Johnson D: The behavioral system model for nursing. *In* Riehl JP, Roy C: Conceptual Models for Nursing Practice, 2nd ed, pp 207–216. East Norwalk, CT, Appleton-Century-Crofts, 1980

Kalisch PA, Kalisch BJ: Nurses on prime-time television. Am J Nurs 82(2):264, 1982a

Kalisch PA, Kalisch BJ: The Advance of American Nursing, 2nd ed. Boston, Little, Brown & Co, 1986

Kalisch PA, Kalisch BJ: The image of nurses in novels. Am J Nurs 82(8):1220, 1982b

Kalisch PA, Kalisch BJ: The image of the nurse in motion pictures. Am J Nurs 82(4):605, 1982c

King IM: A Theory for Nursing: Systems, Concepts, Process. New York, John Wiley & Sons, 1981

Labor Management Relations Act (1947) as amended by Public Laws 86-257 (1959) and 93-360 (1974), Section 2

Muff J: Handmaiden, battle ax, whore. *In* Muff J: Socialization, Sexism and Stereotyping. St Louis, CV Mosby, 1982

National Commission for the Study of Nursing and Nursing Education: Summary, report and recommendations. Am J Nurs 70(2):279, 1970

National Commission on Nursing: Initial Report and Preliminary Recommendations. Chicago, Hospital Research and Educational Trust, 1981

Neuman B: The Neuman System Model: Application to Nursing Education and Practice. East Norwalk, CT, Appleton-Century-Crofts, 1982

Newman MA: Professionalism: Myth or reality. *In* Chaska NL: The Nursing Profession: Turning Points, pp 49–52. St Louis, CV Mosby, 1990

Nightingale F: Notes on Nursing: What It Is, and What It Is Not. (An unabridged republication of the first American edition, as published by D. Appleton and Company in 1860.) New York, Dover Publications, 1954

Orem D: Nursing: Concepts of Practice, 2nd ed. New York, McGraw-Hill Book Company, 1980

Orlando IJ: The Discipline and Teaching of Nursing Process. New York, GP Putnam's Sons, 1972

Pavalko RM: Sociology of Occupations and Professions. Itasca, IL, Peacock Publishers, 1971

Pavelka M: Definition of nursing practice. Issues 3(Summer):3, 1982

Peplau HE: Interpersonal Relations in Nursing. New York, GP Putnam's Sons, 1952

Rogers ME: Science of Unitary Human Beings: A Paradigm for Nursing. Paper presented before the International Nurse Theorist Conference, Edmonton, Alberta, May 1984

Roy C: Introduction to Nursing: An Adaptation Model, 2nd ed. Englewood Cliffs, NJ, Prentice-Hall, 1984

Schlotfeldt RM: Resolution of issues: An imperative for creating nursing's future. J Prof Nurs 3:136–142, 1987

Strauss A: The structure and ideology of American nursing: An interpretation. *In* Davis J: The Nursing Profession, pp 60–108. New York, John Wiley & Sons, 1966

Uprichard M: Ferment in nursing. *In* Auld E, Birum LH: The Challenge of Nursing, pp 24–31. St Louis, CV Mosby, 1973

Wiedenbach E: Clinical Nursing, A Helping Art. New York, Springer Publishing Co, 1964

Winslow-Goldmark Report: The Study of Nursing and Nursing Education in the United States. New York: Macmillan, 1923

FURTHER READINGS

Aaronson LS: A challenge for nursing: Re-viewing a historic competition. Nurs Outlook 37(6):274–279, 1989

Bunting S, Campbell JC: Feminism and nursing. Adv Nurs Sci 12(4), 11–24, 1990

Bullough VL et al: The Emergence of Modern Nursing. New York, Macmillian, 1969

Christy T: Equal rights for women: Voices from the past. Am J Nurs 2(2):288–293, 1971

Christy T: First fifty years. Am J Nurs 9(9):1778–1784, 1971

Christy T: Portrait of a leader: Lavinia Lloyd Dock. Nurs Outlook 17(6):72–75, 1969

Christy T: Portrait of a leader: M. Adelaide Nutting. Nurs Outlook 17(1):20–24, 1969

Christy T: Portrait of a leader: Isabel Hampton Robb. Nurs Outlook 17(3):26–29, 1969

Christy T: Portrait of a leader: Isabel Maitland Stewart. Nurs Outlook 17(10):44–48, 1969

Curran CR: Shaping an image of competence and caring. Nurs Health Care 6(9):371–373, 1985

Dolan JA: Nursing in Society: A Historical Perspective, 14th ed. Philadelphia, WB Saunders, 1978

Gamer M: The ideology of professionalism. Nurs Outlook 27(2):108–111, 1979

Griffin GJ, Griffin JK: Jensen's History and Trends of Professional Nursing, 7th ed. St Louis, CV Mosby, 1973

Hanson KS: The emergence of liberal education in nursing education, 1893–1923. J Prof Nurs 5(2):83–91, 1989

Kalisch BJ, Kalisch PA: The nurse-detective in American movies. Nurs Health Care 3(3):146–153, 1982

Kalisch BJ, Kalisch PA: Heroine out of focus: Media images of Florence Nightingale: I. Popular biographies and stage productions. Nurs Health Care 4(4):181–187, 1983

Kalisch BJ, Kalisch PA, Scobey M: Reflections on a television image. Nurs Health Care 5(5):248–255, 1981

Larisey MM: Attic treasures: A look at nursing history. Nurs Forum 25(1):20–24, 1990

Melosh B: Not merely a profession: Nurses and resistance to professionalization. Am Behav Scientist 32(6):668–679, 1989

Parsons M: The profession in a class by itself. Nurs Outlook 34(6):270–275, 1985

Roberts MM: American Nursing: History and Interpretation. New York, Macmillan, 1954

Sleeper R et al: Issues in Health Care: The Edna A. Fagan Health Care Lecture Series. Publication No. 14-1599. New York: National League for Nursing, 1976

Woodham-Smith C: Florence Nightingale. New York: McGraw-Hill Book Company, 1951

2

Educational Preparation for Nursing

Objectives

After completing this chapter, you should be able to

1. *Describe the educational preparation and role of the licensed practical nurse.*

2. *Discuss the educational preparation provided by a hospital-based diploma program of nursing.*

3. *Discuss the educational preparation provided by a baccalaureate degree program of nursing.*

4. *Discuss the educational preparation provided by an associate degree program of nursing.*

5. *Explain the concept of the external degree.*

6. *Identify the purposes of other forms of nursing education: registered nurse baccalaureate programs, master's preparation, doctoral studies, and nondegree programs.*

7. *Discuss what is meant by articulated programs.*

8. *Define the continuing education unit and discuss the purpose of that unit.*

9. *Present the major points in support of mandatory continuing education and the major points in support of voluntary continuing education.*

It would be less confusing if nursing, like many other professions, had one major avenue of educational preparation for practice; however, the development of nursing as a profession has resulted in three major educational routes that prepare graduates to write the National Council Licensure Examination (NCLEX) for registered nursing. Although this circumstance has offered various alternatives and opportunities to the prospective student, it has resulted in much confusion. The health care consumer is often unable to understand and interpret the vast array of initials (e.g., RN, CRN, MN, or DNS) that can now follow a nurse's name. Some of these credentials represent legal titles, some are earned by education, while others are acquired by demonstrating expertise through examination (certification). The employer has difficulty discriminating among the different types of graduates who, at least initially, enter the hospital work environment with similar behaviors. The educator is charged with the responsibility of graduating a "safe" practitioner but lacks clear direction as to how the professional preparation provided by the various educational routes should differ in purpose, design, and structure. This situation has also provided a springboard for much discussion, debate, and, in some instances, dissension among nurses, educators, and interested lay persons regarding aspects of each program as they relate to professional nursing practice.

The three avenues preparing men and women for registered nursing are the hospital-based diploma programs, the baccalaureate programs located in 4-year colleges and universities, and the 2-year associate degree programs primarily found in junior and community colleges. To further cloud the issue, we are now seeing students begin their nursing education in programs that culminate in a master's degree, and at least one program exists in which a student can earn a doctorate before being eligible to write the state licensing examination for registered nursing. You can better comprehend much of the politics of nursing today if you have an understanding of the historical development of the educational preparation of nurses.

A fourth program, that which prepares the practical nurse, is also an option for the person seeking a health career. It is considered vocational training, and graduates write a separate licensing examination.

PRACTICAL NURSE EDUCATION

Although licensed practical nurses (LPNs), or licensed vocational nurses (LVNs) as they are titled in California and Texas, are not considered within the realm of professional nursing, it seems prudent to discuss the education and role of these health care providers. The controls on licensing of practical nurses and on the accreditation of curricula of practical nurse programs have been slower in evolving than those regarding professional nursing.

The practical nurse is no newcomer to the health care delivery system. In the past the practical nurse was the family friend or community citizen who was called to the home in emergencies. This person, usually self-taught, learned by experience which things were effective and which were not. She would perform basic care procedures such as bathing and also would cook for the family and do light housekeeping duties. Gradually states began enacting licensure laws governing the practice of practical nursing. By 1945, 19 states and one territory had licensure laws but in only one state was licensure of the practical nurse mandatory (Kalisch and Kalisch, 1986). When states began adopting mandatory licensure laws governing the practice of practical nursing, a large number of people who had been functioning in this capacity were granted a license by waiver, thus never really having any formal training (see Chapter 4 on Credentialing). However, attrition brought about by time and retirement has resulted in the removal of most of these people from nursing practice.

It is a little uncertain when the first program to offer formal preparation for practical nursing began. Some suggest training programs were started in 1897 (Kalisch and Kalisch, 1986). More popular is the belief that the first programs were initiated through the YWCA in Brooklyn, New York, around 1892. The school started through the YWCA was known as the Ballard School, after Lucinda Ballard, who provided the funding to operate the school. The course of study was approximately 3 months long. The students, called "attendants," were trained to care for invalids, the elderly, and children in a home setting.

Although the YWCA may seem to many of us to be a strange place for a practical nurse program, we need to remember that in the late 1890s and early 1900s, young women traveled from their homes to large cities seeking new careers and a better life. Many of these women found inexpensive housing at YWCAs. Because most of them were untrained and had no marketable skills, the YWCA provided a natural site for a school.

Other early practical nursing programs included the Thompson School, founded in Brattleboro, Vermont, in 1907; the American Red Cross Program, begun in 1908; and the Household Nursing Association School of Attendant Nursing, begun in Boston in 1918.

Although by 1930 only 11 schools were in existence, the number of programs expanded rapidly during the 1940s. During World War I and especially during World War II the need for people who had some skills, but, more importantly, who could be prepared quickly, became crucial. As this need became more and more critical, the practical nurse, who until this time was primarily found in the home, moved out into the world.

In 1941 the Association of Practical Nurse Schools was founded; in 1942 membership was opened to practical nurses and the name was changed to the National Association of Practical Nurse Education and Service (NAPNES). The first planned curriculum for practical nursing was developed in 1942, and in 1945 NAPNES established an accrediting service for schools of practical nursing. The National Federation of Licensed Practical Nurses was organized in 1949. This group, working in 1957 with the American Nurses' Association (ANA), attempted to clarify the role and function of the practical nurse, just as various groups throughout the nation have worked at delineating the roles of other nursing program graduates. The Council on Practical Nursing was established by the National League for Nursing (NLN) in 1957. In 1966 the Chicago Public School Program became the first practical nurse program to be accredited by the NLN.

The general curriculum, which requires 9 months to 1 year to complete, varies considerably from state to state and even from school to school. In many instances the education is weighed in clock hours instead of credit hours as used in the professional programs. Most of today's practical nurse educational programs stress clinical experiences, primarily in structured care settings such as hospitals and nursing homes. Basic therapeutic knowledge and introductory content from biological and behavioral sciences correlate with clinical practice. Usually about one third of the time is spent in the classroom and two thirds in the clinical areas.

The setting in which the educational preparation of the practical nurse occurs may vary tremendously. A program may be offered by a high school, trade or technical school, hospital, junior or community college, university, or independent agency. There has been a movement to incorporate practical nurse education and associate degree programs in the community college. All students are grouped together for "core" courses during the first academic year. At the end of this time, the student has the option of stopping the educational program and seeking licensure as a licensed practical nurse or continuing for an additional year and seeking licensure as a registered nurse. Many students opt to do both. Graduates of these core programs in practical nursing usually possess a broader and more in-depth understanding of the biological sciences and, in some instances, the social sciences also because these are part of the core curriculum and may be college-level courses that are transferable to a 4-year institution. As issues related to educational mobility and "articulation" between programs has received much attention (see Chapter 3), the combined programs have been popular in areas where they exist.

Graduates of practical nurse programs take the NCLEX-PN. The scope of their practice focuses on meeting the health needs of patients/ clients in hospitals, long-term care facilities, and the home. LPNs or LVNs work with patients/clients whose conditions are considered stable. Their work is supervised by a registered nurse or a licensed physician.

Like the associate degree and the hospital-based diploma programs for registered nursing, the educational preparation and the future of practical nursing has received much discussion. Some would advocate two levels of nursing with one being the practical nurse. Others would eliminate practical nursing altogether. In 1987 North Dakota became the first state (and to date the only state) to require all candidates taking the licensure examination for practical nursing to have completed an associate degree in practical nursing. Most of the fervor regarding educational preparation has cooled as a result of the shortage of adequate numbers of nurses. With the "graying" of America and the increasing need for more of nurses in long-term care facilties, practical nursing is enjoying a renewed importance.

DIPLOMA EDUCATION

Most registered nurses practicing today gained their basic nursing education in a diploma program administered by a hospital. The first hospital with a nurse training school was the New England Hospital for Women, which accepted its first five probationers on September 1, 1872 (Kalisch and Kalisch, 1986). Linda Richards generally is recognized as the first nurse graduated in the United States. Diploma, or hospital, schools of nursing flourished during the late 1800s and early 1900s. These training schools provided free or inexpensive staffing for the hospitals offering the educational program. Until 1888, when the first school for males opened as the Mills School of Nursing at Bellevue Hospital, the students were all female. The first African-American nursing school graduate was Mary Eliza Mahoney, who graduated from the program at the New England Hospital for Women and Children in 1879 (Kalisch and Kalisch, 1986).

Nursing students were, in fact, the primary work force of hospitals. Initially the education was largely an apprenticeship. Although some formal theory classes were conducted, learning was primarily achieved by "doing." There was no standardization of curriculum and no accreditation. Programs were developed to meet the service needs of the hospital rather than the educational needs of the students, and programs varied considerably from hospital to hospital.

In the early schools the responsibility for administration of the educational program frequently was vested in the director of nursing service, who also had the role and title of director of nursing education. Many of the instructors were graduates of the program who undoubtedly possessed nursing skills but knew little of teaching-learning theories, teaching skills and techniques, curriculum design and development, or evaluation processes. In many instances the teacher was also a head nurse on one of the units in the hospital. Formal lectures often were delivered by members of the medical staff.

The curriculum generally was laid out in blocks of study that included medical nursing, surgical nursing, psychiatric nursing, obstetrics, pediatrics, operating and emergency department experience, as well as support courses in anatomy, physiology, nutrition, pharmacology, history of nursing, and often a course titled "professional adjustments." If a

Figure 2–1. Typical application for admission to nursing school.

hospital was unable to provide certain learning opportunities, for example, psychiatric experience, students were sent on "affiliation" to a hospital where they could receive that education. Although the hospital dietitian may have been involved in teaching the nutrition course, nurses usually carried the responsibility for the remainder of the instruction, including the courses in biological sciences. The students usually were assigned to the hospital units during the early and late hours of the day (when the staffing needs were the greatest), working what were known as "split shifts." Lectures were given between 1 and 3 o'clock in the afternoon. Most days were at least 12 hours long.

Almost all the students were single young females who started the program after completing high school. They entered the school as "probies" (short for probationer) for a 6-week to 6-month probationary period. This was a testing time for both the student and the school, a time for the student to seriously look at nursing as a career and a time for the school to examine the student's aptitude for nursing. Although not exactly comparable to the experience of freshmen entering some private colleges, this situation had a few similarities. The probie often could be identified by dress; for example, the apron might be worn without a bib during this period. There was no real hazing at this time; however, the probie might be sent on errands that capitalized on her lack of knowledge and that might result in embarrassment later. (A typical assignment would be to send the probie to the central service area of the hospital for a supply of fallopian tubes.)

The students were housed in dormitories that were attached to the hospital. The dorms generally had a housemother, and codes of behavior were strict and well enforced. For example, students who failed to adhere to 9:30 PM curfews, who were caught smoking in their rooms, or who committed other acts of indiscretion were at risk of expulsion from the school. Usually marriage was not permitted during the time the students were in training. Because the students literally lived with one another, a type of socialization and identification occurred and students had a built in support system through one another. Dress codes were rigid, and students who committed minor infractions of social behavior were reprimanded in a number of ways. The following is a quote from a special publication developed upon closure of a diploma school:

> In 1921, a nurse was discharged for "cigarette habit." Skirts of nurses' uniforms were getting shorter but there was periodic measurement to be sure some were not too short.
>
> The year 1924 would see Deaconess' first student protest. Student nurses were required to wear their hair long in those days. A number of them though made arrangements with a barber in the Victoria Hotel to stay open

Figure 2–2. A student who had committed a minor infraction of the rules might have forfeited an article of apparel.

late one evening and they all went down and had their hair bobbed in the latest style. They were deprived of their caps for several weeks and ordered to wear switches and what-nots, their punishment comparatively slight, since "banks and other business regularly dismissed employees for social offense" (Eighty-One Years of Nursing: 1889–1980, p 10).

Students surviving the probationary period finished the remainder of the year as freshmen. They then became juniors for 1 year, and completed the final year of the 3-year program as seniors. During the senior year the student often had responsibility for supervising the units of the hospital, with perhaps a month spent on each of the work shifts—days, evenings, nights. At the completion of the 3 years the students were awarded a diploma, but this was not recognized as an academic degree. If graduates wanted to continue their education toward a baccalaureate

HOSPITAL RULES VIOLATED

Deaconess Chief Says Hair Bobbing "Plain Insubordination."

"Inasmuch as all our probationers, when they enter training, know the hospital's feeling toward 'bobbed hair,' there is no other way to look at this but as a plain case of insubordination."

Thus did Miss Mary Buob, superintendent of nursing at the Deaconess hospital, comment on the epidemic of 'bobbed hair' which has spread among the undergraduates at the hospital, 15 of the junior class succumbing.

"Each one entering training is impressed with hospital decorum and discipline and when she signs her application blank she agrees to abide by the rules of the institution. If they had consulted me it is quite likely we might have laid aside the rule, as I am perfectly willing to listen to any reasonable requests, but inasmuch as they simply defied the rules, it looks to me like a breach of discipline and a plain case of insubordination."

No drastic punishment will be meted out, but the permanent report cards will suffer by the action, she said.

Figure 2–3.

degree they often encountered problems because academic credit had not been given for the three years of study. Legally, hospitals were not chartered as educational institutions.

Symbolism and ceremony were an important part of these programs. Each school had its own identifiable uniform, cap, and pin. The traditional "capping" ceremony at which the student received a nursing cap after a given period of study (usually 3 months to 1 year) was a high point in the educational program. Parents and loved ones attended these ceremonies, which were often conducted in churches, particularly if the nursing program was sponsored by a hospital supported by a religious group. Today many programs have eliminated the cap entirely, conforming to nursing as it is practiced in hospitals. Many view the cap as interfering with the ability of the nurse to work in confined or congested quarters and around much technical equipment.

Of even greater significance was the pinning ceremony that heralded completion of the program. Among much pomp and circumstance loved ones gathered to observe as the nursing director ceremoniously "pinned" each new graduate. As nursing education has moved into institutions of higher education, some of the traditional ceremonies have been discontinued. Some argue that the ceremony recognizing program completion in the collegiate environment is the college commencement and that "special" celebrations for students of particular areas of study are not appropriate. In other cases, the tradition is continued.

Although the education described above may seem archaic by today's standards, a word must be said in defense of such programs. As a result of the many hours spent in hospital service, the students usually emerged from such programs skilled in "nursing arts" and were able to assume positions as staff or charge nurses without orientation. Although they may have shown weaknesses in knowing why something was done, they were certainly able to "do it." The graduate usually had a fairly good concept of her role as a nurse and was capable of functioning competently in that role, although some nurses today might not agree with some aspects of that role. One often hears older nurses, hospital administrators, and physicians extol the virtues of the "good ol' days" when schools produced graduates "who could do something." Certainly, for more than a century, the diploma schools carried the major responsibility for producing graduates who could meet the health care needs of the nation.

By the late 1940s and early 1950s, many diploma schools had affiliated with nearby colleges and universities, and general education requirements such as anatomy, physiology, sociology, and psychology were offered. At this time also the National League of Nursing Education (later to become the NLN) was assuming an active role in curriculum guidance and accreditation. Programs gained a stronger educational foundation because they were required to align themselves more closely with other types of postsecondary education.

Most diploma schools in operation today have sound educational programs that meet the criteria necessary for accreditation, qualified faculty, and clinical learning experiences that meet the student's learning needs rather than hospital's service needs. Graduates of today's diploma programs have been provided a foundation of study in the biological and social sciences and may have some courses in the humanities. There is a strong emphasis in diploma programs on patient/client experiences, and the course of study also includes experience in nursing management (i.e., being in charge of a nursing unit). Graduates work in acute, long-term, and ambulatory health care facilities.

During the mid 1960s there was a significant decline in enrollments in diploma schools. As the push to move nursing education into institutions of higher education reached new heights (see Chapter 3), many hospital-based schools elected to discontinue their programs. Others merged with local community colleges or universities that assumed the administrative responsibility for managing the program of education and awarded an associate or baccalaureate degree when graduation requirements were satisfied. Elimination of hospital-based programs is particularly true in the western part of the United States where only two or three programs remain in existence.

The downward trend in enrollments in hospital-based programs reversed itself in 1990. Many schools found themselves with more applicants than they could accept. The National League for Nursing indicated that enrollments were up 9% over the level of 1988 (Hawken, 1990). Although there are far fewer students enrolled in these programs than in either associate degree or baccalaureate programs, the increase represents a changing pattern.

BACCALAUREATE EDUCATION

The first school of nursing to be established in a university setting was started at the University of Minnesota in 1909. The program existed as a quasi-autonomous branch of the university's school of medicine. Close inspection of the curriculum would reveal a program little different from the 3-year hospital program; nothing was required in the way of higher general education, and graduates were prepared for the registered nurse certificate only. Education was predominantly apprenticeship in nature, and students provided service to hospitals in exchange for education. However, it did result in nursing education being part of an academic organization. By 1916 programs were reported at 16 colleges and universities.

Most of the early programs offering a baccalaureate degree in nursing were 5 years long. This provided for the 3 years of nursing school curriculum similar to that of the hospital programs, and for the additional 2 years of liberal arts. In 1924 the Yale School of Nursing became the first to be established as a separate department within a university; Annie W. Goodrich was its dean. However, the growth of these schools was not rapid. Although the development of baccalaureate education for nurses may not seem like a major step to young people of today, you need to remember that it was not until 1920 that the 19th Amendment to the Constitution of the United States granted women the right to vote. Nursing was considered by many a less than desirable occupation, vocational in its orientation, overshadowed by militaristic and technical aspects, and confined to women. A liberal education, scholarship, and knowledge were thought to be incompatible with the female personality and possibly posed problems for marriage later. The nursing curriculum, with its emphasis on performance of skills rather than the philosophical and theoretical approaches used in the humanities, was not well accepted by universities. Much opposition to collegiate education for nurses came from physicians who argued that nurses would be "overtrained." They were not certain that a sound knowledge base was as important as the acquisition of technical skills and manual dexterity that could be acquired with brief training at the bedside. Physicians also argued that baccalaureate education for nurses would result in their services being too costly.

Baccalaureate education has been advocated by nursing leaders as the minimum educational preparation for supervisory and administrative nursing roles. Baccalaureate education further provides the background needed for public health positions, including school nursing and the educational base for entry into graduate education in nursing. In 1965 the ANA specified baccalaureate preparation in nursing as the minimum educational preparation for entry into professional nursing practice (see Chapter 3).

Characteristics of Baccalaureate Education

Baccalaureate nursing programs are located in 4-year colleges and universities. When the program of studies includes an upper division (junior and senior years), baccalaureate nursing major that is built on a basis of liberal arts and science courses taken during the freshman and sophomore years, it is known as a *basic* or *generic* baccalaureate program.

Applicants to such programs must meet the entrance (and graduation) requirements established by the university and those of the nursing school. The admission requirements usually specify academic preparation at the high school (or preadmission) level, which includes courses in foreign language, higher-level study of mathematics and science, and a high cumulative grade point average. Relatively high scores on college admission tests may also be necessary.

During the freshman and sophomore years of study, students who pursue a nursing education take liberal arts, biological, and physical science courses with college students who are preparing for other majors. In some schools these courses may be completed on a part-time basis; but if this occurs, the entire course of study covers more than a 4-year span. The number of required liberal arts and science courses may vary from program to program but usually constitutes about one half of the total number of credits specified for graduation from the college or university. Students usually begin their study of nursing content in their junior and senior years, thus the term "upper-division major" in nursing. Nursing theory can be taught that builds on an understanding of the physical and biological sciences and liberal arts studied the previous two years.

In recent years there has been some tendency for schools offering baccalaureate nursing education to introduce nursing content at some point in the sophomore year of study. These courses, if offered at this point, often include an overview of the nursing profession and some of the fundamental nursing skills.

Students in baccalaureate nursing programs learn basic nursing skills. They also learn concepts of health maintenance and promotion, disease prevention, and supervisory and leadership techniques and practices and are provided with an introduction to research. Clinical course work includes experience in community health settings and practice as leaders on a nursing team within the acute care hospital as well as basic care procedures. Emphasis is placed on developing skills in critical decision making, on exercising independent nursing judgments that call for broad background knowledge, and on working in complex nursing situations in which the outcomes are often not predictable. Acting as a patient/ client advocate, the graduate of a baccalaureate nursing program collaborates with other members of the health care team in structured and unstructured settings and supervises those with lesser preparation. The baccalaureate graduates often work with groups as well as with individuals.

In 1979 the NLN Council of Baccalaureate and Higher Degree Programs developed a statement on the "Characteristics of Baccalaureate Education in Nursing." This statement, as revised in 1986, concludes with the following list of activities that the graduate of the baccalaureate programs in nursing is able to do.

- Provide professional nursing care, which includes health promotion and maintenance, illness care, restoration, rehabilitation, health counseling, and education based on knowledge derived from theory and research
- Synthesize theoretical and empirical knowledge from nursing, scientific, and humanistic disciplines with practice
- Use the nursing process to provide nursing care for individuals, families, groups, and communities.

- Accept responsibility and accountability for the evaluation of the effectiveness of their own nursing practice
- Enhance the quality of nursing and health practices within practice settings through the use of leadership skills and a knowledge of the political system
- Evaluate research for the applicability of its findings to nursing practice
- Participate with other health care providers and members of the general public in promoting the health and well-being of people
- Incorporate professional values as well as ethical, moral, and legal aspects of nursing into nursing practice
- Participate in the implementation of nursing roles designed to meet emerging health needs of the general public in a changing society (National League for Nursing, 1987)

Changes in Baccalaureate Education

In recent years there have been changes in the nature of baccalaureate education. Some schools, seeking to add an advanced component, have added courses that permit a degree of specialization at the baccalaureate level (e.g., additional courses in coronary or intensive care nursing). Other schools are providing more grounding in research, either as preparation for graduate school or for a more varied role in nursing. One of the most interesting changes has occurred in California. In that state the rules and regulations for schools of nursing stipulate that all courses required by the Board of Nursing for licensure as a registered nurse be offered within the first thirty-six months of full-time training, the first six academic semesters, or the first nine academic quarters, whichever is shortest (California Board of Registered Nursing, 1976). In essence this means that all educational preparation required for application for licensure of students enrolled in baccalaureate programs in that state must be completed by the end of the junior year. This leaves the senior year to be filled with specialty experience, preceptorships, or whatever the school might deem appropriate education. This change in the licensure law has also caused some problems. Some students complete their junior year and successfully pass the licensing examination. They then elect to drop out of school and work as a registered nurse. Although they are licensed in the state of California, these students have no degree from any school, which creates problems if they seek licensure in another state.

ASSOCIATE DEGREE EDUCATION

The movement for associate degree education began in 1952. It has the distinction of being the first and, to date, the only type of nursing education established on the basis of planned research and experimentation. Three events undoubtedly influenced its beginning. First, it followed in the wake of the community college movement across the United States, which saw the organization and growth of 2-year community colleges that not only offered the first 2 years of a traditional 4-year college program but also brought to the community many vocational and adult education programs. The goal of the community college was to make some form of college education available to all who would desire it. Second, the cadet nurse program was created during World War II and demonstrated that qualified students could be adequately educated in less than the traditional 3 years. Lastly, the development of associate degree education was influenced by the studies conducted about nursing education in the United States, as discussed Chapter 1.

Characteristics of Associate Degree Education

Associate degree education, which had its birth in the Cooperative Research Project in Junior and Community College Education for Nursing, began at Teachers College, Columbia University, and was directed by Mildred Montag. The original project included seven junior and community colleges and one hospital school, located in six regions of the United States. This type of nursing education has expanded from only two schools in 1952 to over 800 in 1991.

There are four basic characteristics of associate degree education. These include (1) encompassing the nursing program as an integral part of the college that controls and finances the program; (2) assuring the members of the nursing faculty the same privileges and responsibilities granted to other faculty; (3) organizing the curriculum for completion in 2 years with a clearly stated philosophy, rationale, and conceptual framework; and (4) assuring that students are treated as are other community college students with regard to admission, progression, and graduation requirements (National League for Nursing, 1973). The programs are designed to award an associate degree on completion and graduates are eligible to write the state licensing examination from registered nursing.

Associate degree education was founded on the premise that the health care delivery system could incorporate a nursing technician whose function would be less autonomous than that of the baccalaureate-prepared nurse but greater than that of the practical nurse. The graduate would be prepared to work "at the bedside" under supervision, performing the routine nursing skills for patients. This would be a new type of worker, the nursing technician, to help meet nursing needs. This caregiver would be educated in a new type of technical education program in nursing that would be completed in 2 years' time in junior and community colleges. One half of the curriculum would comprise general education courses and the other half, nursing courses. Learning experiences were carefully selected to meet specific objectives. Montag believed that most students would conclude their education at this point and would not continue on to earn a baccalaureate degree.

Competencies of the Associate Degree Graduate

In 1978 the NLN published a document entitled *Competencies of the Associate Degree Nurse on Entry into Practice*. Drafts were mailed to all associate degree programs and to individual members of the Council of Associate Degree Program (CADP) for input. This document began with assumptions basic to the scope of practice of the associate degree nurse on entry into practice and continued with a list a competencies. Assumptions with regard to practice were as follows (National League for Nursing, 1978):

- Is directed toward clients who need information or support to maintain health
- Is directed toward clients who are in need of medical diagnostic evaluation and/or are experiencing acute or chronic illness
- Is directed toward clients' responses to common, well-defined health problems
- Includes the formulation of a nursing diagnosis
- Consists of nursing interventions selected from established nursing protocols where probable outcomes are predictable
- Is concerned with individual clients and is given with consideration of the person's relationship within a family, group, and community
- Includes the safe performance of nursing skills that require cognitive, psychomotor, and affective capabilities
- May be in any structured care setting but primarily occurs within acute- and extended-care facilities
- Is guided directly or indirectly by a more experienced registered nurse

- Includes the direction of peers and other workers in nursing in selected aspects of care within the scope of practice of associate degree nursing
- Involves an understanding of the roles and responsibilities of self and other workers within the employment setting

The document then went on to outline specific competencies of the associate degree nurse on entry into practice.

In 1989 and 1990 this document was again reviewed by members of CADP and was updated to reflect current practice. In the revision the assumptions basic to practice were deleted and what had been five defined roles were condensed to three. These are Role as Provider of Care, Role as Manager of Care, and Role as Member within the Discipline of Nursing. The competencies are focused around these three roles and describe the behaviors the associate degree graduate demonstrates on graduation as well as the competencies the graduate would be expected to demonstrate 6 months following graduation. This last set of competencies are identified as "anticipated competencies" (National League for Nursing, 1990).

The advent of associate degree education in nursing has brought with it a change in the kind of students who enroll. Nursing students were traditionally a homogeneous group consisting of mostly single white females ranging in age from 18 to 35 who were usually scholastically in the upper third of their high school class. Associate degree programs (although sometimes adding selective admission policies to the "open door" philosophy of the community colleges) attract older people, married women, minorities, men, and students with a wider range of intellectual abilities. People who already possess baccalaureate or higher degrees in other fields also seek admission to associate degree programs, often because it can be accomplished faster than earning another baccalaureate degree. Many changes have occurred in nursing since the first associate degree programs were established. Many of the programs preparing graduates with an associate degree have veered from the concepts established by the early leaders of associate degree education.

Concerns Facing Associate Degree Education

Over the years associate degree education has changed somewhat. There is a growing tendency to place more emphasis and time on nursing courses than on general education courses. Faculty, prepared with master's degrees in nursing, have difficulty defining *essential content*. They often respond to suggestions from advisory committees that ask for graduates with greater knowledge particularly as it relates to some specialty areas (e.g., coronary care). Some programs, in an attempt to prepare graduates who can meet the demands of employers, have added courses in team leadership or management, and in physical assessment. In some instances, changes in the basic requirements of the college for completion of associate degrees have increased the number of credits nursing students must complete. The concept of "core course" taken by all who graduate from the college has been a popular one. More content and greater credit hours have resulted in programs that can take up to 3 years to complete.

Criteria for accreditation of these programs established by the accredited schools that are members of the Council of Associate Degree Programs of the National League for Nursing have set 108 quarter hours or 72 semester credits as the maximum number of credits for any program. Many schools have difficulty meeting this criteria. (National League for Nursing, 1991). Where the structure of the program would allow completion in 2 years, the selective admission criteria developed by faculty to deal with burgeoning numbers of applicants may not. When enrollments in nursing programs dropped throughout the nation in 1986, associate degree programs were the least affected. Today most programs receive many more applications for admission than there are positions in beginning nursing classes. This has resulted in the need to develop some method for selecting students. In some instances this has been a "waiting list," which honors the concept of "first come—first served." Other schools have used systems similar to a lottery. Also popular are "factoring" systems built around the concept of awarding points for courses completed, past work experience, cumulative grade point average and similar criteria. These factoring systems often result in the student spending at least 1 year in college prior to starting nursing courses in order to secure a position in the beginning nursing class.

An increasing number of graduates are seeking additional education beyond the associate degree, and the "ladder" concept in nursing education is growing. Registered nurse baccalaureate and "two-on-two" programs are increasing as these graduates demand easier matriculation into 4-year institutions of learning. In some states legislation has been passed strongly encouraging, and in some instances mandating, articulation plans allowing graduates to move from one level of nursing education to another with minimum loss of credit. These issues are discussed later in the chapter.

Despite the planning and experimentation that preceded the instigation of associate degree nursing programs, hospital nursing service personnel appeared to be poorly prepared to accept the associate degree graduate. The graduates were sometimes referred to as " 2-year wonders" and were criticized by nursing service personnel for being prepared to function only as beginning practitioners. Only after a period of orientation would they become well indoctrinated with the operations of the hospital and ready to move into staff roles requiring more responsibility. Nursing service levels similar complaints at today's baccalaureate graduate, but nursing service may have the poorest understanding of associate degree education. This is not surprising when one realizes that a major issue in nursing as a whole is the delineation of roles of the various practitioners. What is technical education? How does it vary from baccalaureate programs? What constitutes a professional role?

Another problem involved with associate degree education stems from what might be called "titling." Although technical education for nursing was well delineated by Montag, Matheney, and other leaders in associate degree education, and although it is honored in other fields of study, there has been little acceptance of graduates who are "technicians" in nursing. This resistance has come from the graduates of associate degree programs as much as from the general nursing public. In 1976 the Council of Associate Degree Programs, meeting in Washington, D.C., moved to change the name of the graduate of associate degree programs from "technical" to "associate degree" nurse.

Whereas questions regarding titling, licensure, entry level, and role delineation are yet to be answered, most nursing educators agree that associate degree education in nursing has a permanent place within the educational establishment and within the nursing profession itself.

MASTER'S AND DOCTORAL PROGRAMS THAT PREPARE FOR LICENSURE

In concluding our discussion of the various educational programs that prepare the graduate to write the state licensing examination for registered nursing, we need to mention the generic master's programs.

The history of such programs goes back a number of years, to programs at Yale and several other schools of nursing where students were admitted with a baccalaureate degree in another area. They were granted a master's degree in nursing after completing an established program of study of approximately 2 years that prepared the graduate for registered nurse licensure. In addition, there is one program, located at Case-Western Reserve University, in which the student earns a doctorate in nursing before being eligible to write the licensing examination.

Interest in this type of educational preparation for nursing is increasing. It reflects, in part, the thinking of some nurse leaders that the minimum preparation for professional nursing should be the master's degree. It also provides a higher degree to those persons who possess basic baccalaureate preparation in another area of study and are making career changes. With increasing emphasis being placed on the need for a baccalaureate degree for professional practice, making this type of program an option is certainly credible. When programs offering this option are not available, many students who have degrees in other disciplines have chosen to pursue a 2-year associate degree in nursing. In spite of availability, some persons with degrees in other disciplines opt for the 2-year degree because of time and expense.

SIMILARITIES AMONG PROGRAMS

Currently there appear to be as many similarities in the various avenues to nursing education as there are variances. These similarities may be grouped into several broad classifications that include academic standards, administrative concerns, and areas relating to students.

Academic Similarities

In the academic realm three similarities stand out:

1. All graduates write the NCLEX for registered nursing in their state. All writers must meet the same minimum cutoff score to pass the test and become licensed.

2. All schools must meet the criteria established for state board approval and (in many instances on a voluntary basis) the criteria developed for national accreditation.

3. Members of the faculty are pushed to meet the increasing demands of education, clinical excellence, tenure, and possibly vocational certification. Workloads and the time invested in the performance of professional responsibilities often are disparate with that of instructors from other areas of the campus, even though they are considered colleagues in the educational setting.

Administrative Similarities

From an administrative perspective, two similarities are noted:

1. Adequate financial support is a major concern. All programs are relatively expensive to operate in comparison to other forms of education provided in colleges and universities. Federal and state

agencies are tightening the reins on funding and are demanding greater accountability. Less financial assistance is available to students in the form of scholarships and loans than in the past. Tuition costs are rising.

2. Finding appropriate learning experiences is a challenge. Most programs find themselves searching and competing with other schools for learning experiences in clinical agencies. To some extent this competition is related to changes in societal values and the health care delivery system. Families are electing to have fewer children and, more recently in some societies, to deliver these children at home. The result has been fewer patients in the obstetrical units of hospitals. Pediatric patients are managed on an outpatient basis as much as possible, and hospitalization, when required, is kept to a minimum. The management of the client with psychiatric disturbances is moving from institutions to community mental health centers whenever feasible. Finally, the increase in the number and size of schools in urban areas creates high demand for clinical facilities in those areas.

Similarities Relating to Students

When the area relating to students is considered, three similarities are noted:

1. Selection of students is a major task. All schools must develop sound educational programs while balancing student enrollments against faculty recruitment and retention factors. In many instances the number of applications exceed the positions available in beginning classes. This has resulted in the development of selective admission policies that have been carefully scrutinized by school officials and then reviewed by the school's attorney for correct legal form and for legal ramifications before being accepted by the school's policy-making group.

2. Legal concerns are demanding increased time and attention. Programs are caught up in more legal concerns than in the past, because applicants and students seek their "rights as individuals" and challenge admission and dismissal policies. The NSNA Student Bill of Rights and Responsibilities, which was developed by the National Student Nursing Association, is widely accepted by schools of nursing throughout the country. This bill sets forth the students' basic rights and establishes grievance procedures if a student believes that these rights have been violated (see Chapter

13, Figure 13-4). Another legal concern relates to malpractice coverage for students. Some collegiate programs, now removed from the umbrella coverage of the hospital, ask that students purchase malpractice insurance to provide protection against financial losses that could occur as the result of suits that could be based on errors committed in the learning process.

3. There is greater diversity in the student body. All programs are experiencing a wider diversity in the characteristics of applicants seeking admission to the programs. That is to say, programs are receiving more applications from males, minorities, older adults, and persons who possess degrees in other fields of study. Students with English as a second language are presenting new challenges to nursing faculty in all types of programs.

One usually finds nursing educators united in their efforts to create quality programs that will graduate students who can function satisfactorily in a changing and challenging health care delivery system (Table 2-1).

OTHER FORMS OF NURSING EDUCATION

Educational offerings in nursing have grown tremendously since the 1960s. This is due in part to the changing role of the nurse in health care delivery and to the need for more adequate education to meet the preparation requirements of that role. Another contributing factor is the continuing push to make nursing truly professional. The result is the need for practitioners, with master's and doctoral degrees, who are interested and competent in research techniques and skills. A third significant reason for advancing nursing education relates to requirements placed on the profession for leadership in nursing administration and education. Nurse educators, joining the ranks of other professionals in the academic environment, are required to possess equivalent educational background. Nurses who assume roles in nursing administration have found the need for a solid understanding of management and finance principles that is acquired by study at the master's and doctoral level.

Registered Nurse Baccalaureate Programs

Recent years have seen an increase in the number of registered nurse baccalaureate (RNB) programs. These programs are designed for registered nurses with either a diploma or an associate degree who wish to return to school to complete a baccalaureate degree in nursing. These programs carry various names in different parts of the country, including baccalaureate registered nurse (BRN) programs, two-on-two, and, in the Midwest, capstone programs. There are several reasons for the increase in this form of nursing education. Employers are requiring greater preparation for supervisory roles. Highly qualified young men and women are entering associate degree programs because of cost and time factors and are then planning more education several years after completion of the original program. Nursing as a profession is pushing toward increasing the number of nurses prepared with baccalaureate and higher degrees.

RNB programs vary greatly throughout the United States. In some instances they exist in universities that already offer the generic baccalaureate program. The students may be integrated with generic baccalaureate students, partially separated, or totally separated. Another form of RNB preparation is the two-on-two approach, in which registered nurse students transfer into the college or university with junior standing and complete an additional 2 years of upper-division nursing classes. In some instances, this is the only program in nursing offered by that college or university, that is, the college does not offer a basic program that prepares a graduate for licensure. Some schools offer nurse practitioner preparation in conjunction with the baccalaureate degree, although the growing tendency is to place this at the master's level.

The general trend is to allow the transfer of credits in basic education courses such as psychology, sociology, and in the natural and biological sciences earned at junior and community colleges. Often some transfer credit is given for nursing (e.g., 45 quarter credits), or the courses may be challenged. Distribution requirements of the particular college or university must be satisfied, and upper-division nursing courses must be completed in such areas as physiological nursing, community health, and supervision. A minimum of 2 years usually is required for completion of the program, although the time may be longer, depending on the number of requirements satisfied at the time of entry.

When the programs offering baccalaureate education to registered nurses were first launched, they were criticized by some nurse educators. The criticism seemed to revolve around three central themes. The first was based in the fact that the ladder concept in nursing education was slow to develop. As we discussed earlier, many nurse educators perceived associate degree education as terminal and did not accept it as a stepping-stone to baccalaureate education.

The second concern related to the problems associated with evaluating previous learning and granting credit for that learning. How should one equate nursing process that was taught at the 100 level in the com-

Table 2–1. **Educational Opportunities for Registered Nursing: A Comparison**

	Diploma	Associate Degree	Baccalaureate
Location	Is usually conducted by and based in a hospital	Most often conducted in junior or community colleges, occasionally in senior colleges and universities	Located in senior colleges and universities
Length of Study	Requires generally twenty-four to thirty months but may require three academic years	Requires usually two academic or sometimes two calendar years	Requires four academic years
Requirements for Admission	Requires graduation from high school or its equivalent, satisfactory general academic achievement, and successful completion of certain prerequisite courses	Requires that applicants meet entrance requirements of college as well as of program	Requires that applicants meet entrance requirements of the college or university as well as those of program
Program of Learning	Includes courses in theory and practice of nursing and in biological, physical, and behavioral sciences May require that certain courses in the physical and social sciences be taken at a local college or university	Combines a balance of nursing courses and college courses in the basic natural and social sciences with courses in general education and the humanities	Frequently concentrates on courses in the theory and practice of nursing in the junior and senior years Provides education in the theory and practice of nursing and courses in the liberal arts as well as the behavioral and physical sciences
Clinical Component	Provides early and substantial clinical learning experiences in the hospital and a variety of	Requires as a significant part of the program supervised clinical instruction in	Provides clinical laboratory courses in a variety of settings where health and nursing care are given

	community agencies; these focus on an understanding of the hospital environment and the interrelationship of other health disciplines		hospitals and other community health agencies
Opportunity for Educational Advancement	Little or no transferability of courses unless affiliated with a community college or university	Is structured so that some credits may be applied to baccalaureate degree	Provides the basic academic preparation for advancement to higher positions in nursing and to master's degree
Competency on Graduation	Graduate is prepared to plan for the care of patients with other members of the health care team, to develop and carry out plans for the care of individuals or groups of patients, and to direct selected members of the nursing team. Has an understanding of the hospital climate and the community health resources necessary for the extended care of patients	Graduate is prepared to plan and give direct patient care in hospitals, nursing homes, or similar health care agencies and to participate with other members of the health care team, such as licensed practical nurses, nurses aides, physicians, and other registered nurses in rendering care to patients	Graduate is prepared to plan and give direct care to individuals and families, whether sick or well, to assume responsibility for directing other members of the health care team, and to take on beginning leadership positions. Practices in a variety of settings and emphasizes comprehensive health care, including preventive and rehabilitative services, health counseling and education, and care in acute and long-term illnesses Has necessary education for graduate study toward a master's degree and may move more rapidly to specialized leadership positions in nursing as teacher, administrator, clinical specialist, nurse practitioner, and nurse researcher
Licensure	Must successfully complete state licensing examination	Must successfully complete state licensing examination	Must successfully complete state licensing examination

munity college with nursing process that was taught at the 300 level in the senior university?

The third area that presented difficulties was that of determining what additional courses in nursing should be offered and how they should be offered. A serious question existed as to whether the standards, program objectives, and educational structures that had been developed for the generic student were appropriate for the registered nurse. What learning experience could be included that would help to "socialize" the student for the role of a baccalaureate graduate? What additional nursing courses were needed to form the upper-division major in nursing that would provide a basis for graduate education?

Because the skills of the various graduates were not clearly delineated, it was difficult to develop a curriculum that would enable the RNB graduate to demonstrate specific terminal behaviors. When attempts were made to develop such programs, baccalaureate educators found themselves confronted with another concern: they were working with adult students. This required them to rethink teaching-learning principles to provide effective education. Students were seeking a learning program that allowed for part-time study, provided more evening and weekend classes, and permitted part- or full-time employment while pursuing more education. They wanted the education brought to them rather than going to the educational setting.

RNB education and two-on-two educational programs have recently gained more acceptance. In some instances schools operating both basic and RNB programs report graduating more RNB students than basic graduates. At least three factors are responsible for the change in attitude toward RNB education. change. First, the ANA Commission on Nursing Education has provided a push to increase the availability of baccalaureate programs for registered nurses. As more and more states endorse the ANA position on entry into practice, nurse educators, steeped in the traditional approaches to baccalaureate education, are challenged to create and accept more innovative educational strategies.

The second factor comes from pressure within each state itself. A number of states have enacted legislation, sometimes in response to the nursing shortage, that requires the development of a state-wide plan for articulation between various types of nursing education programs. In most instances the legislation establishes a date by which the plan will be implemented.

The last push for increased development of educational mobility has come from organizations in the health care arena. The American Medical Association (AMA) House of Delegates has suggested career mobility as one way to alleviate the nurse shortage. Members of the National League for Nursing passed a resolution at the convention held in 1989 requiring that the NLN drop entry issue activities and take steps that would increase educational mobility.

Some of the RNB programs currently in operation provide for part-time study or for studies completed through evening courses. The desirability of such an approach for nurses who must work to support their education is obvious. Other innovative RNB programs provide baccalaureate education to people living in areas geographically remote from colleges or universities. These programs have used new technologies available for the electronic transmission of information.

The External Degree

The concept of an external degree is not new. Universities in Australia, the Soviet Union, and England have long recognized independent study validated by examination. The University of London has awarded college degrees earned in this fashion since 1836. The major difference between the external degree and the traditional educational experience is that students awarded an external degree are not required to attend classes or follow any prescribed methods of learning. (They may choose to take some classes.) Learning is assessed through highly standardized and validated examinations. This approach to education had not been developed in the United States until recently. Schools in the United States that were first to recognize the value of this self-directed learning were New York's Empire State College and the University Without Walls consortium.

The New York Regents External Degree (REX) Program of the University of the State of New York has become part of this movement. The New York Board of Regents established the College Proficiency Examination Program in 1961. Similar to the College-Level Examination Program tests developed by the Educational Testing Service, the examinations allow students to gain credit and meet the regents' external degree requirements without attending classes.

In 1971 the New York Board of Regents authorized an external associate degree program in nursing; the external baccalaureate degree in nursing was to follow in April 1976 with the first baccalaureate degrees awarded in 1979. The W. K. Kellogg Foundation provided funds to support the initiation of the program. The programs have grown in popularity, and both the associate degree program and the baccalaureate program are accredited by the NLN programs.

The nursing program, like other external degree programs in arts, science, and business, uses an assessment approach and is primarily— although not exclusively—designed for those with some experience in nursing. It is philosophically based on principles of the adult learner that advocate education that is flexible and learner oriented. Specifically, the responsibility for demonstrating that learning has occurred is placed on the student, and the responsibility for identifying the content to be learned and objectively assessing that this has occurred rests with the faculty. The nursing major is divided into cognitive and performance components. The cognitive learning is documented through five nationally standardized and psychometrically valid written examinations. These examinations are available nationally through the American College Testing Program and are administered six times a year at nearly 200 sites. Clinical skills are evaluated through four criteria-referenced performance examinations. Five regional performance assessment centers have been established throughout the United States to make the performance examinations more accessible to candidates. Because performance examinations are quite different from typical evaluation procedures, the people who administer the examinations must complete a 100-hour training program. The major thrust of the training sessions is to exchange teaching-helping behaviors with those of the neutral observer whose role is to determine that criteria have been met (Lenburg, 1984).

Collaborative relationships have been established with academic institutions that want to assist REX candidates who live in their area. The local colleges advertise the program to area nurses and offer courses designed to assist the student who is preparing for examination. Close collaboration occurs between REX faculty and the local college faculty. Students who want to learn more about this program are encouraged to write to the University of the State of New York, Regents External Degree Program, Cultural Education Center, Albany, New York 12230.

In 1981 the California State University Consortium inaugurated the West Coast's first statewide external degree baccalaureate program in nursing for working registered nurses who have current California licenses. Fashioned after the New York model, the program was developed around self-paced instruction modules and other nontraditional learning options. The program emphasized flexibility in learning methods, pace, and site at which the learning occurs. Critics of the program expressed concern about its ability to maintain prevailing standards of education. Cost was another factor.

Despite objections, alternative and nontraditional avenues to nursing education continue to grow and appeal to the learner. Nursing education, like nursing care, should be tailored to the consumer's needs.

Figure 2–4. Clinical skills are evaluated through performance examinations.

NURSING EDUCATION AT THE GRADUATE LEVEL

The critical need for nurses who have had additional preparation to function in educational settings, in supervisory roles, and as clinical specialists and to fulfill the expanded role of the nurse has resulted in the increase of programs at the graduate level.

Master's Preparation

A variety of models of master's preparation in nursing exist. Most could be classified as traditional in approach, but a study of master's programs found that 36% used nontraditional options (Forni, 1987). Some less traditional approaches include outreach programs; summers-only programs; RN-to-MSN tracks that provide a direct route to master's degrees for registered nurses who have graduated from diploma or associate degree programs; programs for groups with special needs, such as registered nurses with non-nursing baccalaureate degrees or those seeking preparation as technical nurse educators; and programs that admit non-nurses and foreign graduates. Some schools offer off-campus classes, perhaps rotating sites, and some use telecommunication systems to deliver core content by way of television. In at least one school all classes are on Fridays. Several unique programs (e.g., those at Yale University, Pace University, and the University of Tennessee at Knoxville) offer a master's degree in nursing after completion of a baccalaureate degree in another field. Such programs, called generic master's degree programs, were discussed earlier in the chapter.

Most programs require at least 1 full year for completion; many have been expanded to 2 years. Master's programs in nursing are often found in senior colleges and universities that have baccalaureate programs in nursing. They have the option of seeking voluntary accreditation from the NLN.

Persons seeking information about master's degree programs in nursing should be aware of the NLN publication *Master's Education: Route to Opportunities in Contemporary Nursing.*

Doctoral Studies

The number of requests for admission to doctoral study in nursing has greatly increased since the early 1980s. The impetus for this movement stems from the need for advanced study for academic advancement or tenure in the educational setting and reflects the need in nursing research for the advancement of the profession as a whole.

Before doctorates in nursing were offered, doctoral study in other fields allowed nursing into the mainstream of education in the United States. A doctorate outside the area of nursing was often the only doctorate available to the person seeking further education; doctorates in nursing are relatively new to the educational milieu, as opposed to such degrees in psychology, sociology, anthropology, or physiology. Certainly nursing can and has benefited from other disciplines.

Doctoral programs in nursing offer a variety of degrees such as the doctor of nursing science (DNSc), the doctor of science in nursing (DSN), the doctor of nursing education (DNEd), or the doctor of philosophy (PhD) in nursing. Other types of doctorates are also available to nurses, such as the doctor of education (EdD) or the doctor of public health (DPH).

The difference in preparation and function of graduates possessing these various degrees in confusing, but for the most part nurses with doctorates provide leadership roles in education, often serving as a dean or director of nursing programs, or they are involved in the research and development of a body of nursing knowledge.

Although assuming no role in the accreditation of doctoral programs, the NLN has published a pamphlet entitled *Doctoral Programs in Nursing* that provides information about various programs of doctoral study in nursing.

DIRECTLY ARTICULATED PROGRAMS

Another recent innovation in nursing education is a program that provides direct articulation between lower-level and higher-level programs. It is this type of education that many of the legislative mandates are encouraging. The purpose of such a program is to facilitate opportunities for students to start nursing education, stop when some goal (such as practical nurse licensure) is achieved, or keep moving up the educational ladder.

The plan, which is especially attractive to practical nurse and associate degree students, allows them to move up the career ladder from practical nurse to associate degree nurse to the nurse with a baccalaureate degree. Students in an articulated licensed practical nurse/associate degree program would spend 1 year preparing to be an LPN and another year completing the associate degree. If they want to continue after this 2-year period, they can earn a baccalaureate degree at another institution after two more years of study. From that point a student could continue work toward a master's degree.

Such programs usually involve planning between two or more institutions, but, depending on start and stop points, they may occur within a single institution. Of concern to nurse educators today is whether nursing assistants should be included in this ladder approach and, if so, how they can be accommodated.

These multiple-entry, multiple-exit programs are not without problems. Initially they are difficult to develop because of the tremendous amount of joint planning needed. Leveling of content in nursing as well as in the supporting areas of natural and behavioral sciences is critical. Understanding what has been taught and determining how to evaluate current knowledge is also important. Educators need to speak the same language and develop mutual respect.

Figure 2–5. Among innovations occurring in nursing education over the past decade are programs that provide direct articulation between lower-level and higher-level programs.

NONDEGREE PROGRAMS

Specialized programs have been developed to help to prepare individuals for roles of increased breadth and scope. Some of these programs are incorporated into the preparation leading to a particular degree; others exist as part of a school's continuing education program.

The registered nurse anesthesia and the midwifery programs both award a certificate after completion of a standardized and rigorous course of study lasting from 18 months to 2 years. Each program stipulates its own admission requirements, some requiring licensure only, others requiring a baccalaureate degree.

Programs that have been introduced more recently include nurse practitioner and nursing specialist preparation in areas of nursing practice such as pediatrics, gerontology, family health, genetics, and women's health care. Designed to meet the increasing demand of the community, these courses provide concentrated study in specific areas over a period of time lasting from several months to a year or more. Requirements for admission vary tremendously. Some require licensure for admission, others stipulate the baccalaureate degree, while still other programs require that the education occur at the post–master's degree level.

The proliferation of such programs has been so great that a complete listing is impossible. A student interested in pursuing such preparation is encouraged to write to the college or university of choice for information about available programs.

INTERNSHIPS AND RESIDENCIES FOR THE NEW GRADUATE

When nursing education moved from hospital-based diploma programs into higher education, a new problem was created. Employers of the new graduates, who expected these graduates to function as experienced and qualified professionals on the day after graduation, complained that they were not prepared to assume staff nurse positions within their institutions.

The changes that had occurred in nursing education, including changes in diploma education, had resulted in shortened clinical experience. Many graduates of diploma schools of the 1950s would have as much as 4000 clock hours of clinical experience, albeit more as an apprenticeship and a service to the hospital than as a learning experience. Graduates of associate degree programs, with integrated curricula and objective-based learning experiences, emerged into the work world with clinical learning time of 800 or fewer clock hours. Baccalaureate and hospital-based programs also had decreased their clinical hours as curricula were reorganized.

Critics in nursing service were distressed by a new type of graduate who could think, analyze, and synthesize but who was inexperienced in "doing." Most graduates needed an orientation to the work facility and to their new role in that organization and time to become efficient in the administration of their newly learned skills. Although few would question the need for internships and residencies for the new physician, the need for a similar experience for new nursing graduates was viewed as appalling.

The new graduates, unable to live up to the expectations placed on them, became frustrated and discouraged and often opted for a less stressful situation, sometimes even outside nursing. Nursing educators, in defending the education provided, cited other professions, such as law and engineering, in which graduates needed a period of time to adapt to the world of work.

By the 1970s it was apparent that something must be done. Although the cost was a problem, orientation programs, internships, and residencies for new graduates were instituted by hospitals. The programs were intended to ease the transition from the role of student to that of staff by providing the opportunity to increase clinical skills and knowledge as well as self-confidence. Programs can last from several weeks to a year and are designed for graduates of all nursing programs—associate degree, diploma, and baccalaureate. They often include rotations to various units within the hospital, including specialty areas, and they accommodate different shifts. Usually some formal class work is associated with the experience, but the majority of the time is spent in direct patient care, often under the supervision of a preceptor.

Some direct benefits to institutions, other than a better prepared new employee who remains in employment, have resulted from such programs. Inadequacies in policy and procedure books have been uncovered and, as a result, these books have been rewritten. Performance evaluation tools that are more objective in format have emerged. Nursing practice throughout an agency may have become more standardized. Job satisfaction has increased. It is no longer unusual for hospitals to advertise planned orientation and internships as benefits offered to the new graduate who would seek employment at their institution.

CONTINUING EDUCATION

Continuing education programs are widely publicized in today's nursing literature. They are frequently presented just prior to and as part of major nursing conventions. Some professional meetings carry continuing education credit. Other continuing education programs exist as an extension of nursing program at a college or university.

Continuing education in nursing is defined as "planned learning experiences beyond a basic nursing educational program. The learning experiences are designed to promote the development of knowledge, skills, and attitudes for the enhancement of nursing practice, thus improving health care to the public" (American Nurses' Association, 1974).

Like so many other areas of nursing, this is not new. In an article entitled "Nursing the Sick," written around 1882, Florence Nightingale wrote:

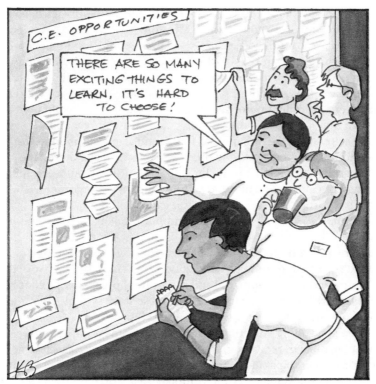

Figure 2–6. Today colleges, universities, hospitals, voluntary agencies, and private proprietary groups are all offering continuing education courses to registered nurses.

> Nursing is, above all, a progressive calling. Year by year nurses have to learn new and improved methods, as medicine and surgery and hygiene improve. Year by year nurses are called upon to do more and better than they have done. It is felt to be impossible to have a public register of nurses that is not a delusion (cited in Seymer, 1954, p 349).

The first continuing education courses for nurses probably would be considered postgraduate instruction today. In 1899, Teachers College at Columbia University instituted a course for qualified graduate nurses in hospital economics. Nursing institutes and conferences were first offered to nurses in the 1920s. Often these were given to make up for deficiencies in basic nursing curricula of the time. Hospital in-service or staff development programs were also beginning to be discussed in nursing literature around this time. Today most hospitals employ someone who is responsible for an in-service education program.

By 1959 federal funds became available for short-term courses, giving much thrust to continuing education. In 1967 the ANA published "Avenues for Continued Learning," its first definitive statement on continuing education; and in 1973 the ANA Council on Continuing Education was established. The Council, which is responsible to the ANA Commission on Education, is concerned about standards of continuing education, accreditation of the programs, transferability of credit from state to state, and development of guidelines for recognition systems within states. In 1974, "Standards for Continuing Education in Nursing" was published by the ANA, and the federal government altered the Nurse Traineeship Act of 1972 to include an option that would provide continuing education as an alternative to taking increasing numbers of students into programs receiving federal capitation dollars.

By the 1970s almost all nursing publications had something to say about continuing education for nurses. Practically all states were organizing or planning to organize some method by which the nurse could receive recognition for continued education. These systems were called continuing education approval and recognition programs, or continuing education recognition programs, and most state systems followed the guidelines and criteria prepared by the ANA.

The continuing education unit (CEU) became a rather uniform system of measuring, recording, reporting, accumulating, transferring, and recognizing participation in nonacademic credit offerings. The definition of a CEU was developed by the National Task Force on the Continuing Education Unit, which represented 34 educational groups. Although nursing was not one of the groups, the definition has been accepted by the profession. Ten hours of participation in an organized continuing education experience under responsible sponsorship, capable direction, and qualified instruction is equal to one CEU.

Today colleges, universities, hospitals, voluntary agencies, and private proprietary groups are all offering continuing education courses to registered nurses. Cost of that education varies tremendously. Nurses attending meetings and conferences may earn a CEU, or part of one, for merely being in the meeting. No attempt is made to assess whether learning has occurred. Professional journals are including sections on programmed instruction that can be completed in the comfort of one's living room. These have an evaluation mechanism. Telecourses are offered by television. Workshops, institutes, conferences, short courses, and evening courses abound. Yet some nurses do not feel the need to keep up with these current offerings.

A system for accreditation and approval of continuing education in nursing was developed and implemented by the ANA in 1975. Accreditation was awarded for a period of 4 years and assured the public that the continuing education offerings provided consistent quality. A new system, put into operation August 1, 1987, allows organizations that offer continuing education to seek accreditation as either a provider or an approver. A provider is any organization that is responsible for the development, implementation, and evaluation of courses. An approver could be the state nurses' associations, a specialty organization, or a federal nursing service that has been designated to approve the continuing education process. Organizations could be both approvers and providers. The advantage of this program is that it made the system more accessible to groups seeking approval of courses or classes in that it brought it closer to the membership and those offering the programs.

An issue today is whether continuing education should be mandatory or voluntary. Mandatory continuing education affects licensure, that is, any nurse renewing a license in a state requiring (mandating) continuing education will have to meet that state's regulations for completing CEUs. Voluntary continuing education is not related to relicensure. Most states are moving toward mandatory continuing education. Government agencies and state legislatures are exerting pressure on nurses, as they have on physicians, attorneys, dietitians, dentists, pharmacists, and other professionals, to provide evidence of updated knowledge before renewal of license.

A position supporting mandatory continuing education raises some other issues. How shall the learning be measured? Who should accredit the programs? How can quality be ensured? By whom and where shall records be retained? Who should bear the cost? What should be the time frame for continuing education? How many hours, courses, and credits should be required?

You can write directly to a state board of nursing for information on specific requirements (see Appendix A for addresses).

CONCLUSION

The development of nursing education in the United States has resulted in three major avenues to preparation for licensure as a registered nurse. In addition, various other nontraditional approaches to nursing education have evolved. Much controversy exists over which of these routes best prepares the graduate to function in the beginning role of a registered nurse and which degrees should be required for the various expanded roles.

The answers are yet to be determined, but one thing is certain: as nursing grows as a profession and as technology expands and influences health care delivery, changes must and will occur in the education of persons prepared to deliver that care.

In addition, continuing education, whether it is represented by further education that results in a higher degree or whether it takes the form of classes, seminars, or workshops that update and increase expertise, is being encouraged by more and more organizations. Staying current in practice is critical to safe patient care.

Nursing education has had a dynamic history. And it will have a dynamic future. It might be well for nurses to stop apologizing for the many and varied approaches to licensure, certification, and continuing education. Instead, it is time to applaud the innovations that exist and to perfect the quality of the education available. Only then will the public reap the benefits of this creativity.

REFERENCES

American Nurses' Association. Standards for Continuing Education for Nursing. Kansas City, MO, American Nurses' Association, 1974

Deaconess Hospital School of Nursing. Eighty-One Years of Nursing: 1989–1980. Spokane, WA, Deaconess Hospital, 1980

Forni PR: Nursing's diverse master's programs: The state of the art. Nurs Health Care 8(2):770–775, 1987

Hawken PL: NLN perspective: News from the President. Nurs Health Care 11(9):486–487, 1990

Kalisch PA, Kalisch BJ: The Advance of American Nursing, 2nd ed. Boston, Little, Brown & Co, 1986

Laws Relating to Nursing Education Licensure: Practice with Rules and Regulations. Sacramento, CA, California Board of Registered Nursing, 1976

Lenburg CB: Preparation for professionalism through regents external degrees. Nurs Health Care 5(6):319–325, 1984

National League for Nursing: Characteristics of Associate Degree Education in Nursing. Publication No. 23-1500, Council of Associate Degree Programs. New York, National League for Nursing, 1973

National League for Nursing: Characteristics of Baccalaureate Education in Nursing. Publication No. 15-1758, Council of Baccalaureate and Higher Degrees. New York, National League for Nursing, 1987

National League for Nursing: Competencies of Associate Degree Education in Nursing. Publication No. 23-1731, Council of Associate Degree Programs. New York, National League for Nursing, 1978

National League for Nursing: Criteria and Guidelines for Accreditation of Associate Degree Program, 7th ed. Publication No. 23-2439, Council of Associate Degree Programs. New York, National League for Nursing, 1991

National League for Nursing: Educational Outcomes of Associate Degree Nursing Programs: Roles and Competencies. Publication No. 23-2348, Council of Associate Degree Programs. New York, National League for Nursing, 1990

Nightingale F: Nursing the sick. In Seymer LR: Selected Writings of Florence
Nightingale. New York, Macmillan, 1954

FURTHER READINGS

Allen VO, Sutton C: Associate degree nursing education: Past, present, and
future. Nurs Health Care 2(9):496–497, 1981

American Association of Colleges of Nursing. Guidelines for Baccalaureate Education in Nursing for Registered Nurse Students in Colleges and Universities. Publication Series 79, No. 3. Washington, DC, American Association
of Colleges of Nursing, 1980

American Nurses' Association: A Case for Baccalaureate Preparation in Nursing,
ANA publication No. NE-6 15M. Kansas City, MO, American Nurses' Association, 1979

Battista-Calderone A: Designing interactive video instruction: An educator's
perspective. Nurs Health Care 10(9):504–510, 1989

Boyle R: Articulation: From associate degree through master's. Nurs Outlook
20(10):670–672, 1972

Brubaker BH: A faculty learns to make self-pacing work. Nurs Health Care 11(2):
74–77, 1990

Cal State launches off-campus program for the working R.N. Am J Nurs 82(6):
893, 904–905, 1982.

Coleman E: On redefining the baccalaureate degree. Nurs Health Care 7(4):
193–196, 1986

Craver DM, Sullivan PP: Investigation of an internship program. J Contin Educ
Nurs 16(4):114–118, 1985

Davids SL, Laeger E: Developing a BSN program across two institutions: Arizona
state university west campus/Glendale community college—the adjuvant
model. Nurs Health Care 11(2):84–87, 1990

Feldman HR, Jordet C: On the fast track. Nurs Health Care 10(9):490–493,
1989

Felton G: Harnessing today's trends to guide nursing's future. Nurs Health Care
7(4):211–213, 1986

Johnston SC: The use of the Rines model in differentiating professional and
technical nursing practice. Nurs Health Care 3(7):374–379, 1982

Kasprisin CA, Young WB: Nurse internship program reduces turnover, raises
commitment. Nurs Health Care 6(3):137–140, 1985

Kurzen CR: Contemporary Practical/Vocational Nursing. Philadelphia, JB Lippincott, 1989

Lenburg C, Johnson W: Career mobility through nursing education. Nurs Outlook 22(2):265–269, 1974

Mead ME, Berger S, Nicksic E: Contracts for continuing education. J Contin
Educ Nurs 16(4):121–126, 1985

Montag ML: Community College Education for Nursing. New York, McGraw-
Hill Book Company, 1959

O'Leary J: What employers will expect from tomorrow's nurses. Nurs Health Care 7(4):207–209, 1986

Parkinson CF, Parkinson SB: A comparative study between interactive television and traditional lecture offerings for nursing students. Nurs Health Care 10(9):498–502, 1989

Schwartz MD: An introduction to interactive video systems. Computers Nurs 2(1):8–13, 1984

Seymer LR: The Nightingale training school: One hundred years ago. Am J Nurs 60(5):658–661, 1960

Smith PL: Non-nurse college graduates in a specialty master's program: A success story. Nurs Health Care 10(9):494–497, 1989

Tanner CA, Hartshorn J, Rosenfeld P: Critical care nursing in baccalaureate programs. Nurs Health Care 10(9):482–488, 1989

Woolley AS: Defining the product of baccalaureate education. Nurs Health Care 7(4):199–201, 1986

3

Perspectives on Nursing Education

Objectives

After completing this chapter, you should be able to

1. *Discuss the importance of the Brown report.*
2. *Identify at least two factors that prompted improvements in nursing education.*
3. *Discuss the development and major points of the ANA Position Paper on Nursing Education.*
4. *Discuss the positions of other nursing organizations in regard to entry into practice.*
5. *Discuss the problems that have been encountered in attempts to implement the ANA position on entry into practice.*
6. *Explain what is meant by a grandfather clause and why it is necessary when licensing laws are changed.*
7. *Discuss the concept of differentiated practice.*
8. *List some changes that may occur in the methods of nursing instruction in the future.*
9. *Discuss the impact of reduced federal funding on nursing education.*
10. *State the reason nursing theories are important to the profession.*
11. *Identify three nursing theories and theorists.*

In our discussion of nursing and nursing education thus far, we have provided a background for understanding the development of nursing as a profession and a discussion of the various educational paths that will prepare you for the practice of that profession. Nursing education, because it prepares the graduates of tomorrow, must be responsive to change. Social, technical, political, and financial factors will affect the way that nursing is practiced and the manner in which students will be educated for the profession in the future.

THE PUSH FOR CHANGE IN THE 1950s

Throughout the years perhaps no aspect of nursing has been more studied than the educational preparation of nurses. You read about some of these studies in Chapter 1.

The Brown Report

One of the important studies about nursing was conducted in 1948 by Esther Lucille Brown, who was not a nurse. She was concerned that young women were not choosing nursing as a profession and believed as a result of her study that the majority of schools were not providing a professional education. Brown, in her report *Nursing for the Future*, recommended that the term *professional*, when applied to nursing education, be restricted to schools able to furnish professional education as that term was understood by educators (Brown, 1948). This meant that nursing education should move away from the system of apprenticeship that predominated at the time and into a planned program of education that would be similar to that offered by other professions. She recommended that the schools be operated by universities or colleges, hospitals affiliated with institutions of higher learning, medical colleges, or independently. She also recommended that programs be periodically examined or reviewed and that a list of accredited schools be published and distributed.

Following the publication of the Brown report a committee was established to implement some of the recommendations, particularly those related to accreditation of programs. The committee eventually became the National Committee for the Improvement of Nursing Services. From a subcommittee of this group a classification system for schools evolved that ranked them according to overall excellence. All the college-controlled schools ranked in the top groups. At the same time the National League for Nursing Education (NLNE, later to become the National League for Nursing) was recommending that hospital schools consider transferring control and administration of their programs to educational institutions. The NLNE also urged that federal grants be provided to nursing schools to allow for their improvement.

The State Board Test Pool

Along with this push for the improvement of nursing education, there was also increased pressure on licensing authorities to establish the State Board Test Pool. The NLNE offered to assist states develop and adopt machine-scored examination questions that would assure greater uniformity in testing. Originally only six states participated in the testing developed by the NLNE, but by 1949 41 states were using it. In 1951 a standard passing score (350) was adopted. The development of the State Board Test Pool helped each school focus and expand on its goals. (See Chapter 4 for more information on the development of licensing examinations.)

National Accreditation of Nursing Programs

By 1952 the National League for Nursing (previously the NLNE) had a temporary accreditation program in place and was helping schools find ways to improve their programs of instruction. The accreditation program had a noticeable effect on standards of nursing education. As a result of accreditation activities, schools were forced to look at the educational preparation of faculty, the workload of faculty and students, the structure of clinical teaching, withdrawal rates, and state board examination scores.

Changes in Nursing Service

While changes were occurring in the education of nurses, equally significant changes were taking place in the activities for which nurses were responsible in the workplace. With the advent of antibiotics and other major advances in medical treatment, the public was seeking care in hospitals as opposed to home treatment. Infants previously born at home were now being born in hospitals. Increased hospitalization practices drove the need for qualified nurses to a new high. Hospitals were often desperate to find nurses to fill the needed positions, which represented half of all hospital personnel.

The role of the nurse was also changing. Nursing staff were assuming responsibilities formerly associated with the role of the physician. Unfortunately, they were also assuming responsibilities that could have been done by housekeeping, dietary, laboratory, and pharmacy departments. Nurses began spending more time managing personnel, delegating responsibilities, and carrying out other administrative activities. These changes in practice required nurses prepared with higher levels of education (i.e., baccalaureate and master's degrees).

In 1955 the first fellowship program was established by NLN to assist nurses working on master's and doctoral degrees. The money to support the program came from a grant from the Commonwealth Fund (Kalisch and Kalisch, 1986).

As attempts were made to increase the number of nursing personnel prepared as registered nurses, the 2-year associate degree programs came into existence (see Chapter 2). These programs, housed in community and junior colleges, prepared a graduate educated in 2 years and skilled in bedside nursing. The number of associate degree nursing programs grew rapidly during the 1960s. These programs appealed to men, minorities, and older students than had traditionally sought educational preparation for nursing. The number of baccalaureate programs also increased during this time.

Figure 3–1. Basic practice and expanded practice require different educational backgrounds.

CONTINUED PUSH FOR CHANGE IN THE 1960s

In 1961 the surgeon general of the United States Public Health Service appointed a group that would advise him on the federal government's role in providing adequate nursing services to the country. This group was known as the Surgeon General's Consultant Group on Nursing.

The Report of the Surgeon General's Consultant Group

A report of the Surgeon General's Consultant Group on Nursing was published in 1963. It emphasized the need for more nurses and pointed to the lack of adequate financial resources for nursing education as a major problem. The report also identified several other concerns, among them the facts that too few schools were providing adequate nursing education, that too few college-bound young people were being recruited into the profession, and that more nursing schools were needed in colleges and universities.

Graduation from a program offering a baccalaureate degree in nursing was recommended as the minimum educational preparation for nurses assuming leadership roles (U.S. Public Health Service, 1963).

The Surgeon General's Consultant Group on Nursing also made recommendations that federally funded low-cost loans and scholarships be made to students in both professional and practical nursing programs. It advocated the use of federal funds to construct additional nursing school facilities and to expand educational programs. The Nurse Training Act of 1964 was an outgrowth of these recommendations (see Chapter 11).

The Push by ANA for Educational Change

By the later 1950s and early 1960s the American Nurses Association (ANA) began to look with concern at nursing education and the delivery of nursing care. The ANA believed that improvement of nursing practice depended on the advancement of nursing education. In 1960, 1962, and 1964 the house of delegates discussed promoting the baccalaureate degree as the basic educational foundation for professional nursing. In 1962 a committee on education was appointed by the ANA board of directors to pursue this goal.

ACTIVITY OF THE ANA RELATED TO NURSING EDUCATION

For 2 years the Committee on Education studied the major changes and trends in and around nursing, especially as the trends affected patient care. This activity culminated in the development and publication in 1965 of *A Position Paper on Educational Preparation for Nurse Practitioners and Assistants to Nurses.*

Premises and Positions of ANA Position Paper

The ANA Position Paper was developed in accordance with basic premises or assumptions. The basic premises are as follows:

1. Nursing is a helping profession and, as such, provides services that contribute to the health and well-being of people.
2. Nursing is of vital consequence to the individual receiving services; it fills needs that cannot be met by the person, by the family, or by other persons in the community.
3. The demand for services of nurses will continue to increase.
4. The professional practitioner is responsible for the nature and quality of all nursing care patients receive.
5. The services of professional practitioners of nursing will continue to be supplemented and complemented by the services of nurse practitioners who will be licensed.
6. Education for those in the health professions must increase in depth and breadth as scientific knowledge expands.
7. In addition to those licensed as nurses, the health care of the public, in the amount and to the extent needed and demanded, requires the services of large numbers of health occupation workers to function as assistants to nurses. These workers are presently designated nurses' aides, orderlies, assistants, attendants, etc.
8. The professional association must concern itself with the nature of nursing practice, the means for improving nursing practice, and the standards for membership in the professional association (American Nurses' Association, 1965, p 106).

Based on these premises the paper took four major positions:

1. The education for all those who are licensed to practice nursing should take place in institutions of higher education.

2. Minimum preparation for beginning professional nursing practice at the present time should be baccalaureate degree education in nursing.
3. Minimum preparation for beginning technical nursing practice at the present time should be associate degree education in nursing.
4. Education for assistants in the health service occupations would be short, intensive preservice programs in vocational education institutions rather than on-the-job training programs (American Nurses' Association, 1965, p 107).

Responses to the ANA Position Paper

In general, the Position Paper was received with mixed feelings in the nursing community. There were three different educational programs that prepared graduates for registered nurse licensure—baccalaureate, associate degree, and diploma. Both the associate degree and the diploma programs were concerned about the impact of the Position Paper on their programs. Advocates of associate degree programs were particularly concerned that their graduates might have to assume the title "licensed practical nurse" as outlined in the paper. In addition, approximately 85% of the 1966 nursing work force was composed of diploma graduates for whom the diploma was the only educational credential. These individuals saw themselves functioning as professional nurses and were concerned that the Position Paper might change that status. The Position Paper also did not differentiate the educational preparation of the "assistants in the health service occupations" and virtually eliminated the 1-year practical nurse program as it was currently known.

Among the more perplexing of the problems was the lack of definitive statements on the competencies of the graduates of each of the programs. The roles, functions, and responsibilities that each would assume within the health care delivery system were not clear. Although the Position Paper was fairly specific in describing the educational expectations of "professional" and "technical" nursing practice, most graduates of programs preparing for registered nurse licensure were employed by acute care hospitals. The role for the registered nurse in these institutions was primarily socialized around the diploma graduate of the 1950s and did not differentiate job responsibilities in regard to educational preparation. All beginning nurses, whether prepared with associate degrees, baccalaureate degrees, or in hospital–based programs, performed similar activities.

In the face of this overwhelming objection to the Position Paper by the nursing community, ANA's newly appointed Commission on Nursing Education turned its focus to concerns about continuing education.

ANA ACTION RELATED TO EDUCATIONAL PREPARATION IN THE 1970s AND 1980s

Many persons serving as members of the ANA House of Delegates believed that the push for baccalaureate education as the minimum credential for entry into professional nursing should continue. Therefore, in 1978 the ANA House of Delegates decided to step up activity that would clarify and strengthen the system of nursing education.

Resolutions Adopted in 1978

At the ANA Convention held in 1978, the House of Delegates accepted three significant resolutions:

1. That by 1985 the minimum preparation for entry into professional nursing practice be the baccalaureate in nursing, that the ANA would work closely with the state nurses' associations to identify and define two categories of nursing practice, and that national guidelines for implementation be identified and reported back to the ANA membership by 1980
2. That the ANA establish a mechanism devising a comprehensive statement of competencies for the two categories of nursing practice by 1980
3. That the ANA actively support increased accessibility to high-quality career mobility programs that use flexible approaches for those seeking academic degrees in nursing (American Nurses' Association, 1979, pp 5–9).

Discussion and activity with regard to educational preparation for nursing continued within the ANA with resolutions and recommendations becoming more and more directive.

A Stronger Push in the 1980s

When the ANA met in June 1984, the House of Delegates again took an aggressive step toward implementation of the Position Paper. Major issues relating to ANA's organizational structure had been settled

2 years earlier. There was no serious shortage of nurses. A number of diploma programs were discontinuing their programs or were placing their programs under the auspices of colleges and universities that granted degrees at the end of the program. Associate degree programs continued to grow in number. The timing was right for activity related to another push for baccalaureate education for registered nurses.

In response, at the 1984 convention, the Cabinet on Nursing Education introduced an initiative and won an unconditional endorsement of its plan to establish the baccalaureate for professional practice in five percent of the states by 1986, in 15% of the states by 1988, in 50% of them by 1992, and in 100% of the United States by 1995. At this time ANA's Board of Directors agreed to commit $100,000 a year over 5 years to assist the state associations to bring this plan into effect. Later an additional $500,000 was allocated for a nationwide public relations campaign to seek support for the changes in the states. The first states to receive these monies were Maine, Montana, Oregon, and North Dakota. Illinois later received a $50,000 grant for a project that would establish two levels of nursing with legislative action slated for 1987 ("ANA Gears Up," 1985).

In 1985, 20 years after the publication of the original Position Paper, the ANA again pushed to make the statement a reality. The 680-member House of Delegates decided that the title "registered nurse" be reserved for the professional nurse prepared with a baccalaureate degree. The title "associate nurse" was adopted as the title to be used for the technical nurse, a graduate of a state-chartered institution that awards an associate degree. The second title was not determined with any ease. Seventeen different titles for the 2-year graduate were considered by the delegates. ("ANA Delegates Vote," 1985).

ACTIVITIES OF THE STATE ASSOCIATIONS

In 1974 the New York Nurses' Association became the first state to adopt a resolution recommending that it be mandatory by 1985 for all applicants for registered nurse licensure in New York State to have the minimum of a baccalaureate degree in nursing, with an upper-division major in nursing. The proposed legislation was also designed to change the educational requirement for the licensed practical nurse to an associate degree. As proposed, the law allowed for "grandfathering" the license of all current RNs and LPNs, and it specified 1985 as the date when new RNs would be required to have a baccalaureate degree and new LPNs to earn an associate degree. This would have eliminated the

1-year practical nursing program. Although the resolution did not move far in terms of legislation, it started movements in other states and became the springboard for vigorous debate in the entire health care field regarding the appropriate educational preparation required of a professional nurse.

Other states were soon to follow with position statements. By August 1986, at least 48 state nurses' associations had taken positions supporting a change in the educational requirements for entry into nursing practice. The change most commonly recommended was to stipulate the baccalaureate degree in nursing as the requirement for licensure at the professional level and the associate degree in nursing as the requirement for licensure at the technical level. This would mean that there would be one entry point for each level of licensure. Boards of nursing would need to redefine the legal scope of practice for each level (Edge, 1986). Some states had settled on titles to be used by nurses prepared at the two levels; few had developed a competency statement for the categories.

In January 1986, North Dakota published and put into effect administrative rules that required nursing programs to develop specific curricula leading to the associate degree for practical nurse programs and the baccalaureate degree for registered nurse programs in order to be approved by the North Dakota Board of Nursing. This requirement became effective January 1, 1987. The North Dakota legislature was not involved in this change because educational requirements for licensure were not a part of the act itself. (They were stipulated in the rules and regulations that do not require legislative activity for change.) The rules were submitted to the attorney general for his review, as required by the laws of North Dakota, and were subsequently approved "as to their legality." They were adopted by the board on January 16, 1986 ("North Dakota Rule," 1986).

North Dakota was an ideal state in which to start these changes. It had five baccalaureate nursing programs, one of which also offered an associate degree and two of which offered a master's degree. The state had only three hospital-based diploma programs and two state-supported associate degree programs. There were seven programs in North Dakota that prepared licensed practical nurses. The state did not need to "import" nurses from other states to meet the health care needs of the state. Because the Nurse Practice Act was not changed, only the rules, it was not necessary to add a grandfather clause. Nurses already licensed were protected because the revised rules set an effective date of January 1, 1987.

Other states that had nurse practice acts that would allow for the changing of educational requirements for licensure through the rules process carefully watched the activities that were taking place in North Dakota. Some states had organized groups dedicated to protecting the role of the associate degree graduate. Oregon became the first state to have a bill passed in the state legislature that would bar the state board of nursing from making any change in entry-level requirements without legislative approval. Utah and Pennsylvania were to follow ("ADNs, Community College," 1985, "Pennsylvania Legislature," 1987).

OTHER NURSES' ASSOCIATIONS AND THE ENTRY ISSUE

Gradually, other nursing specialty groups and associations endorsed the baccalaureate degree as minimum preparation for entry into professional nursing practice. Among the first organizations to support the position was the National Student Nurses' Association (NSNA), which voted in favor of this at its convention in 1976.

In 1979, several associations indicated support of the baccalaureate degree as the minimum educational level for future entry into professional practice. These were the Association of Operating Room Nurses (AORN), the Emergency Department Nurses' Association, the Association of Rehabilitation Nurses, the American Association of Occupational Health Nurses, and the Executive Board of the Nurses' Association of the American College of Obstetricians and Gynecologists. Many of these organizations had stipulations or qualifications on their position that related to regional planning, career mobility, and clarification of concepts of levels of practice. Eventually most of the major nursing organizations supported the position, at least conceptually.

The NLN has perhaps struggled with its position as much as has any nursing organization. Historically, because the composition of the memberships of the NLN includes educational councils representing practical, diploma, associate degree, and baccalaureate and higher-degree nursing programs, the organization voiced its support for all types of programs. A 1981 NLN "Position Statement on Preparation for Practice in Nursing" affirmed its support for all programs, citing the "social reality" of different types of people seeking careers in nursing as its rationale. However, beginning in 1982, that position changed. First, the board of directors approved a "Position Statement on Nursing Roles: Scope and Preparation." Although supporting three levels of nursing (professional, technical, and vocational), it stated that "professional nursing practice requires a minimum of a baccalaureate degree with a major in nursing" ("NLN Calls," 1982, p 154). Many of the members of the NLN, especially those from the Diploma Council, strongly objected to this position. However, it was supported by a vote of the membership at the 1983 convention. From 1983 until the present various proposals and "trial balloons" regarding entry, titling, and examination have been presented to the NLN membership. At the 1987 biennial convention, the membership "postponed indefinitely" resolutions addressing this issue and in 1989 instructed the NLN to put its energies into activities that would promote upward mobility in nursing.

Discussion of the entry issue would not be complete without including decisions made by two other organizations. One of those organizations is the National Council of State Boards of Nursing. At an August 1986 meeting, representatives of the state boards voted without debate and opposition to take a "formal position of neutrality on changes in nursing education requirements for entry" (Hartung, 1986, p 124).

The final group we will consider is the National Federation of Licensed Practical Nurses (NFLPN). During the 1980s this organization was faced with hospital layoffs of large numbers of practical nurses in favor of hiring more highly educated registered nurses. In August 1984 the membership passed a resolution that would support increasing the period of study of the practical nurse program to 18 months and the awarding of an associate degree at the completion of the program of study. It was the intent of the resolution that much of the increased time would be spent in increasing clinical expertise, and the written rationale for the recommendation was openly one of job security. The title of licensed practical nurse would be retained for graduates of such programs who had passed the National Council Licensure Examination for practical nursing (NCLEX-PN) ("NFLPN OKs," 1984). Seven years later only one state had moved toward implementation, but the NFLPN continues to support this position. Because a large number of practical nurse programs exist in vocational-technical schools, the recommendation of the ANA to place all nursing education in institutions of higher education remains unacceptable to the practical nurse group. They emphasize the critical need for the practical nurse in long-term care facilities.

PROBLEMS ASSOCIATED WITH CHANGES IN THE EDUCATIONAL PREPARATION OF NURSES

A number of problems need to be resolved before the ANA position statement can become a reality.

Titling

One of the most controversial problems is that of titles. Although the position statement calls for two levels of nursing practice, the titles to be used by persons working at each level have not been identified by many states. Some state associations have incorporated titles into their position statements, generally using the title "RN" for the baccalaureate graduate and "LPN" for the 2-year associate degree graduate. This has caused widespread dissatisfaction among the ranks of associate degree graduates, students, and educators who believe that this denigrates the associate degree graduate, who currently may use the RN title if successful on state licensing examinations. The use of these titles is also upsetting to graduates of current diploma schools, from which no degree is granted. It would seem that neither title could be used by those graduates.

Following the decision of the ANA to title the associate degree graduate "associate nurse" and the NLN's suggestion to designate the title "registered associate nurse" to the 2-year graduate, there was activity in some states to use those titles. Staunch supporters of associate degree education were not willing to make this compromise, arguing that since the beginning of the associate degree movement in the 1950s, the graduates have held the title "registered nurse." In supporting their stand on titling they pointed to the past success of the associates degree graduates on the NCLEX-RN.

Scope of Practice

Of equal concern to the issue of titling is that which relates to the description and delineation of the scope of practice for the two levels of caregivers. The scope of practice, as discussed in Chapter 4, is that section of the Nurse Practice Act that outlines the activities a person with that license may legally do. As states have moved toward plans for implementing two levels of practice, the process of making nursing diagnoses and developing nursing care plans has been included in the scope of practice of the professional nurse only. Associate degree educators have been adamant in their contention that unless the scope of practice for the 2-year graduate also includes these behaviors, that graduate will be unemployable and able to do less than the LPN of today ("Illinois RNs Seek," 1986).

The Grandfather Clause

Historically, the licensing of professions and occupations has been within the realm of the police power of each individual state. This power to license is used to safeguard the health and welfare of citizens. When a state licensure law is enacted, or if a current law is repealed and a new law enacted, the grandfather clause has been a standard feature that allows persons to continue to practice their profession or occupation after new qualifications that they might not meet have been enacted into law. The legal basis for the process is found in the 14th Amendment to the U.S. Constitution, which says that no state may deprive any person of life, liberty, or property without due process of law. The Supreme Court has ruled that the license to practice is a property right.

The use of the grandfather clause in nursing is by no means a new process. For example, it was not until the mid 1950s that theoretical and practical experience in psychiatric nursing was required in all nursing curricula and that psychiatric content was included in state licensing examinations. When laws changed to make this a requirement, hundreds

Figure 3-2. When a state licensure law is enacted or if a current law is repealed, the grandfather clause has been a standard feature that allows persons to continue to practice their profession.

of practicing nurses had never had a formal course in psychiatric nursing and had not been required to write a psychiatric examination to qualify for licensure. The right of these nurses to continue to be licensed, and thus to practice their profession, was protected by a grandfather clause. (Most of these nurses are now retired from the active practice of nursing.)

When applied to the entry-into-practice issue, the grandfather clause would guarantee registered nurses who had been educated in associate degree or diploma programs before the date of any changes that would require a baccalaureate degree for registered nurse licensure the right to continue to be licensed and practice as registered nurses as long as their practice was safe. As an example of the application of the process, let us assume that changes in a state's licensure laws to require a baccalaureate degree as the minimum educational preparation for registered nurse licensure became effective June 1, 1995. After June 1, 1995, diploma and associate degree graduates would be licensed as technical nurses. All associate degree and diploma graduates licensed before June 1, 1995 would be considered registered nurses, as protected by the grandfather clause. Some people believe that the entry-into-practice resolutions would not have passed in state conventions without the assurance of a grandfather clause. Some voting delegates seemed more concerned "how will this affect me, personally" than about the impact of the resolution on nursing as a whole.

The grandfather clause is limited to the protection of a nurse's license. Additional qualifications can be established for certain jobs for RNs, and these are not included in nurse practice acts. For example, many head nurses, supervisors, and directors of nursing service are currently working in these positions with associate degree and diploma preparation only. Qualifications could be written that would require the minimum of a baccalaureate degree to work in the capacity of a head nurse, supervisor, or director of nursing service. Similar actions have already occurred with regard to qualifications for teachers in nursing schools. Accreditation standards for the Council of Associate Degree Programs now stipulate that nurse educators possess a master's degree in nursing, and the doctoral degree is being recommended for educators in baccalaureate programs. In some areas of the country, changes have also occurred in the educational preparation required of persons working in community health and school nurse positions.

Some nurses believe that the grandfather clause should be conditional. If it were conditional, persons licensed before the changes in the licensure law would continue to use their current title for a stipulated period, for example, 10 years. At the end of that period, if they had not completed the education mandated in the changes (or any other conditions that might have been added), they would have to use the title stipulated in the new law for persons with their educational preparation. Because of the complexity and the questionable status of the issue, there is little likelihood that conditional "grandfathering" will occur.

Interstate Endorsement

Another concern expressed over licensure changes is related to interstate endorsement or reciprocity for licensure among states. Nursing is one of the few professions to have developed a process by which national examinations with standardized scores are administered in each state or jurisdiction. This allows a nurse who has passed the licensing examination in one state to move to another state and seek licensure in that state, without the need to retake and pass another examination. Because nurses have been highly mobile, this has been a great advantage. As states move toward making changes in their practice acts, it is hoped that similar changes will be considered across the nation so that interstate endorsement can be maintained without requiring reexamination.

COMPETENCY EXPECTATIONS AND DIFFERENTIATED PRACTICE

A final and significant concern is the task of describing and differentiating the competencies and the scope of practice of nurses graduating from the various types of nursing education programs. Although this is a concern that must be addressed if the ANA Position Paper were to be implemented, it represents a problem the nursing profession faces without changes imposed by the Position Paper. At the present time, graduates of baccalaureate nursing programs and graduates of 2-year associate degree programs write the same licensing examination for practice as a registered nurse. It seems faulty to suggest that the educational background provided in 4-year programs and that provided in 2-year programs is so similar in outcomes that the same expectations can be made of graduates of both programs. This position fails to recognize the broad range of functions in nursing and the potential for improving the quality of care that can be given to those needing that care. Because 2-year graduates are currently demonstrating success on the licensing examinations, it might also be suggested that the current licensing examinations are not testing those skills that are developed in a 4-year program. Currently, little differentiation exists in beginning staff nurse positions filled by graduates of associate degree or baccalaureate programs.

The need for realistic statements regarding competencies of each level or category of nursing are necessary so that appropriate testing can be developed, and so that each category can be used effectively and efficiently within the health care delivery system. Validated competencies will also provide a basis for the development of curriculum patterns that will ensure adequate preparation of each category of caregiver without running the risk of overeducation or undereducation at any one level. It can also serve as a foundation for the development of educational mobility patterns within the profession.

Some work has been done toward describing the competencies of graduates of the different programs in nursing. In 1978 the NLN published *Competencies of the Associate Degree Graduate on Entry into Practice.* This document was revised and published as a second edition in 1990. (See Chapters 2 and 11 for more discussion of associate degree competencies.) In 1979 an NLN task force presented a working paper on competencies of graduates of nursing programs that included descriptions of practical, associate degree, diploma, and baccalaureate graduates. This paper has been published as *Competencies of Graduates of Nursing Programs;* however, these statements are largely theoretical. Many of the statements, especially those describing the baccalaureate graduate, call for intellectual processes of critical decision making. These processes may be difficult to measure because they may be evidenced only when used inappropriately or not used at all. Recognizing that there is still much work to be done in this area, in 1989 the NLN again appointed a committee to look at competencies across all nursing education programs.

In 1982 two projects sponsored by the Midwest Alliance in Nursing were started. One, entitled "Defining and Differentiating ADN and BSN Competencies and Facilitating ADN Competency Development" was funded by the W. K. Kellogg Foundation. The second, entitled "Continuing Education for Consensus on Entry Skills," was funded by a grant from the Division of Nursing of the Department of Health and Human Services. The goal of these studies was to achieve a regional consensus among nursing service persons and educators from both types of programs on differentiated statements of scope of practice for each level of graduate.

In 1986 the National Council of State Boards of Nursing published a study conducted for the organization by the American College Testing Program. The purpose of this study, entitled "A Study of Nursing Practice and Role Delineation and Job Analysis of Entry-Level Performance of Registered Nurses." was to validate the NCLEX-RN. Five major areas were examined: (1) role delineation, (2) the influence of the setting, (3) the transition from entry level practice to practice beyond entry level for registered nurses, (4) the differences in RN practice as a function of education, and (5) evaluation of the NCLEX-RN test plan. In looking at the role delineation, 17 categories of activities were identified. The study found that there was a high degree of consensus in nursing about the criticality of nursing activities (i.e., which activities may sometimes be omitted and which can never be omitted). It further indicated that the specific setting strongly influenced the activities that occurred, that first-line managers were consistent in indicating that the transition time for a new graduate is about 6 months, and that the influence of educational background on the practice patterns of newly licensed registered nurses was not as great as one might expect. New baccalaureate graduates showed a greater tendency to be involved in some type of research activities than did new diploma and associate degree graduates, but on all other types of activities that were studied, no substantial differences were found (National Council, 1986).

Despite slow movement in the area, there continues to be a push to realistically define the competencies of the graduates of the various programs. Once identified, some hope that differentiated roles can be implemented in the practice setting that will allow graduates to practice as educated. Advocates of differentiated practice believe this is one answer to the nursing shortage.

OTHER FACTORS AFFECTING NURSING EDUCATION

Three decades have passed since the ANA first began activities to require the baccalaureate degree for entry into professional nursing. No issue has so divided members of the nursing profession or created as much dissension. During the 30 years that nurses have been debating educational preparation for nursing a number of other issues have emerged.

The Nurse Shortage

In the early 1990s discussions and debates related to educational preparation were quickly dropped. The United States found itself in a serious nurse shortage. Hospitals that at one time sought to employ only graduates with baccalaureate degrees once again offered positions to associate degree graduates, and those hiring only registered nurses again offered jobs to licensed practical (vocational) nurses.

Two factors were largely responsible for the nurse shortage. The first was an increasing demand for nurses in the expanding health care delivery system. With more people requiring care, with advancing technology, and with Americans living longer there were many more nursing positions to be filled. Also contributing to the increased demand was the drastic change in the nurse's role. Nurses assumed expanded roles of practice and responsibility.

The second factor related to the drop in enrollments in nursing programs that swept the nation around 1986. Some blamed the dissension that existed in nursing with regard to educational preparation as being at least partially responsible for discouraging capable young men and women from choosing a career in nursing. Additional factors that undoubtedly affected the decision of men and women considering a career in nursing were the salaries paid to nurses. The need to provide health care coverage 24 hours a day, 7 days a week may have been unattractive to some. At times nursing was not depicted by the media as a desirable profession. Other professions offered better salaries, better hours, and more status. Many persons sought educational preparation for positions in business.

As a result of dropping enrollments much effort was invested in recruitment efforts, and nurse's salaries took a decided upswing as a result of the shortage. In 1990 the NLN reported that enrollments in nursing had increased 14%. Associate degree programs led with a 15% increase, followed by baccalaureate programs with an increase of 13% and diploma programs that saw a 5% jump in enrollments ("Student Count Soars," 1991). Although people are once again seeking careers in nursing, the increasing need for nurses has kept the shortage alive.

The RCT Proposal

Responding to the nursing shortage, in 1988 the American Medical Association (AMA) put forth a proposal for a registered care technologist (RCT). RCTs, as outlined by the AMA, would be educated in a 9-month program that would prepare each individual to carry out basic care procedures such as bathing, transport, and wound care as well as passing oral medications under supervision. After another nine months of preparation "advanced" RCTs could work in critical care where they would monitor patient status and manage the care of patients on monitors and ventilators. It was planned that the RCTs would report to the nurses but would be licensed under medical boards.

Nurses who for years were divided by the entry issue suddenly united. As a group they saw the move as a clear threat to the quality of care and to the nursing profession. Across the country meetings were held to find other approaches to the nursing shortage. The ANA put money and effort into public education strategies. Support was sought from legislatures, hospitals, health groups, and consumers. Finally, in 1990 the AMA decided to discontinue activity to implement its proposal.

CHANGES IN NURSES' EDUCATION

As nursing advances as a profession, it is critical that the education that prepares individuals for roles within the profession also changes and advances. The earlier sections of this chapter have addressed some of the factors that have encouraged change or predict change for the future. The following section describes some of the changes that have occurred.

Educational Mobility

One of the approaches to the nursing shortage has been an increased emphasis on educational mobility in nursing. Rather than debate which is the appropriate educational preparation, educational mobility recognizes the unique contribution of nurses educated at all levels and serves to facilitate advancement from one level to another with minimal repeat of course work. This movement has received impetus in some states from legislative mandates that stipulate that plans for articulation from one type of nursing program to another must be developed and implemented within a given period of time. In other instances, such activity has occurred without legislative action. Many states are beginning to establish state-wide plans that will facilitate the enrollment of the practical nurse in associate degree programs or the advancement of the associate degree graduate to registered nurse baccalaureate programs.

The Use of Technology in Nursing Education

One of the advances seen in nursing education has been the increased use of technology in teaching. Some of the technological advances used in nursing education facilitates the process of making nursing education more geographically accessible to the student. Outreach programs, which take the educational program to the student rather than requiring the student to come to the college, have been started in many parts of the country. These have been particularly useful in helping to meet the needs of the registered nurse seeking baccalaureate preparation. Cable television and video instruction have extended the perimeter of the classroom.

The use of videotaping and television in the classroom and in the practice laboratory has already proved to be an effective and efficient method to extend the ability of one instructor to assist many students. Videotaped demonstrations eliminate the need for tedious repetitions of basic procedures for small groups. Students can view videotapes at their own convenience and can use videotaped playbacks to assess their own skills, freeing the instructor for other instructional activities. Interactive classrooms allow students at distant learning sites to communicate with an instructor and a class on a university campus.

The computer age has also reached the nursing classroom. Computer assisted instruction and interactive programs allow students to practice decision making skills in a safe environment, learning how to select the best alternative for care without placing the patient in any jeopardy. The development of computer software in nursing education exceeds one's ability to know all the alternatives for instruction. Computer science is no longer a foreign language. Large amounts of money have been invested by groups such as the Helene Fuld Trust Foundation to make computerized education available to nursing students.

Nursing educators are also revising programs of study to address the needs of the adult learner, rather than fashion all educational patterns toward the recent high school graduate. Programs that permit part-time study, and thus allow the student to work while attending school, have also been developed. Classes that traditionally were conducted during peak morning hours are being moved to late afternoon hours or to weekends to appeal to and meet the needs of the working student. Programs designed to accommodate to varying learning rates through self-paced modules respond to individual learning needs. Remedial classes in basic mathematics, grammar, study skills, or English as a second language have been made available to students who may not have had the same educational opportunities as others.

As nurses recognize the need to become more political to bring about the changes they see as necessary in the health care delivery system, courses will need to be developed that will provide the necessary information to allow the nurse to function in this new political role. Politics requires learning about power, a term some nurses want to reject as being incompatible with the aims of the profession. Kalisch and Kalisch (1982, pp 1–2) have defined power as "the ability to affect something or to be affected by something. Power means the capacity to alter behavior." Nurses, because they offer critically needed services, possess much potential power but need a basic understanding of how to make use of that potential to bring about desired change. As nurses assume a stronger patient advocacy role, they must possess better understanding

Figure 3–3. As hospitals, like other industries, put the computer to work in their agencies, the new graduate will be forced to have a beginning understanding of computer language and the operation of the machines.

of the social system, policy formation and implementation, the legislative process, lobbying, and political mobilization. Many programs have made a step in this direction by including courses in assertive behavior in their nursing curricula, but this is only a beginning.

Some nurses see themselves functioning as independent practitioners or in joint practices. This role requires additional understanding of business management and economics and a knowledge of advanced clinical skills. Alternative health care providers will find themselves in a competitive system. Escalating medical costs may mean that as a nation, we need to modify our concepts of health care delivery so that it responds to the needs of persons of all ages and in all economic strata.

Concerns about Funding

One of the gravest problems facing nursing education today is that of funding. In 1964, through the Nurse Training Act, $238 million was authorized for the advancement of nursing education, and $4.6 million was authorized to administer the programs. The programs, five in all, included construction of nursing facilities, improvement of teaching, continuation of traineeship programs that reimbursed students for advancing their nursing education, provision of loans to nursing students, and monies specifically set aside to improve instruction in hospital-based schools. This act was responsive to the recognized shortage of trained health personnel. In 1963 the Consultant Group on Nursing in their final report, *Toward Quality in Nursing*, estimated that we would need 130,000 more nurses in 1970 than were available in 1960. This would mean that nursing schools would need to increase their graduates by 75%. The consultants also urged an increase in the number of nurses with graduate degrees and baccalaureate degree and an increase in the number of licensed practical nurses.

In the years immediately following the passage of the Nurse Training Act, many schools and students were to benefit from these funds. When the Nurse Training Act reached expiration in 1969, the Health Manpower Act continued most of Nurse Training Act's programs. The 1971 Nurse Training Act, which followed, authorized the largest expenditure of funds for nursing in the history of the country—$855 million. After that period the federal funding for nursing saw a constant decrease. The $160 million appropriated in 1973 dropped to $145 million in 1974. Presidents of the United States, both Republican and Democrat, believed that the nurse shortage had ended. They also contended that nursing students could apply for the federal aid made available to students in general (e.g., basic educational grants). All thought that the amount of money allocated to nursing education was "excessive."

In 1979 Congress again was able to extend the Nurse Training Act for one more year, with funding at $103 million. By 1983 the appropriations were cut to $48.9 million. Laws enacted in the late 1980s to reduce the federal budget deficit further affected monies available to nursing.

As funding was reduced, the purposes for which the funds were made available also changed. Fewer dollars were made available for the basic education of nursing students. Emphasis was placed on funding advanced training for nurses and the preparation of nurse practitioners. Funds were also available for nursing research. Student loans were continued, but the total amount was reduced and "forgiveness clauses," which required students to repay only part of the loan if they became actively involved in nursing on graduation, were eliminated. At the same time tuition costs sharply increased. Capitation funding, which provided money to schools based on student enrollment, was eliminated.

We are feeling the impact of the loss of these dollars and the effect on the profession of nursing. Students are having to find other means for funding their education. Greater numbers of students are attending school part time to allow time for employment while attending school. It is hoped that the nurse shortage of the 1990s will result in the federal government once more allocating more funds to nursing and nursing education.

Nursing education has suffered from the same reductions in state and local funding that has burdened other programs in higher education. Budget requests must often be reduced and needs set aside. Most critical to nursing are the dollars allocated to faculty salaries. As the salaries for nurses working in the health care delivery system have reached new highs, it is becoming increasingly difficult to attract well-qualified and highly motivated persons to teaching positions in our nursing education programs. Nurses with the education and expertise to be good teachers and positive role models for students can command much higher salaries outside of the educational environment.

Using Nursing Theories and Work of the Theorists in Nursing Education

One of the innovations in nursing that has been receiving increasing emphasis, and will undoubtedly continue to do so, is nursing theory. As nursing education keeps pace with the advancement of nursing knowledge, there has been a push to develop curricular patterns that also respond to the work of nursing theorists. During the late 1970s and the 1980s, criteria for accreditation of nursing programs as established by the educational councils of the NLN placed importance on the need for a conceptual framework around which a program of learning is developed. Although that may be receiving some decreased emphasis today, the curriculum design of the nursing program in which you are enrolled may be based on concepts outlined by a particular nursing theorist. Perhaps one of the hospitals to which you are assigned for clinical experience also uses the principles of a nursing theory to structure the delivery of care.

A theory is a "scientifically acceptable general principle which governs practice or is proposed to explain observed facts" (Riehl and Roy, 1974, p 3). Because nursing as a developing profession is seriously involved in research on which to build a sound body of nursing knowledge, theories are valuable to us. They provide the bases for hypotheses about nursing practice. They make it possible for us to derive a sound rationale for the actions we take. If the theories are testable, they will then allow us to build our knowledge base and to guide and improve nursing practice. This is explained in the words of Barbara Stevens (1984, p 1):

A nursing theory. . .attempts to describe or explain the phenomenon called nursing. A theory is always a shorthand way to understand or characterize a phenomenon. It points out those components or characteristics that give the phenomenon its identity. It pulls out the salient parts of a phenomenon so that one can separate the critical and necessary factors. . .from the accidental and unessential factors.

She goes on to describe a theory as a map whose purpose is "to give one a handle on the phenomenon with which it deals." Today there are many published nursing theories. In an attempt to structure and organize those theories, various authors have categorized or classified theories. Not all are classified similarly. Included are general classifications such as the art and science of humanistic nursing, interpersonal relationships, systems, and energy fields. Others include groupings that include growth and development theories, systems theories, stress adaptation theories, and rhythm theories.

Figure 3–4. Nursing is in the process of building a body of scientific knowledge.

Some examples of growth and development theories with which you are probably familiar are those of Maslow, Erikson, Kohlberg, Piaget, and Freud. Most basic nursing texts incorporate a discussion of the concepts developed by these theorists. The theories are so named because they focus on the developing person. They have the common characteristic of arranging this development in terms of stages through which a person must pass to reach a particular level of development. From a nursing standpoint they allow us to monitor the progress through the various stages and evaluate the appropriateness of that progress. You will recognize Maslow for his approach to self-actualization, Erikson for his psychosocial development, Kohlberg for his theories of moral reasoning, Piaget for his approach to cognitive development, and Freud for psychosexual theories on which medicine later based the school of psychoanalysis. These theories are not truly theories of nursing, however, because they were not developed for the purpose of explaining, testing, and changing the practice of nursing. They represent some of the "borrowed" knowledge around which we build our profession.

Most nursing theories are developed around a combination of concepts. Among those concepts, four subject areas usually are included: (1) an approach to the total person, (2) an approach to health-illness, (3) an approach to the environment (or society), and (4) an approach to nursing. As mentioned earlier, nursing theories may also be classified with regard to the structure or approach around which they are developed.

Theories that speak to the art and science of humanistic nursing were the earliest purely nursing theories developed. Some authors have looked back at the contributions of Florence Nightingale and have included her in that grouping. Among the others are Virginia Henderson and her *Definition of Nursing*, Faye Abdellah and the *Twenty-one Nursing Problems*, Lydia Hall and her *Core Care and Cure Model*, and Madeleine Leininger's *Transcultural Care Theory*.

Interpersonal relationship theories deal with interactions between and among people. Many of these theories were developed during the 1960s. Included in this grouping could be Hildegard Peplau's *Psychodynamic Nursing*, Joyce Travelbee's *Human-to-Human Relationship*, and Ernestine Wiedenbach's *The Helping Art of Clinical Nursing*.

Systems theories are so classified because they are concerned with the interactions between and among all the factors in a situation. A system is usually viewed as complex and in a state of constant change. It is defined as a whole with interrelated parts and may be a subsystem of a larger system as well as a suprasystem. For example, a person may be viewed as a system composed of cells, tissue, organs, and the like.

The person is a subsystem of a family, which in turn is a subsystem of a community. In a systems approach the person is usually considered as a "total" being or from a "whole" being point of view. Systems theories also provide for "input" into the system and "feedback" within the system. The systems approach became popular during the 1970s.

Stress adaptation models are based on concepts that view the person as adjusting or changing (adapting) in order to avoid situations (stressors) that would result in the disturbance of balance or equilibrium. The adaptation theory helps to explain how the balance is maintained and therefore points the direction for nursing actions. Included in this group one often finds Sister Callista Roy's Adaptation Model and Betty Neuman's work, but both may also be considered systems models.

One of the latest classifications of theories is by energy fields. These theories, although they may have been started earlier, have received increased recognition during the 1980s. Included in this group are the works of such persons as Myra Levine, Joyce Fitzpatrick, Margaret Newman, and Martha Rogers.

It is not our purpose to discuss and critique all the many approaches to nursing theory. The student who wants to pursue nursing theorists further is encouraged to consult the section on further reading at the end of the chapter. A brief discussion of the conceptual approach set forth by four nursing theorists who have developed theories used in nursing education programs follows.

Sister Callista Roy's Adaptation Model

This model is organized around concepts that describe how a person can adapt behavior to allow him or her to deal (cope) with stimuli from the environment that are stressors. Stressors disrupt the dynamic state of equilibrium and result in illness. Four adaptive modes, or ways in which a person adapts, are identified: through (1) physiological needs, (2) self-concept, (3) role function, and (4) interdependence relations. Nursing's role is to assess a patient's adaptive behaviors and the stimuli that may be affecting him or her and manipulate the stimuli in such a way as to allow the patient to cope or adapt.

Dorothea Orem's Self-Care Model

This model has a goal of "constancy" for the person and speaks to the concept of self-care. Self-care is the person's own action that has pattern and sequence and, when effectively performed, contributes to the way he or she develops and functions. Nursing's role is to help the person meet the self-care requisites, thus limiting self-care deficits.

Betty Neuman's Systems Model

Identified as a health care systems model, this approach to nursing is organized around stress reduction. It is primarily concerned with the effects of stress and the reactions to stress and the development and maintenance of health, and therefore also speaks to maintaining equilibrium. The person deals with stressors through "lines of defense" and is protected from stressors through "lines of resistance." Nursing's role is focused on reduction of stress factors and through prevention that is "primary, secondary, or tertiary."

Martha Roger's Unitary Man Theory

Although Martha Roger's theory of nursing may not be used to fashion conceptual frameworks in nursing education programs as frequently as some others, it represents a creative approach to nursing. Much of the language being incorporated into nursing education and practice is an outgrowth of Roger's work. Known as the science of unitary man, the essence of this model is the assumption that the person is a unified energy field that is continually interacting and exchanging matter and energy with the environment. These exchanges result in increasing complexity and innovativeness of the person. Health and illness are not viewed as separate states. Nursing's role is to repattern humans and environment to achieve maximum health potential. This model has been used by the North American Nursing Diagnosis Association (NANDA) in developing the nursing diagnosis taxonomy and the language used within that taxonomy. However, the group substituted the words "human response patterns" for the more unfamiliar "patterns of unitary man."

CONCLUSION

Changes occur in our society almost faster than we can adjust to them. Technical advances have fueled an information explosion. The economy hits peaks and suffers setbacks. Life expectancy increases. Innovations occur in the delivery of health care, but the cost of that care continues to increase. Medical advances make it possible to save many lives that would have been lost a decade ago. Legal, ethical, and bioethical issues surround much of the care that is provided. Nursing education must be responsive to all of these changes. Curriculum patterns need to be scrutinized to ensure that nursing programs prepare their graduates appropriately for roles in the health care delivery system. Nurses need to be educated to deal with both the high-tech and the high-touch roles to be occupied by the nurse. The roles of nurses need to be more clearly defined and delineated to respond to the education provided and to enable the graduate to function effectively in the defined role. Nurse educators will also need to be responsive to new innovations in our society and incorporate these into the teaching methods. Another challenge to nursing education will be accomplishing all of the above while at the same time adjusting to severe cuts in federal funding to nursing programs. Perhaps the biggest problem facing nursing will be that of attracting and retaining qualified and enthusiastic faculty when the salaries to be commanded in the health care delivery system significantly exceed those offered by our educational institutions.

REFERENCES

ADNs, community college bar entry-level rules. Am J Nurs 85(8):921, 923, 1987

American Nurses' Association Commission on Nursing Education: A Case for Baccalaureate Preparation in Nursing, publication No. NE-6 ANS. Kansas City, MO, American Nurses' Association, 1979

American Nurses' Association's first position on nursing education. Am J Nurs 65(12):106–111, 1965

ANA delegates vote to limit RN title to BSN grad; "associate nurse" wins vote for technical level. Am J Nurs 85(9):1016, 1017, 1020, 1022, 1024, 1025, 1985

ANA gears up new drive for entry level change: Despite opposition, some SNAs see success soon. Am J Nurs 85(2):194, 1985

Brown EL: Nursing for the Future. New York, Russell Sage Foundation, 1948

Edge S: State positions on titling and licensure. *In* Looking Beyond the Entry Issue: Implications for Education and Service, NLN publication No. 41-2173. New York, National League for Nursing, 1986

Hartung D: Organizational positions on titling and entry into practice: A chronology. *In* Looking Beyond the Entry Issue: Implications for Education and Service, NLN publication No. 41-2173. New York, National League for Nursing, 1986

Illinois RNs seek compromise on scope of practice. Am J Nurs 86(1):77, 84, 90, 1986

Kalisch BJ, Kalisch PA: Politics of Nursing. Philadelphia, JB Lippincott, 1982

Kalisch PA, Kalisch BJ: The Advance of American Nursing, 2nd ed. Boston, Little, Brown & Co, 1986

National Council of State Boards of Nursing: A Study of Nursing Practice and Role Delineation and Job Analysis of Entry Level Performance of Registered Nurses. Chicago, National Council of State Boards of Nursing, 1986

NFLPN OKs "two nursing levels" 18 month curriculum for LPNs. Am J Nurs 84(10):1303, 1312, 1314, 1984

NLN calls for baccalaureate preparation for professional practice. Nurs Health Care 3(3):154, 1982

North Dakota rule changes require associate, baccalaureate education. Issues 7(2):1–3, 1986

Pennsylvania legislature bars change in entry rules. Am J Nurs 87:113, 126, 1987

Riehl JP, Roy SC: Conceptual Models for Nursing Practice. New York, Appleton-Century-Crofts, 1974

Student Count Soars: NLN Sees "Rejuvenation." Am J Nurs 91(2):ll, 1991

Stevens BJ: Nursing Theory: Analysis, Application, Evaluation, 2nd ed. Boston, Little, Brown & Co, 1984

U.S. Public Health Service. Toward Quality in Nursing: Needs and Goals: Report of the Surgeon General's Consultant Group on Nursing. Washington, DC, US Government Printing Office, 1963

FURTHER READINGS

ADN "mavericks" found national group to fight title change. Am J Nurs 86(1): 79, 82, 1986

A first for the nation: North Dakota and entry into nursing practice. Nurs Health Care 7(3):135–141, 1986

AMA to Pilot RCTs. Am J Nurs 88(12):1717, 1720, 1988

Brower HT: Potential advantages and hazards of non-traditional education for nurses. Nurs Health Care 3(5):268–272, 1982

Chaska NL: The Nursing Profession: Turning Points. St Louis, CV Mosby, 1990

Christ T: Entry into practice: A recurring issue in nursing history. Am J Nurs 80(3):485–488, 1980

Fitzpatrick JJ, Whall AL: Conceptual Models of Nursing: Analysis and Application. Bowie, MD, Robert J Brady Co, 1983

George JB: Nursing Theories: The Base for Professional Nursing Practice, 2nd ed. Englewood Cliffs, NJ, Prentice-Hall, 1985

Marriner-Tomey A: Nursing Theorists and Their Work, 2nd ed. St Louis, CV Mosby Co, 1989

NLN seeks compromise on entry: ADNs hold out for RN licensure. Am J Nurs 87(1):113, 124–125, 1987

NLN members agree to shelve entry issues and call for steps to spur career mobility. Am J Nurs 89(8):1082–1083, 1989

Orem DE: Nursing: Concepts of Practice, 2nd ed. New York, McGraw-Hill Book Company, 1980

Primm PL: Entry into practice: Competency statements for BSNs and ADNs. Nurs Outlook 34(3):135–137, 1986

Roy SC, Roberts SL: Theory Construction in Nursing: An Adaptation Model. Englewood Cliffs, NJ, Prentice-Hall, 1981

State boards declare "neutral stance" in entry-level debate. Am J Nurs 86(10): 1180, 1986

Stull MK: Entry skills for BSNs. Nurs Outlook 34(3):138–139, 1986

Torres G: Theoretical Foundations of Nursing. East Norwalk, CT, Appleton-Century-Crofts, 1986

Unit II
Legal and Ethical Accountability for Practice

As we examine legal and ethical issues in health care, we will first explore the issue of credentials for health care providers. Understanding some of the basic issues related to credentialing and rationale for the existence of credentials, will help to focus your attention on the responsibility of health care providers to the public.

The entire realm of law that governs the practice of any health occupation is a particular concern in a society where individuals often attempt to solve problems in a courtroom. A clear understanding of the rights and responsibilities of both care providers and care recipients is important to you.

Ethical issues associated with health care are constantly before our society. Each new technological advance brings additional concerns to our attention. In this unit we try to provide you with a general background that will help you address ethical concerns. In addition, we have presented some specific ethical problems in the hope that considering them before you become directly involved will help you to address the problems more effectively.

4

Credentials for Health
Care Providers

Objectives

After completing this chapter, you should be able to

1. *Define and discuss the concept of credentialing.*
2. *Differentiate between a diploma, certification, and licensure as credentials.*
3. *Outline the history of nursing licensure.*
4. *Differentiate between permissive and mandatory licensure for nursing.*
5. *Identify the major content areas in laws regulating nursing practice.*
6. *Discuss the process of revocation of a nursing license.*
7. *Outline the role of the state board of nursing as outlined in the model practice act.*
8. *Differentiate between licensure by examination and licensure by endorsement.*
9. *Discuss the historical development of the licensing examination for nursing.*
10. *Discuss future trends in nursing licensure.*
11. *Discuss mechanisms for licensing graduates of foreign nursing schools.*
12. *Discuss the concept of certification in nursing.*
13. *State the problems associated with certification in nursing.*

Credentials are written proof of qualifications. They communicate to others the nature of one's competence and can be used as a tool for evaluating one's ability to perform in a specific occupation. Some people want to know why credentials for health occupations are necessary. The basic rationale is that the public may suffer through receiving care from less competent people if there is no clear way to identify competence. Furthermore, those who are engaged in careers in health occupations want to be assured that the standards of practice in their discipline will remain high and that they will not be replaced by people with less educational preparation who would be willing to work for lower wages.

TYPES OF CREDENTIALS IN HEALTH CARE

There are many types of credentials, for example, diplomas, degrees, licenses, and certificates. Each of these serves a different role. Not all are available for each different health occupation.

Figure 4–1. Various forms of credentialing assure the public of qualified caregivers.

Diplomas and Certificates of Graduation

Those who have a planned education of some kind, whether it be a 6-week program for a nursing assistant or 12 years for a surgeon, receive a diploma or written certificate attesting to that educational attainment. This may be the only credential the person possesses.

When only a diploma or educational certificate is available, it is necessary to know about the educational program itself to evaluate the person's abilities. Education for the various health occupations may vary widely. For groups such as physicians, the program is standardized across the nation. For some of the new allied health workers, such as respiratory technicians, the course of study may not be standardized. Methods of accrediting these programs also vary.

Certification

For some groups there is a standard credential available in the form of certification provided by a nongovernmental authority, usually a professional organization. Workers with this type of credential are referred to as "certified" or as "registered." This type of credential should not be confused with a legal license. Certification usually is granted on completion of an educational program and the passing of a standardized examination, both of which are prescribed by a professional organization.

Some professional organizations provide certification for related occupational groups as well as their own. One such organization is the National Association of Medical Records Administrators, which examines and "registers" medical records administrators and examines and "certifies" medical records technicians.

In some fields a separate, independent organization has been formed with the sole purpose of credentialing in a particular field. The National Accrediting Association for Clinical Laboratory Sciences is such a group. At one time the American Society of Clinical Pathologists was responsible for credentialing people in the laboratory sciences; however, in an attempt to make the laboratory science credentialing system more independent and as objective as possible, a separate organization was formed for that purpose. Members of the various professional groups involved in laboratory science cooperated in setting up this accrediting association. The organization is incorporated as a private, voluntary entity and is not a governmental institution or department. Many states have made certification by this body the required criterion for practice in clinical laboratory sciences. It is recognized by all groups in the field of laboratory science as a professional credential.

Some other bodies that currently accredit are investigating the possibility of setting up independent national entities with the sole purpose of credentialing. One reason for this action relates to the current consumer movement. In general, the public has not trusted the objectivity of people in professional groups. The creation of an independent credentialing body would ensure that those currently practicing a profession would not be the sole arbiters in determining who enters the field. A second reason for this move is financial. By setting up a separate organization, which must be self-supporting through fees for its services, the professional groups are relieved of the financial burden that can result when an accrediting program grows rapidly and costs escalate. A third reason is to provide a broader-based support for the credentialing process. A fourth reason relates to the complex federal laws governing nonprofit organizations and their tax-exempt status. The board members of these organizations commonly include representatives from the profession, the educational setting, the public, and related professions.

Licensing

A license conferred by an individual state is available for some health occupations. Many different health occupations are licensed in different states. Most states restrict licensing to those who have more direct contact with patients or clients. Physicians, dentists, pharmacists, and nurses are licensed in all states. The licensing of other occupational groups varies.

Qualifications required for licensure and the testing for competence also differ greatly from state to state. Most licensing laws specify completion of a state-approved educational program and require, in addition, the successful completion of a written examination prescribed by the state. However, the uniform licensing examination system available to registered nurses is unique in health care. For example, there is a national licensing examination for pharmacy, but California prepares and administers its own examination and does not use the national pharmacy examination. There are national medical board examinations but some states administer independent medical examinations. Even when the same examination is used for licensure, as in pharmacy, some states require that a person new to the state retake the licensing examination when applying for a second license in that state.

In some states the licensing laws require continuing education to maintain competence. The trend toward including this provision in licensure laws is growing. In many states pharmacists have been one of the first groups required to pursue continuing education. Continuing education is required for relicensure of nurses and physicians in many states.

THE HISTORY OF CREDENTIALING IN NURSING

Nursing leaders have historically maintained an ethical position that accountability to the public for quality nursing care is essential. The public, however, often has no method for evaluating the competence of an individual nurse. Therefore, the nursing profession has acted to try to ensure that nurses have credentials that can be evaluated by anyone.

Credentials were not always available for nurses. Before the Nightingale schools became prevalent in England and nursing schools were established in the United States, very little training was available to those who wanted to provide nursing care. Those who had received some training and those who had not worked side by side to deliver care. After schools of nursing became common, a rudimentary means of identifying the qualifications of caregivers was the certificate of completion that was issued by the nursing school. This was the first true credential for nursing practice.

However, because the quality of education that was offered in the nursing schools differed widely—programs varied in length from 6 weeks to 3 years—it became apparent that a completion certificate was not an adequate guarantee of competence. Nursing leaders were concerned about the situation. They believed that the patient had no way to judge whether a particular nurse's education was sound and might suffer from the quality of care administered by a poorly prepared nurse.

In 1896 the Nurses Associated Alumnae of the United States and Canada was created. (This organization later evolved into the American Nurses' Association [ANA].) One of the major concerns of the association was the establishment of a credentialing system that was firmly based in laws passed by a legislative body. This form of credential is called licensure. The route of legal licensing for credentialing was long and difficult. Nurses, legislators, and the public had to be educated about the value of legislation to govern the profession and to be encouraged to support it. Table 4-1 is a chronology of nursing licensure.

Permissive Licensure

The ANA campaigned vigorously for the adoption of state licensure laws. These early laws provided a voluntary process by which a nurse who met predetermined standards would be licensed to practice, and the license would be registered with the state. This is called *permissive* licensure because the person is "permitted" to be licensed if requirements are met. Under this system no one was required to have a license to

Table 4-1. *The History of Nursing Licensure*

1867   Dr. Henry Wentworth Acland first suggested licensure for nurses in England.

1892   American Society of Superintendents of Training Schools for Nurses organized and supported licensure in the United States.

1901   First nursing licensure in the world: New Zealand.

1903   First nursing licensure in the United States: North Carolina, New Jersey, New York, and Virginia (in that order).

1915   ANA drafted its first model nurse practice act.

1919   First nursing licensure in England.

1923   All 48 states had enacted nursing licensure laws.

1935   ANA endorsed mandatory licensure.

1938   First mandatory licensure act in the United States: New York (effective 1947).

1946   Ten states had definitions of nursing in the licensing act.

1950   First year the same examination used in all jurisdictions of the United States and its territories: State Board Test Pool Examination.

1965   Twenty-one states had definitions of nursing in the licensing act.

1971   First state to recognize expanded practice in the nursing practice act: Idaho.

1976   First mandatory continuing education for relicensure: California.

1982   Change to nursing process format examination: National Council Licensure Examination for Registered Nurses (NCLEX-RN).

1986   First state to require baccalaureate degree for registered nurse and associate degree for licensed practical nurse: North Dakota (effective 1987).

practice nursing. However, a nurse who was licensed could legally call herself (there were virtually no male nurses at that time) a registered nurse. An employer or a member of the public could then differentiate between a registered nurse and an individual who used the title "nurse" but had not met the established standard.

The standards for permissive licensure included graduating from a school that satisfied certain requirements and passing a comprehensive examination. Only those who had met these standards could use the title "registered nurse." With standards in place the community benefited because there was an established credential that attested to a level of competence. The licensee profited in regard to job availability and salary if the community differentiated between those who were licensed and those who were not licensed.

The first laws providing for permissive licensure were passed in 1903 by North Carolina. By 1923 all the existing 48 states had permissive

Figure 4–2. A standard credential makes hiring easier.

licensure laws. Alaska and Hawaii passed licensure laws while still territories and continued to recognize these laws when they became states.

Mandatory Licensure

After permissive licensure laws came into being, nurses' activity regarding licensure became less intense because most nurses sought and received licenses to practice. However, there was still concern that some persons were practicing nursing without having demonstrated skill and knowledge. The majority of those functioning without licenses were nursing school graduates who had failed the licensing examinations. They were referred to as graduate nurses, as opposed to registered nurses. In addition, some individuals who had been educated as nurses in foreign countries and did not meet the licensure requirements in the state in which they were residing worked as nurses in health care settings.

To eliminate this situation and provide greater protection to the public, many nurses began to call for *mandatory* licensure, which requires that all those who wish to practice nursing meet the established standards and be licensed. The first mandatory licensure law took effect in New York State in 1947. Throughout the years additional states changed their laws relating to the practice of nursing and required licensure. Today, mandatory licensure is the standard in the United States and Canada as well as many other countries. Only the state of Texas allows for permissive licensure.

Concerns About Permissive and Mandatory Licensure

The continued existence of permissive licensure laws in Texas presents some problems to nurses practicing in that state. One concern is that patients are jeopardized by potentially lower quality care. Another issue is that permissive licensure retards the development of the nursing profession as a whole because the public does not differentiate between those without an appropriate education and standard of practice and those who are more qualified. Still another concern is economic. Those without education and credentials often are willing to work for lower salaries; this tends to hold down the salaries of those who do have credentials.

CURRENT NURSING LICENSURE LAWS

During the late 1970s and the 1980s many states altered their nursing practice acts to reflect the changes in modern nursing practice. New legislation is usually initiated through the nurses' association at the instigation of the nursing community. The association may spend months preparing and planning the content of the bill and gaining the support of legislators.

The proposed law enters the legislative process through an elected member of the legislature who has been persuaded that the change in the law is in the best interest of the public. The proposal must go through the entire legislative committee review, public hearing, and legislative voting procedure before it can become a law. During this process individuals and organizations may affect the content of the bill by influencing the legislators. The originators of the law may either support the proposed changes or favor the original content. For example, in 1974 in New York State a bill was introduced that would have changed the educational requirements for entry into practice to require a baccalaureate degree. During the legislative process changes were made in the bill that were acceptable to some original supporters but distressed others. Overall the support for the bill was diminished. The result was defeat of the bill and the proposed changes in educational requirements did not become law.

Rules and Regulations

Each state has its own set of rules and regulations to carry out the provisions of the law regulating nursing. These rules and regulations are established by the administrative body, usually the board of nursing, that is given responsibility by law. Most states require that public hearings be held in regard to the proposed rules and regulations, but the board has the authority to make the final decision. The rules and regulations must be within the scope outlined by the law. Those that are accepted by the appropriate board have the force of law unless they are challenged in court and are found to be not in accord with the legislature's intent.

In some states the nursing practice act is detailed and specifies most of the critical provisions regarding licensure and practice. In other states the nursing practice act is broad, and the administrative body is given a great deal of power in making decisions through rules and regulations.

One example of the difference between what is contained in the enacted law and what is in rules and regulations in different states is in regard to the educational requirements for licensure. In some states the enacted law specifies that a diploma, an associate degree, or a baccalaureate degree is an acceptable preparation for registered nursing. In those states, in order for the educational requirements to change, the enacted law itself would have to be changed. In other states the educational requirement is not in the enacted law. In those states the educational requirement is established by the board of nursing through rules and regulations. This was the situation in North Dakota when the requirement for the registered nurse license was changed to the baccalaureate degree (see Chapter 1). Thus you will want to investigate both the actual nursing practice act and the rules and regulations governing nursing in your state.

Nursing Licensure Law Content

Early in the 1900s the ANA, as part of its leadership role in nursing licensure, formulated a model nurse practice act that could be used by state associations when planning legislation (Snyder, 1984). This model was revised in 1981 by the ANA Congress for Nursing Practice and a more up-to-date approach to nursing licensure legislation was published (American Nurses' Association, 1981). A year later the National Council of State Boards of Nursing (NCSBN) also developed a model nurse practice act (NCSBN, 1982). The NCSBN continues to update its model act as part of its role in supporting the state boards of nursing with the most recent revision being published in 1988 (NCSBN, 1988). In addition the NCSBN has written a Model Nursing Administrative Rules (NCSBN, 1988).

Most state nurse practice acts are periodically rewritten to more accurately reflect modern-day nursing practice. Usually the state nurses association serves as the primary stimulus for legislators to consider nursing legislation. We recommended that you carefully read the nurse practice act for the state in which you will be practicing. A copy of the act may be obtained from the state board of nursing (see Appendix A for addresses).

In some states one act covers both practical nursing and registered nursing, while other states have two separate, but similar, acts. Historically the role of the nursing assistant was not in law. As federal legislation mandating classes and certification for nursing assistants takes effect, some states are modifying laws and rules and regulations to include the role of the nursing assistant.

The following general topics are usually covered in state licensure laws.

Purpose

The purpose of regulating the practice of nursing is twofold: to protect the public and to make the individual practitioner accountable for actions. Note that the protection of the status of the licensed individual is not the reason for licensure. With this in mind you can better understand the inclusion of some other topics in the act.

Definitions

All the significant terms in the act are defined for purposes of carrying out the law. This is where the legal definition of nursing and the scope of practice are spelled out. The ANA model act suggests the following definition for the registered nurse:

> The practice of nursing means: the performance for compensation of professional services requiring substantial specialized knowledge of the biological, physical, behavioral, psychological, and sociological sciences and of nursing theory as the basis for assessment, diagnosis, planning, intervention, and evaluation in the promotion and maintenance of health; the casefinding and management of illness, injury or infirmity; the restoration of optimum function; or the achievement of a dignified death. Nursing practice includes but is not limited to administration, teaching, counseling, supervision, del-

egation, and evaluation of practice and execution of the medial regimen, including the administration of medications and treatments prescribed by any person authorized by state law to prescribe. Each registered nurse is directly accountable and responsible to the consumer for the quality of nursing care rendered (American Nurses' Association, 1981).

In addition, the NCSBN has stated that "the focus of nursing practice is generally accepted to be individual human response to actual or potential health problems" (Practice Questions, 1989).

Although no state uses the exact wording of any recommendation, among the concepts commonly included are the reference to performing services for compensation, the necessity for a specialized knowledge base, the use of the nursing process (although steps may be named differently), and components of nursing practice. Several states include some reference to treating human responses to actual or potential health problems. This definition first appeared in New York State's license law and was later incorporated in the ANA's *Nursing: A Social Policy Statement* (1980). Most states refer to the execution of the medical regimen, and many include a general statement about additional acts, which has been interpreted to recognize that nursing practice is evolving and that the nurse's area of responsibility can be expected to broaden (LaBar, 1984a).

Definitions of practical (vocational) nursing are more restrictive and usually designate that the individual must function under the supervision of a registered nurse or physician and in areas demanding less judgment and knowledge than is required of the registered nurse. The practical nurse standards usually focus on the assessment and intervention portions of the nursing process. Some states provide a list of specific functions that are appropriate to the practical nurse or list specific functions that are not permitted.

A variety of nursing assistants are employed in health care facilities. They may have other titles such as mental health technician, nurse aide, or medication technician. The preparation of and scope of practice for these individuals is a matter of serious concern to the public. With the current nursing shortage, these individuals may be assigned tasks and responsibilities beyond their educational preparation and competence. Adding legal requirements for education and defining their scope of practice in the law is one mechanism that has been used to control their practice.

Board of Nursing

The board of nursing is the agency that is legally empowered to carry out the intention of the law. The membership of the board, the procedure for appointment and removal, and the qualifications are important aspects of the nurse practice act because the board has the power to write the rules and regulations that will be used in daily operations.

The members of the state board of nursing usually are appointed by the governor. The law specifies the occupational background of the candidates, nominations are often made by nurses, but the final membership is appointed. North Carolina is the only state in which the registered nurse members of the state board are elected by the registered nurses in the state.

Boards of nursing range in size from seven to 17 members. Prerequisites regarding the educational background of nurses who serve as board members vary from state to state. Some states require that the board include nurses from differing occupational areas, such as education and nursing service. Most have at least one public member of the board. A few have at least one physician on the nursing board (LaBar, 1985).

In the majority of states there is a combined board for registered nurses and licensed practical nurses. In the other states two separate boards exist. Each state board has a paid staff that usually is headed by a registered nurse who is employed as the executive director of the state board of nursing. The executive director is responsible for administering the work of the board and seeing that rules and regulations are followed.

The ANA recommends that the board of nursing have the authority to carry out the following:

- Govern its own operation and administration
- Approve or deny approval to schools of nursing
- Examine and license applicants
- Renew licenses, grant temporary licenses, and provide for inactive status for those already licensed
- Regulate specialty practice
- Discipline those who violate provisions of the licensure law through conducting hearings, issuing subpoenas to witnesses, revoking, suspending, or refusing to renew a license, or setting limitations or conditions on practice (American Nurses' Association, 1981).

Some functions are performed by a centralized state licensure agency in the majority of states. These agencies range from those that have responsibility only for housekeeping matters, such as collecting fees, managing routine license renewals, and providing secretarial services, to those that have all decision-making authority, relegating the individual boards, such as the board of nursing, to advisory status.

Each state board must operate within the framework of its own state law regarding the practice of nursing, but all cooperate with one another through the National Council of State Boards of Nursing (NCSBN). They also cooperate with the ANA and the National League for Nursing (NLN) in some matters but maintain the separation that is required of a governmental body. For example, state boards acting together through the NCSBN have contracted with CTB Testing Service to prepare the licensing examinations for registered nurses and practical nurses that are used throughout the United States.

Qualifications for Licensure Applicants

The qualifications for licensure may be described in detail, or only general guidelines may be given, leaving the details up to the board of nursing. The most common basic requirements are graduation from an approved educational program and proficiency in the English language. Some states make the educational requirements more specific, such as requiring high school graduation and either an associate or baccalaureate degree or a diploma in nursing for the registered nurse applicant.

All states require a passing score on a comprehensive examination but do not name the examination in the law. The current licensing examinations are discussed later in this chapter. Many states require that the applicant be of "good moral character" and some require "good physical and mental health" (LaBar, 1985). Those who are licensed in other states must meet the same requirements. The process of obtaining an additional license is called "licensure by endorsement" (for further information, see "Obtaining a License").

Titling

This section of the law reserves the right to use specific titles for those who have met the requirements. In some states only the titles registered nurse and licensed practical nurse are specified. Other states also regulate the used of titles for advanced practice such as nurse practitioner or nurse midwife.

Grandfathering

Whenever a new law is written, a statement is usually included specifying that anyone currently holding the license may continue to hold that license, even if some requirements are changed. Without this provision the enactment of a new law would require that all individuals who are currently licensed reapply and show that they meet the new standards.

When new requirements are instituted that the legislature believes are important for the safety of the public, all currently licensed individuals may be required to meet that standard within a given period of time. For example, the legislature in Washington State passed a bill requiring all licensed health professionals to have evidence of 7 hours of education in the acquired immunodeficiency syndrome (AIDS) that included certain specified topics. New applicants had to meet this requirement before a license would be granted. Current license holders were required to meet this requirement before a license would be renewed.

Renewal

The length of time for which a license is valid is specified in the law, as well as any requirements for renewal. In some states license renewal requires only payment of a fee. In many jurisdictions continuing education is required for renewal. One state (Washington) dropped its continuing education requirement after a brief period. Documenting continuing education may require submission of records or may be attested to by signing a form. In many states where the applicant is not required to submit records at the time of renewal, a procedure for random checking assures compliance with the law. Continuing education requirements vary greatly, for example, from as many as 24 hours every year to as few as 15 hours every 2 years. State requirements for continuing education are outlined in Appendix A.

Financial Concerns

Although the act itself does not usually specify the fees to be charged, general restrictions on the method of calculating fees and on how the fees may be used are often included in the act. The act may specify how the expenses of the board of nursing are to be met and who has legal authority to make decisions regarding the use of funds.

Nursing Education Programs

Some state laws describe the requirements of a nursing education program in only the most general terms, leaving the details up to the board of nursing. In other states the law is specific. It may specify the number of years of education, the courses or content that must be included, and the approval process for a program. If the law is general, then the board sets more specific standards. All nursing education programs in a state must fulfill the requirements of the state law.

Disciplinary Action

Disciplinary action may take the form of license withdrawal, or restrictions may be placed on the license, such as working only in a setting where narcotics are not administered. Such disciplinary action can only be taken based on criteria that are stated in the law. In the past most state acts contained general statements with regard to such matters as immoral and unprofessional conduct. Because of their vagueness, they proved to be unenforceable in court. In addition, most courts have only supported reasons for revocation of the license when the offense was in some way related to performance. Therefore, most modern laws contain specific concerns, such as the following, which are recommended by the ANA:

Fraud in gaining a license

Felony conviction

Addiction to drugs

Harming or defrauding the public

Willfully violating the nurse practice act (ANA, 1981)

Figure 4-3. A nursing license may be revoked by the State Board of Nursing for reasons clearly spelled out in the law. These reasons may include fraud in obtaining a license, conviction of a felony, and conduct likely to harm the public.

Violations and Penalties

Specific power is provided to prosecute those who violate the provisions of the law. The board may be authorized to ask a court to halt a specific practice that it believes is contrary to the law until a full hearing can take place. This is called "injunctive relief." This term refers to the court order called an injunction that is presented to the individual or organization.

Exceptions

Certain provisions may allow those who are not licensed to act as nurses in specific situations. Performing as a student while in an educational program is usually the primary exception. In addition, those who are caring for family members or friends without pay are exempted. Those who are practicing nursing in a federal agency, such as a military hospital, are usually exempted from the local state law as long as they maintain a current license in another state.

Miscellaneous Provisions

Each law requires "housekeeping" details that specify when it will become effective, that the previous act will no longer be in force, and other details pertaining to the individual state. Such provisions are usually of special interest when the law is first passed because nurses want to know when they will be affected by any changes.

Expanded Nursing Roles

Some nurse practice acts provide for the practice of nurses in expanded roles, including nurse midwives, nurse anesthetists, and nurse practitioners. Often the law requires that the person be certified for advanced practice by the ANA or a nursing specialty organization (see section on certification later in the chapter). In some states no specific mention is made of expanded roles, but the board of nursing has approved specialty practice based on the provisions in the basic act. In still other states practice in special roles is not legally sanctioned. Contact the board of nursing for information about specialty practice in each state.

The ANA opposes the inclusion of expanded practice in the licensure law. The association believes that the licensure law should regulate minimum safe practice and that the profession should regulate advanced practice. This is the case in medicine, in which there is only basic licensure because a physician in specialty practice is regulated by specialty boards within the profession. An additional concern is that some of the laws regulating specialty practice have provided for physician review of nursing's scope of practice. This takes away from nursing autonomy and allows medicine to control some aspects of nursing. A third concern is the rigidity, which may not allow for evolving nursing roles.

OBTAINING A NURSING LICENSE

There are two different procedures for obtaining a nursing license, one for applying for an initial license and the other for applying when one is already licensed in another jurisdiction. The initial licensure process is called "licensure by examination." Obtaining a license in a second jurisdiction is called "licensure by endorsement." In both instances, the applicant for licensure must meet all the provisions of the relevant state law such as educational preparation, legal residency status, and other such requirements.

The Nursing Licensing Examination

The establishment of a licensing examination was an important part of early efforts to achieve a high standard for the registered nurse. When each state adopted a licensing law it also established a mechanism for the examination of license applicants. A major achievement in the history of licensure was the formation of the Bureau of State Boards of Nurse Examiners, which eventually led to the use of an identical examination in all states in 1950. The original examination, called the State Board Test Pool Examination, was prepared by the testing department of the NLN under a contract with the state boards. Each state set its own standards for a passing score.

Content of the Examination

Historically, content of the examinations was divided into the subject categories of medical, surgical, obstetric, pediatric, and psychiatric nursing. Because nursing has changed in nature and these topics no longer reflect the totality of nursing practice, the NCSBN adopted a new plan for the examination, which was implemented in July 1982.

The National Council identified nursing behaviors critical to maintaining a safe and effective standard of care (Table 4-2). The Testing Division of the NLN prepared the first test under the direction of the NCSBN. Beginning with the examination in February 1983, the examination was prepared by CTB Testing Service. In addition to preparing the tests, the company scores the examinations and reports scores to the

Table 4–2. **Critical Requirements for Practice**

I. Exercises Professional Prerogatives Based on Clinical Judgment
   A. Adapts care to individual patient needs
   B. Fulfills responsibility to patient and others despite difficulty
   C. Challenges inappropriate orders and decisions by medical and other professional staff
   D. Acts as patient advocate in obtaining appropriate medical, psychiatric, or other help
   E. Recognizes own limitations and errors
   F. Analyzes and adjusts own or staff reactions in order to maintain therapeutic relationship with patient

II. Promotes Patient's Ability to Cope with Immediate, Long-range, or Potential Health-related Change
   A. Provides health care instruction or information to patient, family, or significant others
   B. Encourages patient or family to make decision about accepting care or adhering to treatment regimen.
   C. Helps patient recognize and deal with psychological stress
   D. Avoids creating or increasing anxiety or stress
   E. Conveys and invites acceptance, respect, and trust
   F. Facilitates relationship of family, staff, or significant others with patient
   G. Stimulates, remotivates patient, or enables patient to achieve self-care and independence

III. Helps Maintain Patient Comfort and Normal Body Functions
   A. Keeps patient clean and comfortable
   B. Helps patient maintain or regain normal body functions

IV. Takes Precautionary and Preventive Measures in Giving Patient Care
   A. Prevents infection
   B. Protects skin and mucous membranes from injurious materials
   C. Uses positioning or exercise to prevent injury or the complications of immobility
   D. Avoids using injurious techniques in administering and managing intrusive or other potentially traumatic treatments
   E. Protects patient from falls or other contact injuries
   F. Maintains surveillance of patient's activities
   G. Reduces or removes environmental hazards

V. Checks, Compares, Verifies, Monitors, and Follows up Medication and Treatment Processes
   A. Checks correctness, condition, and safety of medication being prepared
   B. Ensures that correct medication is given to the right patient and that patient takes or receives it

(continued)

Table 4-2. **Critical Requirements for Practice** *(continued)*

   C. Adheres to schedule in giving medication, treatment, or test
   D. Administers medication by correct route, rate, or mode
   E. Checks patient's readiness for medication, treatment, surgery, or other care
   F. Checks to ensure that tests or measurements are done correctly
   G. Monitors ongoing infusions and inhalations
   H. Checks for and interprets effect of medication, treatment, or care, and takes corrective action if necessary

VI. Interprets Symptom Complex and Intervenes Appropriately
   A. Checks patient's condition or status
   B. Remains objective, further investigates, or verifies patient's complaint or problem
   C. Uses alarms and signals on automatic equipment as adjunct to personal assessment
   D. Observes and correctly assesses signs of anxiety or behavioral stress
   E. Observes and correctly assesses physical signs, symptoms, or findings, and intervenes appropriately
   F. Correctly assesses severity or priority of patient's condition, and gives or obtains necessary care

VII. Responds to Emergency
   A. Anticipates need for crisis care
   B. Takes instant, correct action in emergency situations
   C. Maintains calm and efficient approach under pressure
   D. Assumes leadership role in crisis situation when necessary

VIII. Obtains, Records, and Exchanges Information on Behalf of the Patient
   A. Checks data sources for orders and other information about patient
   B. Obtains information from patient and family
   C. Transcribes or records information on chart, Kardex, or other information system
   D. Exchanges information with nursing staff and other departments
   E. Exchanges information with medical staff

IX. Utilizes Patient Care Planning
   A. Develops and modifies patient care plan
   B. Implements patient care plan

X. Teaches and Supervises Other Staff
   A. Teaches correct principles, procedures, and techniques of patient care
   B. Supervises and checks the work of staff for whom she or he is responsible.

(Jacobs A, Fivars G, Fitzpatrick R: What the new test will test. Am J Nurs 82(4):626, 1982) state boards. CTB Testing Service is authorized to sell statistical information related to the examination to the states and individual schools.

The current examination, called the National Council Licensure Examination for Registered Nurses (NCLEX-RN), consists of a single examination for which a single score is given. To ensure that the examination remains relevant to current nursing practice, the NCSBN has supported periodic research studies to identify nursing behaviors that are significant in maintaining a safe and effective standard of care. Newly licensed practicing registered nurses are studied to determine both the frequency and criticality of various behaviors. Frequency refers to how often the behaviors are required of the newly practicing registered nurse. Criticality refers to those actions that if performed incorrectly or omitted could cause serious harm to the client. These studies are called the ''RN Job Analysis'' and are reflected in the *Test Plan for the National Council Licensure Examination* (NCSBN, 1987).

Figure 4–4. Licensing examinations are designed to measure the basic knowledge needed for safe practice.

The NCLEX examination questions are organized into categories based on two sets of factors: client needs and steps of the nursing process. The client needs used are (1) safe, effective care environment (25%–31% of the questions); (2) physiological integrity (42%–48% of the questions); (3) psychosocial integrity (9%–15% of the questions); and (4) health promotion–health maintenance (12%–18% of the questions) (NCSBN, 1987).

The nursing process is divided into the following five steps, each of which is tested in 15% to 25% of the questions: (1) assessing, (2) analyzing, (3) planning, (4) implementing, (5) evaluating. These two sets of behaviors form a matrix for questions (Table 4-3). The multiple-choice questions in the examination are typically based on situations or scenarios that require a nursing response. They are designed to test judgment and decision making, not simply knowledge of facts (NCSBN, 1987.)

Within these categories, then, behaviors that indicate safe practice are tested. For example one question might seek to determine the applicant's ability to assess a given situation to determine whether it was a safe care environment, while another question might determine whether the applicant would implement the correct action to maintain safety. In considering physiologic integrity, a question might focus on the appropriate assessment for a patient with an illness that threatens physiologic

Table 4–3. **Content Distribution of the NCLEX-RN Examination**

	Client Needs			
Phases of the Nursing Process	Safe, Effective Care Environment 25%–31%	Physiological Integrity 42%–48%	Psychosocial Integrity 9%–15%	Health Promotion– Health Maintenance 12%–18%
Assess 15%–25%				
Analyze 15%–25%				
Plan 15%–25%				
Implement 15%–25%				
Evaluate 15%–25%				

integrity and another would focus on evaluating the outcomes of actions taken to preserve physiologic integrity. In this way questions address two aspects of the matrix plan.

The NCLEX-RN examination is offered twice a year, for 2 days in July and for 2 days in February (see Table 4-4 for planned dates). It is given on the same date in all states and territories.

Scoring of the Examination

The score used for determining pass/fail is not a raw score (that is the number right) but one derived from a complex mathematical process. The passing score is 1600 of a possible 3200; the mean is 2000. The exact score obtained by any individual is no longer reported as it once was. The individual is simply notified of "pass" or "fail" status. This was established to prevent the use of scores for rating or grading individuals. The test was not designed for the purpose of differentiating levels of excellence, only for demonstrating basic safe practice and this is what the pass or fail communicates.

Table 4–4. Examination Dates for the National Council Licensure Examination for NCLEX-RN for Registered Nursing

Year	Month	Date	Day
1991	February	5–6	T–W
	July	9–10	T–W
1992	February	5–6	W–Th
	July	8–9	W–Th
1993	February	3–4	W–Th
	July	7–8	W–Th
1994	February	2–3	W–Th
	July	13–14	W–Th
1995	February	8–9	W–Th
	July	12–13	W–Th
1996	February	6–7	T–W
	July	9–10	T–W
1997	February	4–5	T–W
	July	15–16	T–W
1998	February	3–4	T–W
	July	14–15	T–W
1999	February	2–3	T–W
	July	13–14	T–W

To prepare applicants to take the examination, the NCSBN has authorized the preparation of a study book that explains the examination, how it was written, and the scoring system and provides sample questions to familiarize applicants with the way the test is written. Many publishing companies also prepare review books for the licensing examinations. Review courses, both live and videotaped, are available to those who want assistance with preparation.

The Licensure Examination for Practical Nursing

The licensure examination for the practical nurse, the NCLEX-PN has been designed in a similar manner. A new test plan based on the practical nurse job analysis done in 1986 and 1987 was adopted in 1989. New questions were then developed, and the new test plan was effective after 1990 (NCSBN, 1989). Client needs and the nursing process form the basis of this examination also. The practical nurse is expected to be in a dependent role in planning and evaluation and more independent in collecting data and implementing. There is a greater recognition in the new test that a major portion of licensed practical nurses are employed in long-term care settings with clients older than 65 years of age. The percentages of questions in each category are shown in Table 4-5. The test is given in a 1-day period twice each year in April and October.

Table 4–5. **Content Distribution of the NCLEX-PN Examination**

	Client Needs			
Phases of the Nursing Process	Safe, Effective Care Environment 24%–30%	Physiological Integrity 42%–48%	Psychosocial Integrity 7%–13%	Health Promotion– Health Maintenance 15%–21%
Collect Data 25%–35%				
Plan 15%–25%				
Implement 25%–35%				
Evaluate 15%–25%				

Table 4-6 gives the planned dates for the NCLEX-PN examination. The scoring process is similar to that used for the NCLEX-RN examination and a "pass" or "fail" is reported.

Future Trends In Examination

The NCSBN is investigating the potential for computerized testing of nursing licensure applicants. Two types of computerized tests are being developed and tested. Computerized Adaptive Testing (CAT) had its first field trials in 1990. In this computerized test, the multiple choice questions are on a computer screen. The computer will contain a large bank of questions so that different individuals may be presented with different questions. The development of questions and design of the computer program assures that all tests are equivalent even when not identical.

The computer computes the score as the applicant answers questions. Based on the computation made as the applicant progresses, additional questions are presented to clearly determine whether the applicant meets the standards for safe, effective practice. An exceptionally capable ap-

Table 4–6. National Council Licensure Examination Dates For NCLEX-PN for Practical Nursing

Year	Month	Date	Day
1991	April	18	Tuesday
	October	16	Wednesday
1992	April	15	Wednesday
	October	21	Wednesday
1993	April	14	Wednesday
	October	13	Wednesday
1994	April	13	Wednesday
	October	12	Wednesday
1995	April	12	Wednesday
	October	24	Wednesday
1996	April	17	Wednesday
	October	16	Wednesday
1997	April	16	Wednesday
	October	9	Thursday
1998	April	7	Tuesday
	October	20	Wednesday
1999	April	14	Wednesday
	October	13	Wednesday

plicant who answers all questions correctly or one who is having difficulties and answers all incorrectly might be presented with fewer questions. When all areas have been tested and enough questions answered to obtain a clear score (either passing or failing) the examination would be ended.

The second type of computerized test is more complex to develop. It is called Clinical Simulation Testing (CST). In this test a client situation is presented on the computer screen. The applicant is asked to determine the appropriate action and type the answer into the keyboard. The applicant receives points for correct actions and for the order or priority in which actions are chosen. Points are subtracted for inappropriate actions. Actions that might cause harm to the client are especially flagged. Consideration is being given to putting the situations on a videodiskette to provide visual cues as well as written information. This type of testing is much more expensive to develop and administer than a multiple-choice question examination. CST was first field-tested in 1991.

The final decision on the use of computerized testing rests with the state boards of nursing. These two types of computer testing may be combined in some way to create a unique approach to nursing examination. The NCSBN hopes to begin computerized testing in the late 1990s. Some of the concerns being addressed are the cost of the computer systems, security of tests, assistance for applicants in working with computers, and the legal implications of this new testing procedure.

Licensure by Endorsement

Obtaining a nursing license in a state after first being licensed in another state is called licensure by endorsement. There are no reciprocal agreements between states that provide for automatically moving licensure from one state to another. Each case is considered independently, based on the rules and regulations of the state. However, owing to the uniformity of licensing laws throughout most of the United States and its territories, nurses have enjoyed easy mobility between geographical areas.

Because the same licensure examination is used nationwide, no state requires that the examination be retaken. Basic educational requirements as well as additional requirements in the law must be met. Some states require that a nurse moving into the state meet the current criteria for new licensure. In other states a nurse must fulfill the requirements that were in effect at the time of the original licensure. A state may require a nurse to meet other criteria, such as those for continuing education, before granting licensure by endorsement.

A temporary license that allows the applicant for licensure by endorsement to be employed while credentials are being verified and processed is available in some states. This is not permitted in other states; a license must be obtained before any employment is legal in those jurisdictions.

At the time of this writing, North Dakota is the only state where licensure by endorsement is not available to all nurses registered in other states. In North Dakota an associate degree in practical nursing is required for licensure as a licensed practical nurse and a baccalaureate degree in nursing is required for licensure as a registered nurse. This change was made by the North Dakota Board of Nursing without the need for legislative action. This action was challenged in court and upheld as within the power of the North Dakota State Board according to their licensure law. All nurses currently registered in North Dakota retained their licenses when the change occurred in 1987. This also applies to nurses who were licensed in other states prior to 1987. Nurses whose initial licensure is after 1987 are eligible for temporary licensure in North Dakota while they work towards the required degree.

Licensure of Graduates of Foreign Nursing Schools

Nurses who have graduated from a nursing school in a foreign country and want to practice nursing in the United States must satisfy the board of nursing in their state that their education meets the requirements of the state and take the NCLEX-RN examination. To prevent the exploitation of foreign graduates who come to the United States to practice nursing and fail to pass the licensing examination, and to help assure safety in health care for the U.S. public, the ANA and the NLN have sponsored an independent organization called the Committee on Graduates of Foreign Nursing Schools (CGFNS), which administers an examination to foreign-educated nurses. The examination covers proficiency in both nursing and English and helps the foreign-educated nurse to determine the possibility of passing the actual licensing examination. Nurses may take the CGFNS examination while still in their own country, although it is also given in the United States.

To obtain a nonimmigrant preference visa from the U.S. Immigration and Naturalization Service or a work permit from the U.S. Labor Department, the foreign-educated nurse must first pass the CGFNS examination. The majority of states also require the CGFNS examination as a preliminary step for foreign-educated nurses before taking the NCLEX examination for licensure.

In addition to its role in preparing and administering the CGFNS examination, the CGFNS organization also investigates and validates credentials held by graduates of foreign nursing schools for boards of nursing and other appropriate organizations. Nursing education throughout the world is varied and offers differing titles and types of education. Those who are not familiar with a foreign nursing education and licensure system may have difficulty determining whether the credentials presented are the equivalent of the licensed practical nurse or of the registered nurse in this country. CGFNS maintains current data on nursing from around the world as well as having a staff who are involved full time with this process. This enables this organization to provide an accurate evaluation of credentials of graduates of foreign nursing schools (Schaefer, 1990).

Fees

All states charge a fee for processing an application for licensure. At the time of initial licensure there are also fees for taking the licensing examination and a fee to the company that prepares and scores the examination. The total cost for initial examination and license is usually more than $100. In addition, there is a fee each time a license is renewed. For specific information on licensure fees, temporary permits, and continuing education requirements, write to the board of nursing of the state in which you are interested.

REVOCATION OF A LICENSE

A license to practice any occupation becomes a property right of the individual after the state has awarded it. As long as the individual renews by paying the appropriate fees and meets any requirements, such as continuing education, a license cannot be revoked without cause. The possible reasons for revoking a license are spelled out in the law. (The common reasons are listed earlier, in the discussion of disciplinary action.)

The procedure for revoking a license includes the right of the individual to have a hearing, which functions in many ways like a court proceeding. The state board or a specially designated hearing board is responsible for conducting the hearing and handing down a decision. The board may revoke the license completely or may put a variety of conditions on the person. For example, an individual being faced with charges based on chemical dependency might be directed to enter a treatment program, to not be employed in any nursing position with direct responsibility to clients or access to drugs, and to be monitored for compliance. If these conditions are met, the individual may then be reinstated to full rights and privileges of licensure. The board's decision may be appealed to a court of law in most states. The individual being threatened with revocation of a license should have an attorney for legal counsel throughout the proceeding.

Sunset Laws

Most laws remain in effect until the legislature votes to rescind or replace them. Because this has resulted in archaic laws remaining in effect for years and years, some states have passed what are known as "sunset laws." Sunset laws provide that any regulatory act, such as the nurse practice act, will automatically be rescinded if not reauthorized. In states with sunset laws, nurses cannot wait for an opportune time when they would like to support changes in the nurse practice act. Instead they must identify when sunsetting will occur and work in advance to bring a positive vote just to retain the current law. The advantage of sunset laws is that they guarantee that the legislature will review and evaluate agencies and programs.

CERTIFICATION IN NURSING

As discussed earlier, certification is a professional, not a legal credential. The definition of certification adopted by the Interdivisional Council on Certification of the ANA states: "Certification is the documented validation of specific qualifications demonstrated by the individual registered nurse in the provision of professional nursing care in a defined area of practice"(ANA, 1978). Certification is available from a variety of professional nursing and health care organizations.

ANA Certification

Currently, ANA certification is a method of recognizing nurses who provide direct patient care. Applicants must demonstrate current practice that is beyond that which is required for licensure as a registered nurse. The applicant must take a national examination and submit evidence of completing any other requirements for the specific clinical area. Certificates are valid for a period of 5 years, after which the nurse must meet specific criteria to renew the certification for another 5 years. Table 4-7 lists the various certification credentials available from the ANA.

Other Certification Programs

The Nurses Association of the American College of Obstetricians and Gynecologists (NAACOG) established a joint certification procedure

Table 4–7. ANA Certification Areas Available

Clinical Specialist Certifications (Require Master's Degree)

Clinical Specialist in Adult Psychiatric/Mental Health Nursing
Clinical Specialist in Child/Adolescent Psychiatric/Mental Health Nursing
Clinical Specialist in Medical-Surgical Nursing

Nurse Practitioner Certification (Require Specific Specialty Educational Program)

Adult Nurse Practitioner (BSN required)
Family Nurse Practitioner (BSN required)
Gerontological Nurse Practitioner
Pediatric Nurse Practitioner
School Nurse Practitioner (BSN required)

Other Nursing Specialty Certification (No Specific Specialty Educational Program Requirement)

Child and Adolescent Nurse
Community Health Nurse (BSN required)
Gerontological Nurse
High-risk Perinatal
Maternal Child Health
Medical Surgical Nurse
Nursing Administration (BSN required)
Nursing Administration, Advanced (master's degree required)
Psychiatric and Mental Health Nurse

For further information about any of these programs, write to Certification Unit, American Nurses' Association, 2420 Pershing Road, Kansas City, MO 64108.

with the ANA for the maternal-gynecological-neonatal nurse. The NAA-COG withdrew from joint sponsorship of this program in 1979 and began providing independent certification in 1980. The National Association of Pediatric Nurse Associates Practitioners (NAPNAP) offers certification for the pediatric nurse practitioner. Thus there are currently two certificates being awarded in the same area by two organizations. NAPNAP and the ANA have had joint conferences regarding certification, and it was hoped that one jointly sponsored certification might result. Fundamental differences still exist, however, between the two organizations on how authority for determining standards should be established.

The American College of Nurse Midwives provides a certification program for nurses specializing in nurse midwifery. Nurses graduating from approved midwifery programs apply for certification through this organization. Approved programs may be at a basic level or at a master's degree level. The license to practice as a midwife depends, however, on the state licensure laws. Some states do not allow the practice of nurse midwives; in other states the law recognizes the certification as an appropriate credential for practice; and in still other states no decision has been made.

Certification as a registered nurse anesthetist is provided by the American Association of Nurse Anesthetists (AANA). Since 1952 the AANA, with the approval of the American Hospital Association, has accredited programs for preparing nurse anesthetists and has administered an examination for certification of graduates of these programs. According to the AANA, certified registered nurse anesthetists administer more than half of all anesthetics. Nurse anesthetists were the first nurses to be certified beyond the basic level.

Many other specialty organizations in nursing have certification programs (Table 4-8). Most of these are administered by a separately titled and funded certification organization that is closely related to the specialty organization. This administrative structure is set up to protect the

Table 4–8. Certification Available Through Other Organizations

Nurse Practitioner Certification

Nurse Midwife (ACNM)
Pediatric Nurse Practitioner (NAPNAP)
Ob/Gyn Practitioner (NAACOG)

Nursing Specialty Certification

Critical Care Nurse (CCNA)
Emergency Room Nurse (EDNA)
Enterostomal Therapy (ETA)
Hemodialysis Nurse (AANNT)
Infection Control Specialist (APIC) (not exclusively nurses)
Inpatient Obstetric Nurse (NAACOG)
Neonatal Intensive Care Nurse (NAACOG)
Neonatal Nurse Clinician (NAACOG)
Neurosurgical Nurse (AANN)
Nurse Anesthetist (AANA)
Nursing Home Administrator (ACHCA) (not exclusively nurses)
Occupational Health Nurse (AOHN)
Operating Room Nurse (AORN)
Rehabilitation Nurse (ARN)
Urological Nurse (AANNT)

For further information on certification in any of these areas, contact the organization shown in parentheses. Addresses appear in Appendix B.

sponsoring organization from economic liability, to preserve tax-exempt status, and to provide a more objective approach to the credentialing process. Information on any of these specialty certification programs can be obtained by writing directly to the organization (see Appendix B).

Some health care organizations offer credentialing to individuals in specific occupations that may include nurses. For example, the Society of Gastroenterostomal Assistants offers certification to individuals employed in gastroenterology laboratories. This certification is available to both registered nurses and licensed practical nurses. The Association for Practitioners in Infection Control certifies individuals who are professionals in infection control and include nurses in this group.

Certification as a Basis for Licensure

Some states are using some certification as a means of identifying competence in an expanded or specialized role for the registered nurse, and thus are giving legal status to the certification. The requirements and methods for obtaining certification remain under the control of the organization granting the certification. The nurse receives a license from the state to practice in the expanded role. This is true of certified nurse anesthetists who are all certified through the American Association of Nurse Anesthetists but who receive legal status to practice in anesthesia by the appropriate authority in their state. This may be the board of nursing, although in some states nurse anesthetists practice under the board of medicine

Titles being used in these expanded roles vary from state to state. Some current titles are advanced registered nurse (ARN), specialized registered nurse (SRN), nurse practitioner (NP), independent nurse practitioner (INP), advanced registered nurse practitioner (ARNP), and certified registered nurse (CRN). In some states the specialized nurse uses the title of the specific certification, such as family nurse practitioner (FNP) and pediatric nurse practitioner (PNP).

Problems Related to Certification

The problems associated with certification have yet to be resolved. Programs that prepare nurses in these various specialties lack uniformity. The situation is reminiscent of the early years of nursing education. Some advanced programs accept any registered nurse and are completed in 6 to 9 months. Other programs that prepare nurses for the same specialty may be at the master's degree level. Thus the title awarded by the program is not a reliable indication of the degree of competence achieved by the nurse specialist. It is hoped that the certification program will improve the situation by defining the common standard of performance that must be demonstrated to attain the certificate.

Another concern is the disparity from state to state in credentialing nurses in specialty areas. This can hamper mobility and interfere with meeting the health care needs in areas of the United States where these nursing specialists are not recognized. Some believe that the certification program will be of help because it sets national standards that states may adopt. When different states adopt certification as an appropriate way of credentialing, reciprocity between those states is facilitated.

A third problem is related to the equivalency of certificates in different specialties. Not all specialists have the same educational, testing, or practice requirements. Some certify persons in independent areas of primary care, while others certify persons in what are essentially specialty areas of hospital nursing. To identify the exact meaning of a certificate in a nursing specialty, one would have to investigate the specific requirements of that certificate. Certification has not solved the problems related to credentialing in nursing specialties.

The Future of Certification In Nursing

Both the public and nurses have been confused because credentialing in nursing involves so many aspects related to both licensure and certification. Because the ideal credential clearly communicates qualifications and competence, it is important for nursing to create a more uniform credentialing system.

To clarify the matter, the ANA, in cooperation with 47 other interested groups, funded a major research study on credentialing in the field of nursing. The major recommendation of the study was that an independent, free-standing center for nursing credentialing be established. This would be similar to the organization for credentialing in laboratory sciences previously mentioned. The study committee believed that this move toward an independent center would provide the checks and balances necessary to preserve equity for all in the system and would be an efficient, cost-effective service that would avoid duplication of efforts and provide for geographical mobility for nurses (ANA, 1978).

Although the recommendation for a central credentialing center for nursing was made in 1978, and further study and discussion resulted, all the various nursing organizations that provided credentialing in specialty practice could not agree on how to accomplish this goal. The threats to organizational autonomy and power involved in giving up an existing certification program were great.

In 1988 the ANA independently established a credentialing center titled the American Nurses Credentialing Center, bringing together all of its credentialing activities. They invited all other organizations providing credentialing to join. Some organizations joined but most retained their individual programs.

Then in 1991, eight national nursing certification programs joined to establish the American Board of Nursing Specialties. These organizations were the American Nurses Credentialing Center of the ANA, the American Board for Occupational Health Nursing, American Board of Neuroscience Nursing, Association of Rehabilitation Nurses, Council on Certification of Nurse Anesthetists, National Board of Nutritional Support Certification, Nephrology Nursing Certification Board, and the Orthopaedic Nurses Certification Board. According to their report these eight organizations represent more than 65% of the total number of RNs certified in specialty practice (Specialty certification. . ., 1991). The goal of this board is to assure quality in specialty nursing and to increase the public's ability to identify individuals who bring a consistent standard of education and experience to their practice. This is a major breakthrough in the entire certification process for nursing.

THE FUTURE OF CREDENTIALING IN HEALTH CARE

Numerous new health care occupations related to new procedures and processes in medical care are developing. This has created pressure to license each new occupation. Educational programs vary, and a considerable amount of overlapping has occurred between occupational groups, creating a complex situation.

There continues to be pressure to license additional health care providers by those who believe the state should take positive action to protect the public. Those who oppose credentialing of additional individual groups of health care workers believe that modern-day employers are able to assess workers and differentiate between them on the basis of competence and that reliance on formal credentialing procedures limits career mobility and adds to the cost of health care. Because individual health care consumers seldom contract with individual health care workers, the consumer can rely on the institution's judgment regarding the health care workers' competence. Additionally, licensing is very expensive for the state. Some of those who oppose credentialing of individual health occupations believe that licensing the institution that hires the employees would be an adequate safeguard for the public. Credentialing in the various other health occupations will remain an important concern.

CONCLUSION

Understanding the process by which health care occupations are credentialed will provide you with a background to interact more effectively with others in the health care environment. An awareness of the various credentials in use in the field of nursing will help you to plan more effectively for your own future in nursing. Whether the future holds a credential other than that of a registered nurse, understanding the extent of the issue and the significance of credentialing for the future of the nursing profession will help you to respond in a more knowledgeable way. Certainly the debate regarding credentials is not finished. Students of today will be responsible for shaping the health care practice of tomorrow.

REFERENCES

American Nurses' Association: Nursing: A Social Policy Statement. Kansas City, MO, American Nurses' Association, 1980

American Nurses' Association: The Study of Credentialing in Nursing: A New Approach, Vol 1, The Report of the Committee. Kansas City, MO, American Nurses' Association, 1978

American Nurses' Association Congress for Nursing Practice: The Nursing Practice Act: Suggested State Legislation. Kansas City, MO, American Nurses' Association, 1981

LaBar C: Boards of Nursing: Composition, Member Qualifications, and Statutory Authority. Kansas City, MO, American Nurses' Association, 1985

LaBar C: Statutory Definitions of Nursing Practice and Their Conformity of Certain ANA Principles. Kansas City, MO, American Nurses' Association, 1984a

LaBar C: Statutory Requirements for Licensing of Nurses. Kansas City, MO, American Nurses' Association, 1984b

National Council of State Boards of Nursing: Model Nurse Practice Act. Chicago, National Council of State Boards of Nursing, 1988

National Council of State Boards of Nursing: Model Nursing Administrative Rules. Chicago, National Council of State Boards of Nursing, 1988

National Council of State Boards of Nursing: Model Nursing Practice Act. Chicago, NCSBN, 1982

National Council of State Boards of Nursing: Test Plan for the National Council Licensure Examination for Practical Nurses. Chicago, NCSBN, 1989

National Council of State Boards of Nursing: Test Plan for the National Council Licensure Examination for Registered Nurses. Chicago, NCSBN, 1987

"Practice Questions: A Framework for Thinking." *Issues* Vol 10(3), pp. 3-5. Chicago, National Council of State Boards of Nursing, 1989

Schaefer B: International credentials review: Crucial and complex. Nurs Health
Care 11(8):431–432, 1990
Snyder ME, LaBar C: Issues in Professional Practice, Vol 1, Nursing: Legal
Authority for Practice. Kansas City, MO, American Nurses' Association,
1984
Specialty certification groups form organization. Am Nurse 23(4):20, 1991

FURTHER READINGS

American Nurses' Association: Questions and Answers: Sunset Laws and Nursing.
Kansas City, MO, American Nurses' Association, 1984
Bullough B: Nurse practice acts: How they affect your expanding role. Nurs '77
17(2):73–81, 1977
Fickeissen JL: Getting certified. Am J Nurs 85(3):265–269, 1985
Grinberg E: Why form a certification corporation? Oncol Nurs Forum 12(May/
June):89–93, 1985.
McCarty P: Certification allows nurses to show their competence Am Nurse
17(3):6, 1985
Providing for the needs of handicapped candidates. Issues 10(5):8–9, 1989
Spanier A: The development process of NCLEX-PN and NCLEX-RN pools.
Issues 9(3):3–6, 1988
Task force proposed timetable: Five activities identified for credentialing center.
Am Nurs 12(5):3, 1980

5

Legal Responsibilities for Practice

Objectives

After completing this chapter, you should be able to

1. *Differentiate between common law and statutory law.*

2. *Explain the role of institutional policy in legal decision making.*

3. *Differentiate between civil law and criminal law.*

4. *Define negligence and malpractice.*

5. *Explain the standard of the reasonably prudent nurse.*

6. *Define liability.*

7. *Identify situations in which liability is shared by employers or supervisors.*

8. *State points to be considered in the purchase of professional liability insurance.*

9. *Discuss the nurse's responsibility in the specific issues that can constitute malpractice.*

10. *Identify factors that contribute to a suit being instituted against a health care professional.*

11. *Discuss a variety of actions by the nurse that might prevent the initiation of a suit.*

12. *Explain the various aspects of testifying for a legal proceeding.*

Discussion about the individual nurse's responsibility and accountability for personal actions is appearing more frequently in nursing literature. Certainly as a nurse you will need to be very aware of your responsibilities. You will also want to clearly understand to whom you are accountable for your actions. Your professional responsibilities rest on a dual framework of legal and ethical constraints.

ETHICS VS. LAW

Ethics are the principles of conduct governing one's relationships with others—basic beliefs about values for right and wrong. For example, ethics are at the basis of a decision to go to work in the morning, even if you do not want to. It is possible to pretend to be sick and stay home in bed for the day. There are no laws governing your action in such a situation. What is right is a personal decision. However, because the community as a whole would agree that to pretend illness to escape work was inappropriate behavior, the employer would be supported in a decision to dismiss you from your job if you should do this on a continuing basis. Ethical decisions, therefore, have consequences both for oneself and for others. In this very simple case the employer did not have anyone to do the necessary work, patients were deprived of care, and you lost your job.

Law includes those rules of conduct or action recognized as binding or enforced by a controlling authority such as the local, state, or national government. Ethics and the law may go hand in hand, with one supporting the other. Situations in which this occurs are the easiest to understand. For example, if you choose to steal money from your employer, that would be considered unethical behavior. It would also be a violation of the law. Many laws were written to provide a basis for the community to enforce those ethical principles of conduct that were believed to be essential to the well-being of the majority of people.

In some instances ethics may address entirely different questions than the law does. The first example of reporting to work as expected is an instance that would not be addressed by laws, although most people would have a similar view of right and wrong in that instance.

In still other situations some people will find that the law and their own ethics are divergent. These are the most difficult circumstances to face. An example of the law setting different standards than those set by ethics occurs in the case of a member of the armed forces killing an enemy soldier during a war. No country considers this to be an illegal

---

Karine Gvard, R.N., M.N., J.D., served as a consultant regarding the legal material presented in this chapter.

act, but some people believe that such action is unethical and have therefore become conscientious objectors during times of war.

The purpose of this chapter is to show how the law affects nursing practice. Ethics are discussed more completely in Chapters 6 and 7. Examples are given throughout this chapter to help you understand the concepts discussed. The example situations were chosen to help you understand a specific concept. In an actual incident many more factors were considered than can be presented in a brief paragraph. It is the interaction of these multiple factors that makes it impossible to make absolute predictions regarding legal outcomes in specific situations that occur in the real world of practice. Another point that you need to understand is the importance of the specific factual data in each case. Often cases appear to be similar on the surface but some precise facts that differ may contribute to differing decisions in the apparently similar cases. Different judges and juries may also interpret facts and law differently, resulting in very different outcomes for similar cases. To help you see how actual cases occur, summaries of actual legal cases are presented for your consideration throughout the chapter.

If you have a question about a specific personal situation, you would be well advised to consult an attorney who is experienced in medicolegal matters. The facility where you are employed may have a legal counsel who is available to you. Another source of legal aid is your nurses' association attorney. If you desire private counsel, suitable names may be recommended by your local bar association.

SOURCES OF LAW

There are two general sources of law: statutory law and common law.

Statutory Law

Statutory law comprises two groupings. One, enacted law, contains those laws enacted by legislative bodies such as a county or city council, a state legislature, or the Congress of the United States. Nurse practice acts are in this category and are passed by state legislatures. Laws enacted by legislative bodies carry the greatest weight in a court (Bernzweig, 1987).

The second group of statutory law, regulatory law, includes the rules and regulations established by governmental agencies such as licensing boards and other rule setting bodies. Rules and regulations formulated by the state board of nursing are in this category. These agencies are authorized through enacted laws to establish regulations. These rules and regulations have the same force as enacted law unless found by a court to be outside the scope of or contrary to the intent of the enacted law.

Common Law

Common law derives from common usage, custom, and judicial decisions or court rulings. Previous judicial decisions or court cases are used to establish precedents for interpretations of statutory and common law. These decisions are binding within the jurisdiction of that particular court but are used in a more general way for guidelines in other jurisdictions. Common law is fluid and cannot be defined with precision. In general, statutory law carries more weight in the court than does common law.

The circumstance of abandoning a patient demonstrates how common law applies to nursing. There are no statutory laws dictating that nurses cannot leave a seriously ill patient unless they assure that someone else will provide care, but common practice and custom, which could be supported through testimony of nurses and other health care workers, require this of a nurse. Failure to meet this standard might be deemed a violation of common law.

Rulings

A ruling made by a state attorney general is an attempt to provide guidelines based on an interpretation of the statutory and common law relative to a specific situation and is not a final legal decision. Different attorneys general might vary in their opinions. The validity of an opinion only stands until a court rules on the situation. The final decision in any legal issue rests with a court.

The Role of Institutional Policy

Institutional policies provide guidance as to the proper actions to be taken in specific situations. These policies do not simply restate laws but offer much more concrete direction. Established hospital policies may be considered by the court as indications of common usage (common law) and therefore may become important as a basis for legal decisions. They may protect the institution itself and the employees of the institution from legal difficulties if they are based on current practice and sound legal advice.

Most often policies are developed by members of the hospital staff who have expertise in the practice area under consideration. An attorney may also be consulted to ensure that policies and protocols conform to legal requirements. Final approval of policies often rests with the board of trustees, directors, or commissioners who have ultimate responsibility for the financial and legal management of the organization.

Institutional policies are changed in response to new situations and new expectations occurring in society. Usually there is an established institutional route for the change or expansion of hospital policy. Nurses may be in a position to recognize the need for such a change as they use policy or protocol and compare it with the latest professional information.

CLASSIFICATION OF LAWS

Law can be divided into civil and criminal components. Both statutory law and common law may be subdivided in this way.

Criminal Law

The term *criminal law* applies to law that affects the public welfare as a whole. A violation of criminal law is called a crime and is prosecuted by the government. On conviction, a crime may be punished by imprisonment, parole conditions, a loss of privilege (such as a license), a fine,

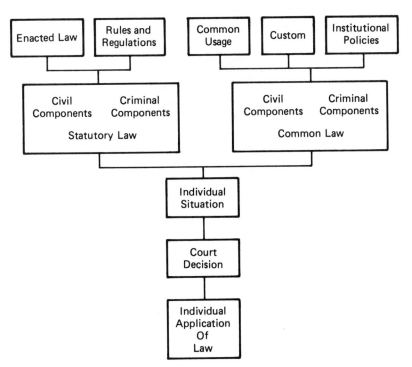

Figure 5–1. Civil law and criminal law both may affect a nursing situation.

or any combination of these. The punishment is intended to deter others from committing the crime as well as to punish the violator.

Civil Law

Civil Law applies to laws that regulate conduct between private individuals or businesses. A tort is a violation of a civil law in which another person is wronged. Private individuals or groups may bring a legal action to court for breach of civil law. Judgment of the court results in a plan to correct the wrong and may include a monetary payment to the wronged party. Because a private wrong has occurred, there is a private remedy. Nurses may find themselves involved with both civil and criminal laws, either separately or within the same situation.

CRIMINAL LAW AND NURSING

Because a violation of any law governing the practice of any licensed profession may be a crime, you must be aware of the extent of the nurse practice act. In instances in which the nurse practice act restricts functioning to acting under the direction of a physician or other licensed person, that explicit authorization must exist.

Violation of a State Practice Act

Bowland, a registered nurse, served as the primary care provider for a woman in childbirth. She was found to be practicing midwifery without the proper certification, and the court ordered a trial on a misdemeanor complaint for the illegal practice of medicine. Practicing nurse midwives in California had to have a certificate in midwifery in order to provide primary care in cases of normal childbirth. The court noted that California's statute specifically prohibited individuals without the appropriate credential from treating, diagnosing, operating on, or prescribing for a woman undergoing normal pregnancy or childbirth.

Rowland v. Municipal Court of Santa Cruz County, 556 P.2d 1081.1089 (1977) California

Standing orders that refer to specific situations as well as the usual orders written for an individual patient may be adequate authorization. However, custom or usual practice will not substitute for the specific authorization required by law. A violation of a professional practice act may be prosecuted as a crime even if no actual harm occurred to the patient.

Situation: Violation of a Practice Act

A nurse in a physician's office is contacted by a patient. The patient describes an urgent problem that the physician commonly treats. The physician is unavailable, and there are no standing orders. The nurse proceeds to give the medication she believes the physician would have prescribed.

The nurse practice act does not give the nurse the authority to diagnose disease and prescribe the medication to treat regardless of whether this is an urgent situation. The medical practice act contains this authorization. This, then is a violation of the law and is a crime, even though the patient was not harmed.

Violation of laws related to the care and distribution of controlled substances is also a crime.

Situation: Violation of Narcotic Laws

In making the routine check of the narcotic record before going off duty, the night nurse notes that the record does not match the actual count in relationship to the morphine in the supply. She is tired and does not wish to spend the time searching the record and correcting the mistake. Instead she makes a false entry for a patient who did not receive a narcotic so that the record appears correct.

Because the laws regulating the controlled substances are quite rigid, this would be a violation of the law.

It is costly to the state to undertake criminal prosecution; therefore, even when discovered, some violations of criminal law are not prosecuted in court. Knowing this, some nurses make the error of believing that "minor" violations are acceptable. Even when not prosecuted in court, criminal action could result in the loss of a job and in loss of a license to practice nursing.

Nurses have also been charged with such serious crimes as murder and assault that were committed while in the role of caregiver. These serious crimes are investigated, prosecuted, and tried by the criminal courts. A license to practice nursing may be temporarily withdrawn while such charges are investigated and tried. If the individual is found innocent, the license may then be restored. If the individual is convicted of the crime, the nursing license may be revoked along with other sentencing and penalties being assigned.

CIVIL LAW AND NURSING

Civil law relates to legal disputes between private parties. Malpractice actions brought in health care situations involve civil law.

Torts

Torts are civil wrongs committed by one person against another (Bernzweig, 1987). The wrong may be physical harm, psychological harm, or harm to reputation, livelihood, or some other less tangible value. The action that causes a civil wrong may be either intentional or unintentional. An intentional tort is one in which the outcome was planned although the person acting may not have believed that the intended outcome was harmful to the other person.

Situation: Intentional Tort

An elderly, oriented, and competent patient decides to leave the hospital in the evening without medical consent, although additional treatment has been planned.

The evening nurse decides that this patient needs the planned treatment and should not be allowed to leave. She removes the patient's clothes from the room, disconnects the telephone so that the patient cannot call for a taxi, and tells the patient that he will not be allowed to leave.

The patient expresses anger and states that he will leave as soon as he finds a way. The next morning he makes a call to his son and leaves the hospital.

The nurse purposefully acted to keep the patient in the hospital against his will. This was her planned intent. Even though she thought it was in the patient's best interests, the patient felt wronged by losing his liberty and freedom of action. A court would generally agree that loss of liberty is a wrong. If legal action is taken, the nurse may be found to have committed an intentional tort (that is a planned wrong to another person occurred).

An unintentional tort is a wrong occurring to another person or property, although it was not intended to happen. The most common cause of an unintentional tort is negligence.

Negligence

Negligence is the failure to act as a reasonably prudent person would have acted in a specific situation (Guido, 1988). If harm is caused by negligence, it is termed an *unintentional tort* and damages might be recovered. *Negligence* is a broad term that has many applications throughout society. All negligence has the following four essential characteristics (Fiesta, 1988):

1. Harm must have occurred to an individual.
2. One person must be in a situation where he or she had a duty toward the person harmed.
3. The person must be found to have failed to fulfill his or her duty. This is called "breach of duty." This might include either doing what should not have been done (commission of an inappropriate action) or failing to do what should have been done (omission of a necessary or appropriate action).
4. The harm must be shown to have been caused by the breach of duty.

Each of these points must be addressed in any legal action. The presence of harm is often very clear. For example, if a person has a fractured hip, no one would dispute that this was harm. When the harm is so clear that anyone would agree on it, the term *res ipsa loquitur* is used. This is Latin for "the thing speaks for itself." In this case the harm does not need to be "proved" to the court because all would agree that a fractured hip is a harm. However, all harm is not so straightforward. For example, when a person claims emotional suffering, the court must determine whether harm actually occurred.

Situation: Negligence

A homeowner fails to repair a broken step at the entrance to his home. He fails to warn a guest of the broken step and the guest trips on the broken step in the dark and is injured.

Negligence could be charged. The injury is the harm; the homeowner has a duty toward a guest to safeguard that guest from foreseeable harm; a reasonably prudent person would have repaired the step or at least warned the guest; and the injury can be shown to be a direct result of the homeowner's failure to act prudently.

Res Ipsa Loquitur

The patient underwent an appendectomy and awakened with sharp pain between his neck and his right shoulder. He received diathermy treatments, but the pain increased and then radiated down his right arm. Eventually he was unable to lift or rotate muscles on the right. After the patient brought suit, two physicians testified that the injury was caused by a trauma or strain applied to his right shoulder and neck during surgery. At the time of the trial no operating room personnel offered any reason for the injury. It could not be proven that the patient was under one person's exclusive control when the injury occurred.

The court found that in the case when an unconscious patient receives injury during the course of treatment, all of those involved in the treatment may be found negligent under the doctrine of *res ipsa loquitur* (the thing speaks for itself). In other words, the injury occurred and the hospital personnel were responsible for the patient during the time when it occurred; therefore hospital personnel were responsible for the injury.

Ybarra V. Spangard 154 P.2d 687 (1945) California

Malpractice

Malpractice is a term used for a specific type of negligence. It refers to the negligence of a specially trained or educated person in the performance of his or her job. Therefore, *malpractice* is the term used to describe negligence by nurses in the performance of their duties.

The definition remains the same with some modification. The professional must have had a *professional duty* toward the person injured. For example, the nurse is acting as a nurse for the person (this may be either a paid or volunteer activity). Additionally the harm occurred to another person or to the property based on failure to act as a reasonably prudent *professional* would have acted in the situation. This is a higher standard than required of the general public (Bernzweig, 1987).

Just as all parts of the situation are very clear in some general negligence situations and not in others, the professional duty is similarly clear in some instances and not in others. The nurse who is assigned to care for a patient in a hospital clearly owes a duty to that patient. Whether a supervisor, another nurse on the unit, or a nurse visitor has a professional duty might be in dispute. In some situations duties overlap and more than one nurse might have a duty toward the same patient. Again the court would decide whether a duty was present.

A breach of duty is a failure to act according to the standards of the profession for that situation (Fiesta, 1988). To determine that a breach of duty was present, the court would have to determine what represents the standard of professional practice for that situation.

The final question then becomes one of identifying the cause of the harm that occurred. Malpractice is only present if the breach of duty was the cause of the harm. In the case of a fractured hip, if the nurse failed to raise the side rail and turned the patient to the side of the bed and off onto the floor, the failure to safeguard the patient (breach of duty) could be shown to be a direct cause of the fall and fractured hip (the harm). The cause of harm is not always so clear and may be part of the dispute in a legal action.

Situation: Omission of Correct Action

An elderly, disoriented person is admitted to an acute care facility. The nurse fails to establish a plan for monitoring and maintaining safety for this person. The patient falls out of bed, sustaining a fractured hip.

This could be found to be malpractice. The nurse was working in a professional capacity and had a duty to this patient. The patient can be shown to have an injury. It may be demonstrated through testimony by

Figure 5–2. A reasonably prudent nurse uses common sense as well as nursing theory.

nurses and by reference to standard nursing texts that a reasonably prudent registered nurse would have been expected to take action to protect this patient from falls. It was this failure to act that caused the fall and fracture. This failure to act could then constitute malpractice.

Situation: Commission of Inappropriate Action

A postoperative patient has an order to ambulate. The nurse assigned to this patient finds that the patient's condition has changed drastically since the order was written. The patient has a fever and a rapid pulse and is complaining of severe acute abdominal pain. The nurse proceeds to have the patient ambulate. The patient faints, sustaining a head injury in the fall. This necessitates additional hospitalization, x-ray films, and diagnostic procedures.

Again, this could be found to be malpractice. The nurse was working as a professional with a duty to this patient. The patient can be shown to have sustained injury. It may be demonstrated that a reasonably prudent nurse would have recognized that the change in the patient's condition called for altering the plan of care and not ambulating at this time. This was the breach of duty. Ambulating the patient in that condition was the cause of the fall and the head injury. Therefore malpractice could be found owing to inappropriate action on the part of the nurse.

Direct Causation of Harm in Malpractice

A patient developed a postoperative infection of the eye following cataract surgery. Scarring of the cornea developed, and after years of unsuccessful treatment for the infection the eye was removed. The patient and a witness both stated that a nurse had picked up an eye patch that had fallen on the floor and applied it directly to the patient's eye. The infection that developed after this event was due to the cultured organisms of *Enterobacter* (a common bowel pathogen) and *Staphylococcus albus* (a common skin pathogen). In spite of the testimony about the nurse's action, the patient lost his suit because he was unable to prove that the organisms came from the floor (a lack of causality between the act and the harm that resulted).

DeFalco v. Long Island College Hospital, 393 N.Y.S. 2d 859 (1977) New York

LIABILITY

A person found guilty of any tort (whether intentional or unintentional) is considered legally liable, or legally responsible, for the outcome.

The person legally liable usually is required to pay for damages to the other person. This may include actual costs of care, legal services, loss of earnings (present and future), and compensation for emotional and physical stress suffered.

Personal Liability

As an educated professional, you are always responsible or liable for your actions (Bernzweig, 1987). Thus, if a physician or supervisor instructs you to do something that is contrary to your best professional judgment and says, "I'll take responsibility," that person is poorly informed about the law. The physician or supervisor giving the directions may also be liable if harm results, but that would not remove your personal liability.

Situation: Personal Liability

The registered nurse giving medications on a large medical unit notes that an order for digoxin (a heart medication) is considerably larger than the usual dose. She looks up the medication in a reference book and finds her view of the dose size confirmed. The ordered dose is several times the usual dose. The RN then calls the supervisor and explains the situation.

The supervisor double checks the order with the RN and then states: "Dr. Jones is an outstanding physician. I am sure he has a good reason for ordering this dose. Go ahead and give the medication as ordered." The RN then gives the medication, and the patient suffers a toxic reaction.

The RN would very likely be held liable for giving the incorrect amount of medication. She had the knowledge and judgment to recognize the dose as erroneous and failed to check with the physician. A statement by the supervisor does not remove the nurse's personal responsibility for her own actions. Because even a competent physician might make an error, the nurse had a responsibility to clarify that order. The supervisor and the physician could be held liable in addition to the nurse but not instead of her.

Although each person is legally responsible for his or her own acts, the example above illustrates that there are also situations in which a person or organization may be held liable for actions taken by others.

Employer Liability

The most common situation in which a person or organization is held responsible for the actions of another is the employer–employee relationship. In many instances the employer can be held responsible for the torts committed by an employee. This is called the doctrine of respondeat superior (let the master respond). The law holds the employer responsible for having hired qualified persons, for establishing an appropriate environment for correct functioning, and for providing supervision or direction as needed to avoid errors or harm. Therefore, if the nurse, as an employee of the hospital, is guilty of malpractice, the hospital may also be guilty of malpractice. The employer's liability may exist even if the employer appears to have taken precautions to prevent error.

It is important to understand that this doctrine does not remove any responsibility from the individual nurse but it extends responsibility to the employer in addition to the nurse. If, for example, a hospital has a procedure that does not conform to good nursing practice as you know it and you follow that procedure, you will still be liable for any resulting harm. You are expected to use your education and training to make sound judgments regarding your work.

Situation: Employer Responsibility for a Staff Nurse

A nurse working in a long-term care facility is giving medications at night. In an attempt to not disturb the patient, she gives an injection in a darkened room, gives it in the wrong location, and hits a nerve.

Both the RN in this situation and the long-term facility might be found liable for the harm that resulted. The RN had a personal, professional responsibility in giving medications. The facility also had a responsibility for making sure that employees carry out procedures safely and correctly.

Charitable Immunity

In some states nonprofit hospitals have "charitable immunity." This means that the nonprofit hospital cannot be held legally liable for harm done to a patient. The employees of that nonprofit hospital are still legally liable for their actions. The trend in legislation is toward the repeal of laws providing for charitable immunity. Those active in the consumer movement have argued that no institution should be relieved of responsibility in such a blanket fashion. If you are employed by a nonprofit institution, it is important that you know whether the law in your state provides for charitable immunity.

Supervisory Liability

When a nurse is in the role of charge nurse, head nurse, supervisor, or any other category in which the job involves supervision or direction of other persons, there is a potential for liability for the actions of others. The supervising nurse is responsible for exercising good judgment in a supervisory role. This includes making appropriate decisions about assignments and delegation of tasks. If an error occurs and the supervising nurse is shown to have exercised sound judgment in all decisions made in that capacity, the supervising nurse may not be held liable for the error of a subordinate. If poor judgment was used in assigning an inadequately prepared person to an important task, the supervisory nurse might be liable for resulting harm. The extent of the subordinate's responsibility would rest on his or her level of education and training. Persons without education or training might not be liable for some errors. The more education subordinates have, the more likely they will be liable also. (Again whenever an individual employee is found guilty of malpractice, the employer may also be found liable.)

Situation: Supervisory Responsibility for an Educated Staff Member

Two sudden admissions to the coronary care unit create a situation in which additional help is needed to care for the patients in the unit.

The staff supervisor calls the person whose name appears first on the list of temporary-placement RNs. This nurse agrees to come in immediately. The nurse is not asked whether she has education or experience in coronary care, nor does she volunteer this information. She has no background or experience in coronary care.

While working in the coronary care unit, the temporary RN is assigned to complete care of two patients. Because of her lack of ability to read the monitors, a potentially life-threatening problem is not identified until the patient "arrests." Resuscitation efforts are successful, but the patient suffers some brain damage.

Both the staffing supervisor who placed the inadequately prepared RN in the unit and the temporary nurse herself could be found liable—the supervisor for incorrectly placing the nurse and the nurse for not recognizing her own limitations. The educational preparation of the temporary nurse gave her the background to understand that expertise was needed in this situation and that she herself did not possess that expertise. If that situation were changed so that the temporary nurse was reviewed for expertise in coronary care and found to the have that expertise, then the supervisor might not be liable for the error of the temporary nurse. The supervisory function of ascertaining level of preparation and ability to meet the standards of the job would have been carried out.

Situation: Supervisory Responsibility for Staff Member with Limited Education

The evening nursing supervisor is responsible for adjusting personnel assignments when employees are absent. She decides to send an extra aide to the emergency department to assist. This aide has never been assigned to the emergency department before and has no education or training other than the orientation to direct care given by the hospital. The supervisor instructs the aide to take care of the desk and answer the phone while others are busy.

While the aide is at the desk alone, a family enters the emergency department with an infant in acute distress. The aide instructs the family to sit down and wait until a nurse comes out of one of the rooms.

It is a long time before the nurse appears and care for the infant is instituted. The infant has a complicated recovery that later could be shown to be due to the delay in initial treatment.

The supervisor might be found negligent in this case for assigning the aide to emergency department duties without proper direction or supervision. The aide might not be found negligent because she had no basis for recognizing the seriousness of the situation nor for recognizing her own lack of ability to meet the responsibilities involved in being at the desk in an emergency department.

LIABILITY INSURANCE

Liability insurance transfers the risk of the costs of being sued and of any settlement from the individual to a large group. The expectation is that most individuals will not be able to afford such costs and that the pool of premiums will adequately cover the costs plus a profit for the insurance company that manages the financial plan.

There is currently a liability insurance crisis in the United States. The cost of liability insurance has escalated at an extraordinary rate. Some of the factors that have caused this to happen are the large judgments that have been made, the number of suits that have been brought, the large fees that attorneys receive, and the high profits of insurance companies. Regardless of the causes, the problem is a very real and serious one for all professionals. Nurses in advanced practice have been especially affected by the increase in premiums because their incomes have traditionally been quite moderate and they cannot raise fees enough to cover insurance costs that may match those of physicians.

The American Nurses Association (ANA) has initiated a data bank related to legal claims against nurses. They are asking all registered nurses to provide information to them regarding legal action in which they have been named as a defendant. Their purpose is to have adequate records to support the contention that the low level of suits against nurses should translate into low cost liability insurance.

Some states have initiated legislation that allows for awards to cover actual losses and costs of care, but that limits awards for pain and suffering and other nontangible factors. Sometimes this has been accompanied by restrictions on insurance company rates. Some laws are also being amended to restrict the monetary liability of any party to the percentage of responsibility. For example, if damages were set at $10,000 and each of two defendants were determined to be responsible for 50% of the problem, one party could not be made to pay more than $5000, even if the other party had no assets and could not pay. Liability laws continue to be a major concern for nurses because nurses are being named in an increasing number of suits.

Institutional and Individual Insurance

Liability insurance pays for attorney's fees and the costs of defending yourself when a suit is brought as well as for a settlement or judgment up to the limits of the policy. Many hospitals or other institutional employers carry liability insurance that covers both the institution and its employees. Some hospitals may limit the coverage that their policies provide for individual employees in an effort to hold down costs.

Even if an employer carries liability insurance, it is often advisable for the individual professional to carry an independent policy. An independent policy may cover the person in voluntary activities as well as on the job. It also will follow the person who moves from one employer to another. If a legal action is instituted against the professional, the individual liability insurance policy may provide independent legal counsel.

Some nurses state that they do not carry insurance because it might encourage people to bring suit against them. They are under the mistaken assumption that persons will not sue if it means financial hardship for the person being sued. This is an error because most individuals who sue do not know whether the nurse carries individual insurance. In addition, insurance is not the only source of payment for a judgment. Judgments may be levied against most tangible assets, such as a house, a car, or savings, as well as against future earnings. Married nurses who reside in community property states should realize that one half of the assets of the family may be vulnerable to a judgment reached. Community property states at this time include Arizona, California, Idaho, Louisiana, Nevada, New Mexico, Texas, and Washington. These factors combine to support the need for the individual professional to carry liability insurance that will provide legal counsel and protection in the case of any judgment.

Analyzing Insurance Coverage

Individual liability insurance for registered nurses is available from a variety of insurance companies directly through their agents and through professional organizations that offer coverage as a service to members. When investigating individual liability insurance, ask yourself the following questions:

1. In what situations would I, as an individual, be covered?
2. In what situations would I not be covered?
3. How is my coverage affected by my actions? For example, if I failed to follow hospital policy, would I still be covered?
4. What are the monetary limits of the policy?
5. Does the policy provide me with an attorney?
6. Is the policy renewable at my option? What factors affect renewability?
7. Does the insurance cover incidents that occurred while the policy was in force, regardless of when the claim is brought (claims occurred coverage), or does it cover incidents only if I am currently insured (claims brought coverage)?
8. What is the cost compared with other policies?

Liability insurance coverage, which is carried by the hospital, should be carefully investigated by the nurse employee. "Full coverage" is not a very informative statement. Questions 1 through 4 above apply to institutional policies as well as to individual policies. In addition, you should ask the following questions in regard to an institutional policy?

1. Does the policy provide me with an individual attorney, or will the same attorney be working for the hospital?

2. At what point would the hospital no longer be responsible and I would be personally responsible?
3. How would my job be affected if a lawsuit is filed or payment is awarded based on the action against me? (Check institutional policy as well as the insurance company policy.)
4. Does the insurance company have the right to seek restitution from me if it pays a claim based on my actions?

It is important that you have accurate answers to these questions so that you can make an informed decision regarding your need for an individual policy.

Insurance Cost and Coverage

The ANA has a group policy providing $500,000 per claim and $1 million total in 1 year as basic coverage for the registered nurse. Optional higher limits are available. The cost for such coverage in 1991 was approximately $69 per year. Inflation can be expected to increase this cost. Since the 1970s the cost of the basic coverage provided by the ANA rose from approximately $12 per year to its current amount. Liability insurance is available from other sources.

Liability insurance coverage for specialty practice as a nurse practitioner, nurse anesthetist, or nurse midwife is a much greater problem. Some insurance companies have refused to cover these groups. Others have dramatically increased costs. Nursing organizations are working to resolve this problem. Group policies are available for some of these individuals through professional organizations. Other individuals are covered by institutional policies and do not try to maintain individual policies.

LEGAL ISSUES IN NURSING

Some individual issues recur continually in nursing practice. It is wise for the nurse to consider and try to understand these particular issues as they relate to individual practice.

Duty to Report or Seek Medical Care for a Patient

A nurse who is caring for a patient has a legal duty to assure that the patient receives safe and competent care. This duty requires that the nurse maintain an appropriate standard of care and also that the nurse take action to obtain an appropriate standard of care from other professionals when that is necessary. For example, if a nurse identifies that a patient needs the attention of a physician and fails to make every effort to obtain that attention, the nurse has breached a duty to the patient.

Situation: Failure to Seek Medical Care for Patient

The registered nurse is caring for a postoperative patient during the night. The patient's blood pressure begins to drop and the pulse to rise. The nurse's assessment indicates that the patient may be bleeding internally. The nurse institutes a plan for close nursing monitoring and calls the surgeon to describe the situation. The surgeon gives a telephone order to increase the intravenous fluid rate and states that he will see the patient in the morning. The patient's condition continues to deteriorate, but the nurse does nothing further to ensure that a physician examines the patient.

If there is an untoward outcome, the nurse can be found to have breached a duty to the patient. The patient relies on the nurse to provide appropriate care and to identify when a physician is needed. The nurse could have made other telephone calls to the surgeon and failing the success of that could have followed the facility's procedure for asking another physician (such as the emergency department physician) to see the patient.

The nurse has a duty to continue all efforts to try to obtain appropriate medical care for the patient. If the nurse had followed all procedures, sought another physician, and continued efforts when initial attempts were unsuccessful, the nurse would not have breached a duty. The nurse cannot guarantee a physician's care but can guarantee that the patient will not be left without an advocate.

Confidentiality and Right to Privacy

Confidentiality and the right to privacy with respect to one's personal life are very basic concerns in our society. This right has been inferred from interpretation of the federal constitution, but is explicitly stated in some state laws. With increased computerization of records, which can result in easier retrieval and cross-referencing of records from a variety of sources, the general public is becoming more concerned about potential invasions of privacy.

All information regarding a patient belongs to that patient. A nurse who gives out information without authorization from the patient or from the legally responsible guardian can be held liable. If you have any question about who the legally responsible guardian is, be sure to consult with your administrative authority. There may be a court-appointed legal guardian, or the situation may be governed by specific state laws regarding who becomes the responsible guardian when the person is unable to give personal consent. The hospital administration should be able to ascertain the correct guardian.

Only those professional persons involved in the patient's care who have a need to know about the patient can be allowed routine access to his record. A physician who is not involved in the patient's care or who does not have an administrative responsibility relative to that care is not allowed routine access. Persons not involved in care can be allowed access to the record by specific written authorization or by court order.

You should be cautious about what information you share verbally and with whom. In some instances, especially those involving treatment for alcoholism, drug abuse, and acquired immunodeficiency syndrome, even revealing the diagnosis or reasons for hospitalization would be considered a legal violation of confidentiality.

A directory information policy has been adopted by many acute care hospitals. This policy gives specific guidelines about what must be revealed according to freedom of information laws but will not violate confidentiality. Usually you are allowed to reveal the patient's name and sex and a general statement of condition (satisfactory, serious, and so on). If your hospital has no written policy, this is a wise standard to follow.

Situation: Breach of Confidentiality

A well-known political figure is hospitalized for a hysterectomy. The registered nurse in charge on the evening after the surgery answers the telephone. The call is from a man who identifies himself as a reporter from the community newspaper. He states that he has heard of the hospitalization and wonders how the patient is doing. The nurse responds that the patient is doing as well as could be expected for someone who has just had a hysterectomy for possible cancer. The column written in the paper suggests that because the political figure has cancer, she is an inappropriate candidate for office in the next election, and this becomes a major campaign issue.

The nurse could be held liable in a suit charging breach of privacy and confidentiality for revealing this information to the press.

Defamation of Character

Any time that shared information is detrimental to the person's reputation, the person sharing the information may be liable for defamation of character. Written defamation is called libel. Oral defamation is called slander. Defamation of character involves communication that is malicious and false. Sometimes such comments are made in the heat of anger. Occasionally statements written in the chart are libelous. Severely critical opinions may be stated as fact. An example of such a statement might be "The patient is lying," or "The patient is rude and domineering." The patient may charge that these comments in the chart adversely affected his care by prejudicing other staff against him. The prudent nurse will chart only objective information regarding a patient and give opinion in professional terms, well documented with fact. In conversations the prudent nurse avoids discussing patients.

Situation: Slander

Two registered nurses are leaving the floor for their coffee break. They are discussing the patients in their care as they wait for the elevator. They enter the elevator with a number of other people and continue their conversation. The first RN says: "That Mrs. Johnson in Room 201. I don't know whether I can take another day of her! She's impossible!" The other RN replies: "I know just what you mean. I had her last week and she was just on the bell all the time. If you ask me, there's nothing wrong with her that a good swift kick wouldn't cure!" First RN: "Do you really think she's faking?" Second RN: "I'm sure of it. Have you ever watched her when her husband comes to visit?"

A relative of the patient is one of a group of people in the elevator who were there to visit Mrs. Johnson and overhears the conversation. The relative reports the conversation to the patient.

If the patient brings suit, the RNs involved might be found guilty of slander. The nurses were discussing the patient in a place where others could hear the conversation. The comments clearly identified the patient, reflected opinions that were not supported with fact, and potentially would jeopardize the patient's reputation and standing in the community.

Defamation of character may also be charged by a health care provider who believes that statements made by another professional are false, malicious, and have caused harm. There are accepted mechanisms for confidentially reporting inappropriate care or errors and these should be used rather than making critical statements to uninvolved third parties. In many states licensed professionals are required to report poor practice or illegal acts on the part of other professionals. Criticism reported without malice and in good faith through appropriate channels is protected from legal action for defamation of character.

Defamation of Character

A nurse in an emergency department made derogatory remarks about certain hospital physicians during a committee meeting. She was asked to resign because of her statements. She filed suit stating that this was an infringement of her rights of free speech. The court upheld the hospital in asking for her resignation because it was not her complaints but the place in which she voiced them that was inappropriate.

Bach v. Mount Clemens General Hospital, Inc., 449 F. Suppl 686 (1978)

The federal government is now maintaining a National Data Bank on all physicians. All convictions for malpractice or situations in which privileges to practice are curtailed or withdrawn must be reported to this data bank, and all institutions must consult this data bank for information before giving a physician privileges. The plan is to expand this data bank to cover other licensed health professionals as well as physicians. The purpose of the National Data Bank is to protect the public from incompetent professionals who continue to practice by moving from one place to another.

Privileged Information

Privileged communication refers to information shared with certain professionals that does not need to be revealed even in a court of law. All states consider certain types of communication between client and attorney, between patient and doctor, or between an individual and a member of the clergy as privileged. Not all states recognize the nurse–patient relationship as one in which privileged communication exists. Even in those states that recognize nurse–patient communication as potentially being privileged, all communication between patients and nurses is not considered privileged. It is important that you understand that privilege is a very limited concept. Only a court can determine if privilege exists in any specific case. If the court does not determine information to be privileged, then you are legally obligated to testify about the communication.

Informed Consent

Everyone has the right to make decisions about oneself. Part of the right to make one's own decisions is the right to either consent to or refuse medical treatment.

Legal Requirement

The law requires that the person give voluntary and informed consent. *Voluntary* means that no coercion existed; *informed* means that the person clearly understood the choices being offered. Included in the discussion must be the alternatives for treatment, the risks of any treatment proposed, the relative value of any treatment proposed, and the risks of not having treatment. This consent may be either verbal or written. Written consent usually is preferred in health care in order to have a record of consent, although a signature alone does not prove that the consent was informed. A blanket consent for "any procedures deemed necessary" is not usually considered adequate consent for specific procedures. The form should state the specific proposed medical procedure or test.

The patient's medical condition is usually not accepted by the courts as a valid reason for not giving complete and accurate information. Currently there are no clear guidelines as to what constitutes complete information. Courts have generally supported the idea that usual risks need to be disclosed, but that rare or unexpected risks do not have to be discussed.

The law places the responsibility for obtaining consent for medical treatment on the physician. It is the physician's responsibility to provide appropriate information, and he or she is liable if the patient charges that the appropriate information was not given.

The nurse may present a form for the patient to sign, and the nurse may sign the form as a witness to the signature. This does not transfer the legal liability for informed consent for medical care to the nurse. If the patient does not seem well informed, it would be prudent for the nurse to notify the physician so that further information can be given. Although the nurse would not be legally liable for the lack of informed consent, the nurse has ethical obligations relative to assisting the patient to exercise his or her rights and to assisting the physician in providing appropriate care.

Responsibility for Informed Consent

An elderly woman came to the hospital for cataract surgery. She signed the usual hospital consent form. After the surgery the woman became blind. She brought suit against the physician and the hospital contending that she had not been informed that this was a possible complication of the surgery. The court held that the hospital was not liable because the responsibility for informed consent rested with the physician.

Cooper v. Curry, 589 P.2d 201 (New Mexico, 1978)

Consent for Nursing Measures

Nurses must obtain consent for nursing measures undertaken. This does not mean that exhaustive explanations need to be given in each situation, because courts have held that patients can be expected to have some understanding of usual care. Consent for nursing measures may be verbal or implied. The nurse may ask, "Are you ready to ambulate now?" The patient answers, "Certainly," providing verbal consent. Alternatively the nurse may state: "I have the injection the doctor ordered for you. Will you please turn over?" If the patient turns over, this is implied consent.

It is well for the nurse to remember that the patient is free to refuse any aspect of care that is offered. However, just as in the case of the physician, the nurse is responsible for making sure that the patient is informed before making a decision. Good nursing care requires that you use all of the means at your disposal to help the patient comprehend the value of the proposed care. For example, the postoperative patient needs to understand that getting into a chair is part of the plan of care, not a convenience for the nurse or simply a change to prevent boredom. Thus a patient's refusal of care is accepted after the patient has been given complete information so that an informed decision was made.

Right to Refuse Treatment

A twenty-three-year-old woman who was a Jehovah's Witness refused to have a blood transfusion because of her religious beliefs. The hospital asked the court to require that she have the transfusion because it was necessary to save her life. The court upheld her right to refuse the transfusion because an adult of sound mind has a right to refuse treatment.

St. Mary's Hospital v. Ransey, 465 So2d 666 (Fla. App. 1985)

The confused or disoriented patient presents a different problem in terms of consent. If the person truly is not capable of making decisions, then the nurse should attempt to present necessary nursing actions in a way that elicits cooperation and avoids confrontation over decisions. When this is not possible, consent may be obtained from the legal guardian for carrying out nursing care measures.

Withdrawing Consent

Consent may be withdrawn after it is given. People have the right to change their minds. Therefore, if after one intravenous infusion the patient decides not to have a second one started, that is his or her right.

As a nurse you have an obligation to notify the physician if the patient refuses a medical procedure or treatment.

Consent and Minors

For a minor, consent usually is given by a parent or legal guardian. You should also obtain the minor's consent when he or she is able to give it. Courts are emphasizing increasingly that minors be allowed a voice in their own lives when it concerns matters that they are capable of understanding. This is especially true for the adolescent, but you need to consider it with any child who is 7 years of age or older. When the minor refuses care and the legal guardian has authorized that care, you should not proceed until legal clarification is given. Your nursing supervisor should be consulted.

Minors who live apart from their parents and are financially independent or who are married are termed *emancipated minors.* In most (but not all) states an emancipated minor can give consent to his or her own treatment. Some states have additional specific laws allowing minors to give personal consent without also obtaining parental consent for treatment of sexually transmitted disease or for obtaining birth control information and supplies. You would need to be sure of the law in your own state if you practice in an area where this would be a concern. An institution should develop policies to guide employees in making correct decisions in this and other areas dealing with consent.

Consent and the Mentally Incompetent

For a person who is legally determined to be mentally incompetent, consent is obtained from the legal guardian. A difficult area involves those for whom no legal determination of competence has been made but who do not seem able to make an informed decision. This might include the unconscious person, the very confused elderly person, or the inebriated person. The law in each state specifies who is allowed to give consent in such situations. There are also guidelines to follow in making the decision that the person cannot give his or her own consent. Your facility policy should contain directions to guide you in obtaining a legal consent. If it does not, you should consult an administrative person for a decision. Determining who is able to give legal consent is not a nursing responsibility.

Emergency Care

Care in emergencies has many legal repercussions. If a true emergency exists, consent for care is considered to be implied. The law holds that if a reasonable person were aware that the situation was life threatening, he or she would give consent for care.

An exception to this is made if the person has explicitly rejected such care in advance, such as a Jehovah's Witness who is carrying a card stating his personal religion and that he did not wish to receive blood or blood products. This is one reason emergency department nurses should check a patient's wallet for identification and information related to care. If this is done with another person and a careful inventory of contents is made and signed by both, there should be little concern for liability for taking such an action.

Institutional Emergency Care

The judgment that an emergency exists is important, because certain actions may be legal in emergencies and not legal in other nonemergency situation. As just discussed, the issue of consent is affected by the determination that an emergency exists. Standards of practice for emergencies also differ from those for nonemergency situations.

Most facilities that provide emergency care have policies designed to ensure that there is adequate support for claiming that an emergency exists. Thus the policy will often state that in the emergency department at least two physicians must examine the patient and concur that there is an emergency that requires immediate action without waiting for consent. This ensures maximum legal protection for the physician and the institution.

In hospital emergencies the nurse sometimes may be in the position of identifying an emergency and that the needed action is one that only a physician usually performs. If "life or limb" is truly in danger, the courts have held that the nurse can do those immediate things necessary even if they usually are considered a medical function, provided the nurse has the essential expertise to perform the action safely and correctly. The hospital would be expected to have a policy, which the nurse would follow, to verify and document the situation fully. This usually involves consultation with a supervisory nurse and verification of the emergency situation as well as attempts to obtain medical assistance.

Situation: Nursing Action in An Hospital Emergency

In an orthopedic unit it is common to care for patients with new casts. A young man with a newly applied long-leg cast is admitted by way of the emergency department at 6 PM. The nurse assigned to this patient's care carefully makes all the appropriate observations throughout the evening and documents his findings. He notes that the leg is beginning to swell and that the edges of the cast are beginning to cut into the skin. At that time the RN notifies the supervisor that a problem is developing and that the nurse thinks the physician should be notified. The supervisor agrees and the nurse begins to try to contact the physician. Continuous observations are made, noting increasing swelling, color changes in the exposed toes, and loss of sensation. The physician cannot be reached and no other physician is immediately available. After consultation with the supervisor, the RN decides that an emergency exists and that the cast needs to be cut open to relieve the pressure. The RN has been taught to use a cast cutter and is familiar with the procedure. Cutting a cast open is considered a medical procedure in this hospital. The RN, with the concurrence of the supervisor, cuts open the cast and secures it in place with an elastic bandage. All observations made, consultations carried out, attempts to notify the physician, and the final action taken are carefully documented in the chart. Hospital policy was followed throughout the situation to make sure that all necessary steps had been taken.

Although this was going beyond the usual nursing practice, this would not be considered a violation of either the nursing or the medical practice acts because an emergency existed and the results of inaction would have been serious. Additionally, the nurse had the expertise and was prepared to carry out the necessary action in a safe manner. This emergency care is usually limited to specific technical procedures that the nurse has learned. It does not include diagnosing disease or prescribing medication unless there are specific standing orders relative to the situation.

Noninstitutional Emergency Care

Emergencies encountered outside the health care environment present other problems. Anyone rendering aid in an emergency is expected to behave as a reasonably prudent person would in such a situation. The nurse rendering aid in an emergency must behave as a reasonably prudent nurse in that situation. Thus the standard is higher than for the nonprofessional person, although the nurse is not expected to perform as if he or she were in an institutional setting. The physical situation and the psychological situation are both considered when determining what is reasonably prudent nursing action.

All states and Canadian provinces have "good Samaritan" statutes that encourage health care professionals to give aid in emergency situations. The first of these statutes was enacted in California in 1959 (Bernzweig, 1987). These statutes vary in content and comprehensiveness but relieve a professional of some liability when reasonable care is used. These laws often make people feel more secure when rendering aid.

In 1968 Vermont enacted a statute that requires all persons to provide assistance to others exposed to "grave physical harm." There are penalties for violation. Since that time Minnesota and the province of Quebec have passed legislation requiring people to render assistance in similar situations. Most European countries have such laws (Bernzweig, 1987).

Each nurse must make an individual decision about rendering emergency aid in a specific situation. This involves ethical as well as legal considerations. If the profession of nursing is a public trust and nurses are truly involved in the business of caring, then failure to come to the aid of an individual who is in serious danger is an ethical violation of that trust. To this date there has been no instance of a nurse being sued for coming to the aid of someone in an emergency situation (Bernzweig, 1987; Fiesta, 1988). Professional liability insurance does provide coverage when the nurse assists in this way and may make you feel more comfortable about rendering emergency aid.

Fraud

Fraud is a deliberate deception for the purpose of personal gain and is usually prosecuted as a crime. Situations of fraud in nursing are not common. One example would be trying to obtain a better position by giving incorrect information to a prospective employer. By deliberately stating that you had completed a nurse practitioner program to obtain a position for which you would otherwise be ineligible, you are defrauding the employer. This may be prosecuted as a crime because you also put members of the community in danger of receiving substandard care. You may also commit fraud by trying to cover up a nursing error to avoid legal action. Courts tend to be more harsh in decisions regarding fraud than in cases involving simple malpractice because fraud represents a lack of trustworthiness that could be damaging to other patients for whom you are responsible.

Situation: Fraud

A registered nurse is giving medications to the patients to whom she is assigned. In the course of the morning she presents a patient with his pills. He states that he was sure the doctor had discontinued the red pill because he had a reaction to it the evening before. The nurse states that she is sure these are the correct medications. The patient takes the pills and the nurse charts the medications. The patient subsequently has a reaction. The nurse becomes frightened, goes back, and alters the medication record to make it appear that the medication was not given.

This situation could be considered fraud. The deception was the changing of the record and the personal gain was freedom from responsibility for the error.

Assault and Battery

Assault is saying or doing something to make a person genuinely fear that he or she will be touched without consent. Battery is unconsented or unlawful touching of a person. Neither of these terms implies that harm was done. Harm may or may not have occurred.

For an assault to occur, the person must be afraid of what would happen even if the threatening person would not or could not carry out the threat. "If you don't take this medication, I will have to put you in restraints" is an example of an assault. The nurse who resorts to threats to achieve an end is in danger of being charged with assault.

For battery to occur, the touching must take place without consent. As you already have learned, implied consent is acceptable. Therefore, if the patient extends an arm for an injection, he cannot later charge battery, saying that he was not asked. But if the patient agreed because of a threat (assault), the touching would still be considered battery, since the consent was not freely given.

If you have an order to give a patient an iron injection and the patient says, "No. I had one of those before and they hurt!" and you persist and give the injection, a charge may be filed against you for battery. This is true even though the iron greatly benefited the patient and was a valid physician's order. The patient always has the right to refuse treatment.

Assault and Battery

A patient was involuntarily committed to a mental hospital. She was a practicing Christian Scientist. When she refused to take medications, she was held down and given an injection by a nurse. She brought suit and recovered damages for assault and battery because the court found she was not dangerous to herself or others and had not been found incompetent and therefore she could not be compelled to take medication.

Winters v. Miller, 446 F 2d 65 (1971)

False Imprisonment

Making a person stay in a place against his wishes is false imprisonment. The person can be forced to stay by using either physical means

Figure 5–3. The improper use of restraints may constitute "false imprisonment."

or verbal means. It is easy to understand why restraining a patient or confining a patient to a locked room could constitute false imprisonment if proper procedures were not first carried out.

Keeping a patient confined by nonphysical means is perhaps less clear. If you removed a patient's clothes for the express purpose of preventing his leaving, you could be liable for false imprisonment. Threats to keep a person confined, such as "If you don't stay in your bed, I'll sedate you," can also constitute false imprisonment. Any time a patient needs to be confined for his or her own safety or well-being, it is best to help the person understand and agree to that course of action. If the patient is not responsible, the guardian or legal representative may give permission. (This returns to the issue of who may give consent.) The third alternative is to objectively document the need in the patient's record and obtain a physician's order as soon as possible. Be sure to follow the policies of the facility.

In the conventional care setting you cannot restrain or confine responsible adults against their wishes. All persons have the right to make decisions for themselves, regardless of the consequences. The patient with a severe heart condition who defies orders and walks to the bathroom has that right. You protect yourself by recording your efforts to teach the patient the need for restrictions and by reporting the behavior to your supervisor and the physician.

In the same context the patient cannot be forced to remain in a hospital. If a patient wants to leave against medical advice, that is the patient's right. Again, you document your efforts in the record and follow applicable policies to protect the facility, the physician, and yourself from liability. The example of an intentional tort given earlier in this chapter involved false imprisonment.

A hospital may not detain a patient for nonpayment of a bill. The hospital is free to take legal action against the person who does not pay, but refusing discharge would also constitute false imprisonment.

False imprisonment suits are a special concern in the care of the psychiatric patient. Some particular laws relate to this situation. In the psychiatric setting you may have patients who have voluntarily sought admission. The same restrictions on restraint or confinement that apply to the patients in the general care setting apply to these patients. Other patients in the psychiatric setting may have been committed involuntarily through the applicable laws of the state. Specific measures may be used to confine the involuntarily committed patient. These are usually defined by law in terms of situations covered, type of restraint allowed, and length of time restraining may be used. If you work in a psychiatric setting, you should review the specific policies that have been developed about restraint to protect clients and assist staff in functioning within the legal limits.

FACTORS THAT CONTRIBUTE TO MALPRACTICE CLAIMS

When poor results or harm do occur in the course of nursing practice, they usually are not followed by a suit. An understanding of some of the factors that enter into whether a suit is instituted may help you.

Social Factors

Much is being written about changes in the public's attitudes toward health care personnel. Health care is big business, and patients complain increasingly of not being known individually. This results in a patient being more willing to bring suit against someone who is part of the large, impersonal system.

Health costs are high, and some people see hospitals and physicians as having the ability to pay a large settlement, whether directly or through insurance. If the patient's own income is lessened or disrupted by the illness, he or she might bring suit as a solution to economic difficulties. Increased public awareness of the size of monetary judgments that are awarded in some instances may also be an economic incentive to instituting a suit.

In the past, nurses' salaries were low, and therefore there was little economic incentive to bring suit against a nurse. As nurses achieve better economic conditions, they, too, face the possibility of suit.

Suit-Prone Patients

Some people are more likely to bring suit for real or imagined errors. If these people are recognized as being suit-prone patients, it is possible for you to protect yourself through increased vigilance in regard to care and by special emphasis on thorough record keeping. Although we would warn you to guard against stereotyping, these general descriptions may help you to prevent problems. The suit-prone patient usually is identified by overt behavior in which he or she is a persistent fault finder and critic of personnel and of all aspects of care. He or she may be uncooperative in following the plan of care and very sensitive to any perceived slight.

The person who exhibits a hostile attitude may extend his or her hostile feelings to the nurses and other health care persons with whom he or she has contact. The nurse who becomes defensive in the face of hostility only widens the breach in the nurse–patient relationship. It is necessary to pay careful attention to those principles for care learned in psychosocial nursing that dealt with how to help the hostile patient. Assisting the patient to solve his or her own problems and supporting the patient are the best protection for the nurse.

Another type of patient who appears more suit-prone is the very dependent person who uses projection to deal with anxiety and fear. This person tends to ascribe fault or blame for all events to others and is unable to accept personal responsibility for his or her own welfare. Again, meeting this patient's needs in a well-considered plan of care is the answer.

A common error when confronting a suit-prone patient is for staff to become defensive and withdraw. This is done partly because the situation is unpleasant and partly because staff members feel personally threatened by the patient's behavior. This increases the likelihood of a suit if a poor result occurs.

Another possible nursing response to the suit-prone patient is to become more directive and authoritarian. This tends to increase the patient's feeling of separation and distance from the staff and again increases the likelihood of suit.

If the staff is helped to view the patient as a very troubled person who manifests his or her problems in this manner, sometimes they find it easier to be objective. The patient is in need of all the nursing skill that the well-prepared nurse can bring to the emotional problems. The suit-prone patient does not always end up suing. Much depends on the response of health care personnel.

Suit-Prone Nurses

Nurses may also be suit-prone. A nurse who is insensitive to patients' complaints, who does not identify and meet patient's emotional needs, or who fails to identify the limits of his or her own practice may contribute to suits instituted not only against the nurse but also against the employer and the physician. The nurse's self-awareness is critical in preventing suits.

PREVENTING MALPRACTICE CLAIMS

The most significant thing you can do to prevent malpractice claims is to maintain a high standard of care. To do this you may work at improving your own nursing practice and also the general climate for nursing practice where you work. You can do this in a variety of ways.

Self-Awareness

Identify your own strengths and weaknesses in practice. When you have identified a weakness, seek a means of growth. This may include education, directed experience, or an opportunity for discussion with colleagues.

Be ready to acknowledge areas of weakness to supervisors, and do not accept responsibilities for which you are not prepared. The nurse who has not worked in pediatrics for 10 years and accepts an assignment to a pediatric unit without orientation and education is setting the stage for an error to occur. Lack of current familiarity with the area is not a defense against liability. As a professional you should not accept the position if you cannot meet the criterion of being a reasonably prudent nurse in that setting. In instances of true emergency (e.g., disaster, flood), courts may be more lenient, but "we need you there today" is not an emergency.

Figure 5-4. There are things that can be done to prevent malpractice suits.

Adapt Proposed Assignments

In the current nursing shortage, nurses may find themselves assigned to units where they have little or no experience with the types of patient problems they will encounter. It is reasonable to be assigned to assist an overworked nurse in a special area if you can assume duties that are within your own competence and allow the specialized nurse to assume the specialized duties. It is not reasonable for you to be expected to assume the specialized duties. Thus, if you are not prepared for coronary care, you might go to that unit, monitor the intravenous lines, take vital signs, and make observations to report to the experienced coronary care nurse. The experienced nurse would then be able to check the monitors, administer the specialized medications, and make decisions. Note that this does fragment the patient's care and would not be appropriate as a permanent solution but could alleviate a temporary problem in a safe manner. It would be unsafe to assign you to total care of patients in that unit because you do not have the skills needed to plan and carry out that care.

Following Policies and Procedures

It is your responsibility to be aware of policies and procedures of the employing institution. If they are sound, they can be an adequate defense against a claim, providing they were carefully followed.

For example, the medication procedure may involve checking all medications against a central medication Kardex. If you have done this and there was an error in the Kardex, you might not be liable for the resulting medication error. You had followed all appropriate procedures and acted responsibly. The liability would rest with the person who made the error in transcribing the medication from the physician's orders to the Kardex. If, however, you had not followed procedure in checking, you might also be liable because you did not do your part in preventing error. As discussed previously, policies are often designed to provide legal direction.

Changing Policies and Procedures

As nursing evolves, changes are needed in procedures. Part of your responsibility as a professional is to work toward keeping all procedures up to date. These are part of nursing expertise. Are there written policies to deal with emergency situations? Statements such as "Oh, we've always done it this way" are not adequate substitutes for clearly written, officially accepted policies. Often facilities that are reluctant to make changes based on the suggestions of individual nurses are much more receptive to new ideas when the legal implications are noted.

Documentation

Nurses' records are unique in the health care setting. They cover the entire period of hospitalization, 24 hours a day, in a sequential pattern. Your record can be the crucial factor in avoiding litigation. Documentation in the record of observations made, decisions reached, actions taken, and the evaluation of the patient's response is considered much more solid evidence than verbal testimony, which depends on the vagaries of memory.

For legal purposes observations and actions that are not recorded may be assumed not to have occurred. Properly kept records may also protect you from becoming liable for the error of another by demonstrating that you did all in your power to prevent harm, including consulting with others. Because each case is determined by the facts as well as by the applicable law, a clear documentation of all relevant data is important.

One concern expressed regarding problem-oriented records and charting "by exception" are that these formats may provide less detailed information and may be less helpful in defense against litigation. This does not have to be the case. You can use any system of charting and record keeping to provide appropriate and adequate documentation of care. If you identify something that needs to be recorded and cannot find a provision within your system to make that recording, you can be sure that others have experienced the same difficulty. Rather than shrugging it off with the assumption that this means the record does not have to be kept, you might begin inquiries toward establishing a clear mechanism for the record keeping that concerns you. When nurses serve on committees to review and plan charting procedures, it is wise for them to seek consultation with the attorney for the facility. This would help ensure that the plan for record keeping is legally sound and professionally useful.

THE NURSE AS WITNESS

In the course of your practice as a registered nurse a time may arise when you will be asked to serve as a witness in a legal proceeding. There are two kinds of cases that would involve the nurse as a witness to the facts in a specific case.

The first type is a personal injury action in which a person has been injured, for example, in an automobile accident and you or your organization has been involved in the care of that person. Your testimony in that case might be on behalf of the person to help describe his or her injuries and care received for those injuries. For example, you may be asked to testify regarding the care given in a burn center to a victim of an electrical accident who received considerable nursing care during the recovery period.

The second type of lawsuit that involves the nurse as witness to specific facts is one in which a patient brings a lawsuit against persons or organizations who have provided health care that the patient believes was below the standard of the community. Medical malpractice is therefore alleged. The nurse may be included in those who are charged with malpractice. For example, you may have to give evidence regarding medical record notes or care given to the patient in the days before the alleged malpractice occurred. In both of these situations the concern is with the specific factual details of the particular case in which you were involved.

The nurse may also be involved in a lawsuit as an expert witness. An expert witness, under Rule 702 of the Federal Rules of Evidence, accepted in the federal courts and many state courts, is defined as "a witness qualified as an expert by knowledge, skill, experience, training, or education" who may testify in the form of an opinion or otherwise. The purpose of testimony as an expert witness is to provide information and opinion that can be used by the court in making a decision. When you appear as an expert nursing witness, your testimony provides an opinion that will assist the judge or jury to understand complex areas of nursing care. This includes an opinion on the appropriate care for a given situation. In this situation you would be giving a professional opinion about the facts of the case as they relate to your area of expertise. For example, if you are an operating room nurse, you may be given medical records from another hospital and asked to render an opinion, on the basis of your expertise, whether the standard of nursing care given at the first hospital was within the standards of the community. Your role as an expert may not be accepted without question in a legal action. You may have to clearly state the qualifications, both education and experience, that enable you to make a judgment.

In any case when you become involved in any legal action, you should be sure that you understand both your rights and your obligations in regard to legal action.

Discovery

In a civil lawsuit, one between parties for the recovery of money damages, there is a lengthy discovery process that leads up to the trial itself. Often cases are settled before trial by the testimony developed in the discovery process. Discovery involves gathering information through document examination, interrogatories (written questions answered under oath), and depositions.

A deposition is a formal proceeding in which each attorney has an opportunity to question the witness, and a sworn verbatim record is made by a court reporter (Guido, 1988). Depositions are often held in attorneys' offices or in the health care facility for the convenience of the health care providers. Sometimes depositions are taken to preserve the testimony of a witness for trial under certain circumstances and are used in place of live testimony at trial. Most depositions in which you would participate, however, would be depositions for discovery purposes.

Testimony as a Witness in Deposition or at Trial

It is wise always to consult an attorney before talking to anyone about a matter in which you have been asked to testify, especially a malpractice action. Many people believe that because they have done nothing wrong they do not need legal counsel. The law is complex, and you could jeopardize the position of an institution for which you work, or even jeopardize yourself and your professional future, with unwise statements. It is possible for the person who is bringing suit to alter or amend the original complaint to involve new defendants including you. If you have liability insurance, you should advise your insurance company and an attorney will be assigned to talk with you. If you are covered by an employer's policy, you should consult with the appropriate administration representative immediately to obtain counsel.

When you are being asked to consult as an expert witness, or to testify as a witness in a personal injury matter, the attorney who asks you to testify should be able to provide you with information you need about your testimony. Feel free to inquire of that attorney what your role is in the case and in which areas your testimony is expected. The attorney is likely to discuss at length what questions will be asked of you and ask you what your answer would be to those question.

As a witness, you will be required to swear or affirm to tell the entire truth. Failure to do this is perjury. You are expected to answer the questions asked of you to the best of your ability; however, you do not have to provide an answer that would incriminate yourself, nor do you have to answer a question for which you do not remember or know the answer. It is perfectly permissible to state "I do not remember" if you do not.

It is helpful if you use words and terms that can be understood by those who are not familiar with medical terminology or explain medical terminology where its use is essential. If hypothetical situations or cases are presented for your response, be sure to note the differences between the hypothetical case and the one currently under consideration before you respond.

Be brief and direct when answering questions. Do not volunteer additional information that has not been asked for by the attorney. You may open up entire areas of inquiry that would not be considered without your comments. It is the attorney's job to ask the question so as to bring out the facts to which he or she wants you to testify. The opposing attorney will have an opportunity on cross-examination to ask you additional questions that the attorney believes are necessary for the facts of the case.

Figure 5–5. When testifying in court you should answer only the questions asked. Do not introduce other information.

CONCLUSION

As a registered nurse, you will have a considerable legal responsibility for your own practice. It is important that you understand all the many ramifications of this responsibility. In addition, you are an important factor in preventing legal action against yourself, your employer, and other professionals with whom you work. Knowledge of the many factors involved in legal questions will be important to you in your career as a nurse.

REFERENCES

Bernzweig EP: The Nurse's Liability for Malpractice, 4th ed. New York, McGraw-Hill Book Company, 1987

Fiesta J: The Law and Liability, 2nd ed. New York, John Wiley & Sons, 1988
Guido GW: Legal Issues In Nursing: A Source Book For Practice. Norwalk, CT, Appleton-Lange, 1988
Vermont Statutes Ann, Title 12, Section 519, Supp 1971

FURTHER READINGS

American Nurses' Association: Guidelines for Boards of Inquiry. Publication No. L-05. Kansas City, MO, American Nurses' Association, 1979
Bernzweig EP: Why you need your own malpractice policy. RN 48(3):59–60, 1985
Bernzweig EP: How to spot the suit prone patient. RN 48(6):63–64, 1985
Carey KW: Refusing to follow orders: What's the cost of saying no? Nurs Life 5(7):53–56, 1985
Creighton H: Law Every Nurse Should Know 5th ed. Philadelphia, WB Saunders, 1986
Creighton H: The nurse as an expert witness. Nurs Manage 19(8):22–23, 1988
Cushing M: The legal side: How a suit starts. Am J Nurs 85(6):655–656, 1985
Fink JL: Legal implications of drug errors. Am Health Care Assoc J 10(7):37–40, 1984
Hemelt MD, Mackert ME: Dynamics of Law in Nursing and Health Care, 2nd ed. Reston, VA, Reston Publishing, 1982
Horty JF: Healthcare law. Mod Health Care (regular column)
Lawsuits: An ounce of prevention. Nursing 20(5):146, 1990.
The legal side. Am J Nurs (regular feature)
Northrop CE: The in's and out's of informed consent. Nursing 15(1):9, 1985
Regan Reports on Hospital Law. Providence, Medica Press (quarterly publication)
Regan Reports on Medical Law. Providence, Medica Press (quarterly publication)
Regan Reports on Nursing Law. Providence, Medica Press (quarterly publication)
Regan WA: Legally speaking. RN (regular column)
Regan WA: OR nursing law. AORN J (regular column)
Rubbert TE: What to do if you are sued. Nursing 15(3):64D–64E, 64G, 64L, 1985
Rx: Avoid "speculation" & "admissions" in charting. Regan Reports on Nursing Law 30(10):2, 1990
Varga K: How to protect yourself against malpractice. Imprint 36(5):33–34 and 36–37, 1989

6

Ethical Concerns in Nursing Practice

Objectives

After completing this chapter, you should be able to

1. *Discuss reasons why ethical concerns are prominent in nursing.*

2. *List common bases used for ethical decision making and discuss their impact on the nurse.*

3. *Identify the basic concepts central to most ethical situations.*

4. *Describe four ethical theories that may be used when working on ethical problems.*

5. *Explain how sociocultural factors affect ethical decision making for nurses.*

6. *Discuss how ethics relates to commitment to the patient/client, commitment to personal excellence, and commitment to nursing as a profession.*

Concerns about right and wrong and good and evil are ethical issues that relate to fundamental beliefs in our society. These concerns have always been with us, and each generation has examined its own issues and the setting in which they occur and has made its own decisions. Today we find it difficult to understand the view of those in the 1800s who believed, based on their interpretation of the Bible, that it was wrong to alleviate the pain of childbirth because pain was meant to be a part of childbearing. Two hundred years from now people may have a similar difficulty understanding the positions that we take on ethical issues.

Because of a number of societal factors that have placed these problems squarely before us, ethical issues are being intensively discussed and debated. Many of the issues discussed in this chapter and the next are controversial and emotionally charged. Controversy often creates conflict. Conflicts may exist in values, in opinions, in solutions, and in judgments. As you read about these issues and discuss them in your classroom or with a classmate, we urge you to respect others by carefully listening to them and honestly attempting to understand their position with its accompanying values and beliefs. Only by considering all aspects of an issue can we seek and find understanding for ourselves. Understanding the issues involved allows us to deal more positively with the personal stress we may experience in our own lives as we attempt to find answers to ethical questions.

Throughout these chapters we emphasize personal decision making as the basic task when confronted with an ethical question. Ethical decision making cannot be avoided in nursing. Issues constantly confront us. Some nurses are tempted to back away and say, "That is not my concern," but the old saying "Not to decide is to decide" was never more true. Doing nothing is indeed making a decision. Decisions are often uncomfortable because we are left with a choice between alternatives, of which none are good or desirable. Dealing with the pain as well as the joy of life is part of being human. As we personally confront difficult decisions we can become more supportive and caring toward the clients, families, and coworkers with whom we work.

A BASIS FOR DECISION MAKING

All persons must determine their own basis for making ethical decisions. Some people rely on formal philosophical or religious beliefs that define matters in relation to truth or to good and evil. Others make a decision in each situation by attempting to weigh what is the greatest good for the greatest number. Still others reach a decision on the basis of personal life experience or on the basis of the experience of someone dear to them. By these and other mechanisms people come to different conclusions when confronted with ethical problems.

A dilemma may be created when individuals come to different ethical conclusions. Many times it is possible and appropriate for you to accept another person's ethical decision as appropriate for them; however, there are other times when your own position will cause you to say, "I must oppose this action." This may bring you into direct conflict with others. When this occurs, we urge you to be constructive not destructive in the methods you choose to work toward your personal goals.

Personal Religious and Philosophical Viewpoints

Your personal viewpoint certainly will be a major factor influencing your ethical decision making. Achieving self-understanding in values is a lifelong learning task, and undoubtedly your position on various issues will change as you move through life. Values represent the concepts, ideals, behaviors, social principles, and major themes that give meaning to our personal life and make us unique. Values are the product of our life experiences and are influenced by family, friends, culture, environment, education, and many other conditions. Because of this our values may change.

Recognizing your own value system is a goal of the classes, seminars, and books on the topic of values clarification. *Values clarification* is a growth-producing process that includes assessing, exploring, and determining personal values. It also includes identifying the priority a particular value holds in our process of personal decision making. Often we do not fully explore our own values until we are confronted with a specific situation in which a decision is necessary. Although you should not feel pressured to alter your personal value system, it is important for you to seriously explore your own feelings and beliefs about various issues.

Religious beliefs form the basis for some of the decisions a person may make. However, a person who is a member of a particular religious group may not abide by all the rules of that faith. Individuals make their own decisions with regard to each situation, and that attitude may not parallel the doctrine of their religious group. For example, some Muslims maintain that women should be completely separated from men and wear veils when in the presence of men. They would find any health care setting that did not respect this belief to be in conflict with basic values. Other Muslims do not adhere to this strict interpretation of Islamic law, and women wear modest clothing but do not wear veils. They would be

Figure 6-1. Decisions made in relation to one aspect of an ethical situation will affect all other aspects of the problem.

more comfortable in most Western health care settings because they would not feel a conflict with their personal values.

Nursing offers a wide variety of job opportunities to the new graduate. Before you accept a position, you may want to consider whether it holds the potential to create conflict with your basic beliefs. Most employers are willing to recognize this as a valid criterion for accepting or rejecting a position. Certainly you cannot expect to avoid all conflict or problem situations, but you probably would want to avoid working in an area in which there was constant conflict. For example, if you are ethically opposed to abortion, it would be wise to avoid employment on an obstetrical unit where therapeutic abortions are routinely performed. In this situation, making your views known and refusing certain assignments after you had begun employment might result in termination because the employer may justifiably assert that you agreed to fulfill all the responsibilities of the position when accepting employment.

Similarly, your personal value system might lead you to work in a particular area in which you have identified a strong ethical commitment. For example, the hospices for the dying in England were begun by religious groups who saw value in the life of the person who was dying. Their religious beliefs were and have continued to be part of their approach to care. If you strongly value your own ethnic or cultural approach to health care, you might choose to work in a health care setting where that approach is part of the philosophy.

Codes for Nurses

Nurses, through their professional organizations, have developed some common guidelines to use in making ethical decisions. They are contained in the American Nurses Association's (ANA) "Code for Nurses," and the International Council of Nurses "Code for Nurses." Each attempts to outline the nurse's responsibilities to the client and to the profession of nursing (Figs. 6-2 and 6-3).

The ANA code is somewhat unique among professional codes because it addresses fairly specific issues and does not confine itself to matters of etiquette or broad general statements. Warren T. Reich, editor in chief of the *Encyclopedia of Bioethics,* was quoted as stating, "This is probably the most interesting and responsive code I have ever read" (New Encyclopedia, 1977, p 8). Tentative codes were presented by nurses in the 1920s, the 1930s, and the 1940s. Finally, in 1950, a code of ethics was adopted. It has been revised several times since then, most recently in 1976. Early versions stated that the nurse had an obligation to carry out physician's orders; later versions, however, stress the nurse's obligation to the client. This includes protecting the client from incompetent, unethical, or illegal practice.

The International Council of Nurses' Code was most recently revised in 1973. The introductory section of this code speaks of the general responsibilities of the nursing profession. Five sections follow, dealing with the more specific concerns of people, practice, society, coworkers, and the profession. In addition, the International Council of Nurses' has written a "Pledge for Nurses." The pledge is a statement of affirmation and acceptance of the personal and ethical responsibilities of being a member of the nursing profession. Both of these documents can serve as guidelines for ethical conduct.

A. N. A. CODE FOR NURSES

1. The nurse provides services with respect for human dignity and the uniqueness of the client unrestricted by considerations of social or economic status, personal attributes, or the nature of health problems.
2. The nurse safeguards the client's right to privacy by judiciously protecting information of a confidential nature.
3. The nurse acts to safeguard the client and the public when health care and safety are affected by the incompetent, unethical, or illegal practice of any person.
4. The nurse assumes responsibility and accountability for individual nursing judgments and actions.
5. The nurse maintains competence in nursing.
6. The nurse exercises informed judgment and uses individual competence and qualifications as criteria in seeking consultation, accepting responsibilities, and delegating nursing activities to others.
7. The nurse participates in activities that contribute to the ongoing development of the profession's body of knowledge.
8. The nurse participates in the profession's efforts to implement and improve standards of nursing.
9. The nurse participates in the profession's efforts to establish and maintain conditions of employment conducive to high quality nursing care.
10. The nurse participates in the profession's effort to protect the public from misinformation and misrepresentation and to maintain the integrity of nursing.
11. The nurse collaborates with members of the health professions and other citizens in promoting community and national efforts to meet the health needs of the public.

(Reprinted by permission of the American Nurses' Association)

Figure 6–2. ANA Code for Nurses.

The Patient's Rights

The patient's rights are another consideration in decision making. Ideally we have always recognized this in some ways. As early as 1959 the National League for Nursing formulated a statement regarding patient's rights. However, for many years health care professionals assumed the attitude that they knew what was best for patients and made many decisions without consulting with or considering the rights of the patient/ client. For example, the patient with an enlarged thyroid gland was not offered information about possible treatment alternatives, although alternatives did exist. The patient's physician made the decision regarding

1973 CODE FOR NURSES

Ethical Concepts Applied to Nursing

The fundamental responsibility of the nurse is fourfold: to promote health, to prevent illness, to restore health and to alleviate suffering.

The need for nursing is universal. Inherent in nursing is respect for life, dignity and rights of man. It is unrestricted by considerations of nationality, race, creed, colour, age, sex, politics or social status.

Nurses render health services to the individual, the family and the community and coordinate their services with those of related groups.

Nurses and People

The nurse's primary responsibility is to those people who require nursing care.

The nurse, in providing care, respects the beliefs, values and customs of the individual.

The nurse holds in confidence personal information and uses judgment in sharing this information.

Nurses and Practice

The nurse carries personal responsibility for nursing practice and for maintaining competence by continual learning.

The nurse maintains the highest standards of nursing care possible within the reality of a specific situation.

The nurse uses judgment in relation to individual competence when accepting and delegating responsibilities.

The nurse when acting in a professional capacity should at all times maintain standards of personal conduct that would reflect credit upon the profession.

Nurses and Society

The nurse shares with other citizens the responsibility for initiating and supporting action to meet the health and social needs of the public.

Nurses and Co-Workers

The nurse sustains a cooperative relationship with co-workers in nursing and other fields.

The nurse takes appropriate action to safeguard the individual when his care is endangered by a co-worker or any other person.

Nurses and the Profession

The nurse plays the major role in determining and implementing desirable standards of nursing practice and nursing education.

The nurse is active in developing a core of professional knowledge.

The nurse, acting through the professional organization, participates in establishing and maintaining equitable social and economic working conditions in nursing.

(Reprinted with the permission of the International Council of Nurses)

Figure 6–3. 1973 Code for Nurses.

A PATIENT'S BILL OF RIGHTS

Approved by the House of Delegates of the American Hospital Association February 6, 1973

The American Hospital Association presents a Patient's Bill of Rights with the expectation that observance of these rights will contribute to more effective patient care and greater satisfaction for the patient, his physician, and the hospital organization. Further, the Association presents these rights in the expectation that they will be supported by the hospital on behalf of its patients, as an integral part of the healing process. It is recognized that a personal relationship between the physician and the patient is essential for the provision of proper medical care.

The traditional physician–patient relationship takes on a new dimension when care is rendered within an organizational structure. Legal precedent has established that the institution itself also has a responsibility to the patient. It is in recognition of these factors that these rights are affirmed.

1. The patient has the right to considerate and respectful care.
2. The patient has the right to obtain from his physician complete current information concerning his diagnosis, treatment, and prognosis in terms the patient can be reasonably expected to understand. When it is not medically advisable to give such information to the patient, the information should be made available to an appropriate person in his behalf. He has the right to know by name, the physician responsible for coordinating his care.
3. The patient has the right to receive from his physician information necessary to give informed consent prior to the start of any procedure and/or treatment. Except in emergencies, such information for informed consent, should include but not necessary be limited to the specific procedure and/or treatment, the medically significant risks involved, and the probable duration of incapacitation. Where medically significant alternatives for care or treatment exist, or when the patient requests information concerning medical alternatives, the patient has the right to such information. The patient also has the right to know the name of the person responsible for the procedures and/or treatment.
4. The patient has the right to refuse treatment to the extent permitted by law, and to be informed of the medical consequences of his action.
5. The patient has the right to every consideration of his privacy concerning his own medical care program. Case discussion, consultation, examination, and treatment are confidential and should be conducted discreetly. Those not directly involved in his care must have the permission of the patient to be present.
6. The patient has the right to expect that all communications and records pertaining to his care should be treated as confidential.
7. The patient has the right to expect that within its capacity a hospital must make reasonable response to request of a patient for services. The hospital must provide evaluation, service, and/or referral as indicated by the urgency of the case. When medically permissible a patient may be transferred to another facility only after he has received complete information and explanation concerning the needs for and

(continued)

Figure 6–4. The Patient's Bill of Rights.

A PATIENT'S BILL OF RIGHTS *(continued)*

alternatives to such a transfer. The institution to which the patient is to be transferred must first have accepted the patient for transfer.

8. The patient has the right to obtain information as to any relationship of his hospital to other health care and educational institutions insofar as his care is concerned. The patient has the right to obtain information as to the existence of any professional relationships among individuals, by name, who are treating him.

9. The patient has the right to be advised if the hospital proposes to engage in or perform human experimentation affecting his care or treatment. The patient has the right to refuse to participate in such research projects.

10. The patient has the right to expect reasonable continuity of care. He has the right to know in advance what appointment times and physicians are available and where. The patient has the right to expect that the hospital will provide a mechanism whereby he is informed by his physician or a delegate of the physician of the patient's continuing health care requirements following discharge.

11. The patient has the right to examine and receive an explanation of his bill regardless of source of payment.

12. The patient has the right to know what hospital rules and regulations apply to his conduct as a patient.

No catalogue of rights can guarantee for the patient the kind of treatment he has a right to expect. A hospital has many functions to perform, including the prevention and treatment of disease, the education of both health professionals and patients, and the conduct of clinical research. All these activities must be conducted with an overriding concern for the patient, and, above all, the recognition of his dignity as a human being. Success in achieving this recognition assures success in the defense of the rights of the patient.

Figure 6–4. *(Continued)*

which treatment method was preferable, and that was the only one presented to the patient. Today we consider this an example of paternalism.

As the health consumer movement became more active, greater attention was paid to the rights of the patient. Today patients may expect to be informed of all alternatives for treatment and often want to participate in making the decision about type of treatment, including both the possible benefits and the risks of the treatment methods presented. The law has also supported the right to informed decision-making.

In 1973 the American Hospital Association published "A Patient's Bill of Rights," which outlines the rights of the hospital patient and serves as a basis for making decisions about hospitalized patients (Fig. 6-5). Some have criticized this document, saying that it is rather innocuous because it simply reminds patients of their rights (such as privacy, confidentiality, and informed consent) but says nothing of hospitals that fail to act in accordance with these rights. The heaviest criticism levied against this paper is that "A Patient's Bill of Rights" fails to recognize explicitly the patient's right to adequate medical care (Kroeger-Mappes, 1986). Another criticism might be focused on the fact that this statement has not been updated since it was written in 1973.

Other groups have also formulated statements regarding rights of the health consumer, nurses' associations among them. In some states, rights of the health consumer are being formalized into legal statements.

BASIC ETHICAL CONCEPTS

Basic concepts that are involved in most ethical situations include beneficence, nonmaleficence, autonomy, justice, fidelity, and veracity. Identifying how they apply to a particular situation and balancing their competing claims often present a challenge.

Figure 6–5. The nurse in providing care respects the beliefs, values, and customs of the individual.

Beneficence and Nonmaleficence

Beneficence refers to the obligation to do good, not harm, to other people. Further it is to act in the best interests of another person (Cohen, Cohen, and Thomasma, 1988). It is difficult to decide who will determine what is good for a person. In most instances we expect that people will make their own decisions. But who decides for the infant, the mentally incompetent, and others who are unable to make decisions? Another problem centers around what is good. Is all life good, or are there situations when not living is better than life? Is it better to sustain life in the face of all disability, or is it better to allow a person to die and have suffering ended? There are no simple answers, and the answers may not be the same for everyone.

A term related to beneficence is *nonmaleficence.* Nonmaleficence means to do no harm. As far back as Hippocrates, physicians were entreated to do no harm. Florence Nightingale stated that the patient should be no worse for having been nursed. In health care we recognize that sometimes we do harm to individuals, although that is not intended. Nosocomial infections, adverse drug reactions, and side effects of such treatments as irradiation and chemotherapy for cancer are certainly harmful to the individuals who experience them. The ethical mandate is that we refrain from *intentionally* inflicting harm. Differentiating situations when harm is intended from situations in which we know harm will occur but that is not the intent (such as in irradiation) is sometimes very difficult.

Autonomy

Autonomy refers to the right to make one's own decisions and, conversely, to respect the choices that others make for themselves (Cohen, Cohen, and Thomasma, 1988). However, there are limitations on the right to choose. What should those limitations be? How is autonomy affected by interpersonal relationships and strong familial ties? Are there instances when people with more background and understanding should make decisions for others? In what instances should the legal system interfere with personal decision making? How does autonomy relate to professionals as well as to patients and their families? For some individuals autonomy may be a less central value than are values related to the family. Is this acceptable? Who decides how much autonomy is "enough?"

Justice

Justice refers to the obligation to be fair to all people. We must ask "How is fairness defined?" Does fairness mean that people should be treated the same? Is it just for one person to receive more resources than another? If so, what makes it "just" and how does that relate to the distribution of scarce medical resources? Does age make a difference in what we consider just? Should it? Does justice imply that the government should provide what individuals cannot provide for themselves? What are the rights of one person when those rights affect the rights of another? Can we measure fairness in any objective sense? These issues will be discussed in greater detail in Chapter 7.

Fidelity

Fidelity refers to the obligation to be faithful to the agreements and responsibilities that one has undertaken. What are the responsibilities of health care personnel to individuals, employers, the government, society, and self? When these responsibilities conflict, which should take priority? In reality, which does take priority? Do circumstances alter which should have priority? What if the health care provider and the client disagree as to the obligations and responsibilities? Who makes the decision as to what constitutes fidelity?

Veracity

Veracity refers to telling the truth. From childhood we are all admonished to tell the truth and to avoid lying. When we are children this seems very straightforward. As we become adults, we see more and more instances where the choices are less clear. For example, do you tell the truth when you know it will cause harm to an individual? If you do, you have then abandoned the principle of nonmaleficence. Do you tell a lie when it would make someone less anxious and afraid? You might see this as beneficence (doing good), but then you have abandoned the principle of veracity.

Sissela Bok, an ethical philosopher, has written an extensive treatise entitled *Lying: Moral Choice in Public and Private Life* (Bok, 1978). In this book she explores the ethical principles that relate to lying and then relates these to specific areas of concern, one of which is lies to the sick and dying. Her conclusions are that lying, by its very nature, is detrimental to the liar as well as to the person to whom the lie is told. She recognizes that justification for lying does exist in some situations. These situations are when the truth will cause greater harm than the lie.

Her conclusions are that there are rarely any instances when lying to the sick and dying is justified. The loss of trust in caregivers, the anxiety created by not knowing the truth, the loss of opportunity to deal with personal and family concerns, and other adverse consequences of not being told the truth far outweigh the perceived benefits of lying. She points out that the damage associated with sad news or risks is usually less than physicians or other caregivers perceive it will be. She states that lying should be seen as an unusual step and one that requires reasons to be set forth and debated and alternatives to be carefully weighed.

As we present a variety of ethical concerns, try to relate these concepts to the problem and identify which ethical concept is presenting the greatest difficulties. Identify whether the conflict is one in which two general values conflict. Try to determine from your own viewpoint which value should have greater weight in that particular situation.

ETHICAL THEORIES

It is not our intent to delve with any depth into the writings of early philosophers. However, some ethical theories are mentioned frequently enough in the literature that surrounds bioethical issues that some background seems appropriate.

An ethical theory is a moral principle or a set of moral principles that can be used in assessing what is morally right or morally wrong in a given situation. Over the years we have called on the theories of philosophers to guide us in considering the various factors affecting our decision making.

Utilitarianism

Utilitarian ethics is found most prominently in the works of Jeremy Bentham (1748–1832) and John Stuart Mill (1806–1873). Utilitarian philosophy is also referred to as a "teleological theory," for the Greek word *teleos*, which means "end." The basic concept is that an act is right if it is useful in bringing about a good outcome or end. Furthermore, when issues compete they are weighed to determine which will bring the greatest good for the greatest number. The act is preferable that produces more total good.

This ethical theory would encourage us to act in ways that would produce the greatest balance of good over evil and is sometimes said to be "the greatest happiness principle." The philosophers who used this term did not consider happiness to be a superficial concept but rather one that reflected true well-being. Using this theory would lead one to weigh consequences of actions. The action with the most positive consequences and the least negative consequences would be the preferred action. People use this approach when they support budget decisions to provide vaccines to thousands of children instead of an organ replacement to one.

Deontology

Another prominent ethical theory is based on a concept of moral duty or obligation. This is termed *deontology* (from the Greek word for duty). Immanuel Kant (1724–1804), who is associated with this position, strongly opposed utilitarianism. He argued that the moral rightness or wrongness of human action should be considered independently of the consequences of the action. According to Kant it is not the consequences that makes an action right or wrong but the principle or motivation on which the action is based that determines right or wrong.

As a society, we use this theory when we determine the motivation for taking a person's life before charging an individual with the crime. For example, a householder may shoot an intruder who is personally attacking him. In another situation, a robber may shoot a store clerk in the course of a robbery. Although the consequence of both acts is the same (a person is dead), the motive is the deciding factor in whether the state charges a person with murder. The householder who shot the intruder would be found to be motivated by self-defense and therefore not guilty of murder. The robber would be found to have been motivated by criminal intent and therefore be charged with murder.

According to Kant, individuals should be guided by concepts of duty to others in determining what actions to take. He believed that some duties are binding. To be considered binding a duty must be universal (i.e., applicable to every individual), unconditional (i.e., acted on without reservation), and imperative (i.e., demanding of action). These three aspects of duty can be applied to an individual situation. For example, when determining the moral action when seeing an automobile accident, you would determine universality by asking "Should every individual be asked to help those injured in an automobile accident?" You would determine the unconditional situation by asking "Should this action apply in every such accident?" Whether action was imperative would be determined by asking "Does this situation require action by those present?" If you answered yes to all of these questions, you would have a binding moral duty to act.

Another fundamental principle of Kant's work is what he called the "categorical imperative." A person, according to Kant's imperative, should always be considered as an end, never as a means to achieve another end. Therefore, according to Kant, we are not justified in using people as research subjects without their knowledge even if the result would be great scientific advance. That would be using them as means and failing to respect their fundamental humanness.

Major concepts of Kant's work are its universal application and its respect for the person. Those using this theory would seek to determine their duty toward others in a given situation regardless of who that individual was.

Natural Law

The "natural law theory" is found in the writings of St. Thomas Aquinas (1223–1274). The fundamental concept of his theory is that actions are morally right when they are in accord with our nature and end as humans and are morally wrong when they are not in accord with our nature and end as humans. Basically this states that good should be promoted, evil should be avoided, and ethics should be grounded in our concern for human good. The word "good" was not defined in a way that might be clear to all of us, but Catholic theologians conceive of natural law as inscribed by God, endowing all things with potentials that serve to define their natural end. Thus there are natural rules that can be discovered that should be used to guide action.

Social Equity and Justice

Rawls proposed a concept of social equity as an approach to justice. He believed that if people of reason were placed in a situation of ethical choice without knowing which position they had in society (a situation he called the original position), they would choose the alternative that supported the most disadvantaged person. Using this approach, the concern of society should be directed toward the most disadvantaged, since they are the ones who are least able to speak for themselves.

SOCIAL FACTORS THAT INFLUENCE ETHICAL DECISION MAKING

Ethical decisions are not made in a vacuum. Many factors exert pressure and demand response as we search for appropriate answers to the dilemmas that face us. All facets of today's world are experiencing change, and nursing is no exception. The "truths" of yesterday are being challenged by the realities and new problems confronting us today.

In studying ethical issues it is important for you to understand the many forces that are operating. These forces are not independent or mutually exclusive but act and react on one another in a constantly changing milieu, causing evolutionary changes in all segments of society.

Social and Cultural Attitudes

Changes in the attitudes of society as a whole profoundly influence each of its segments. For example, the shifting roles of women and of attitudes toward marriage and the family and the changing status of minorities have all required nurses to reexamine their personal feelings and alter their way of providing nursing care.

Ethical concerns are the by-products of a number of factors at work in our society today. The rights of the individual have been increasingly emphasized in all aspects of living and, more recently, in dying. In the health care field this is most pointedly illustrated by the use of the terminology "health care" as opposed to "medical care." Health care suggests much greater involvement of others and places the client in the center of the activity, whereas medical care places the physician in the key role. The meaning of "consumer unit" is shifting from an individual to a total family, or even a whole community. The focus of care also has changed from one that was primarily disease oriented to one that is strongly preventive.

The size of the group being affected by ethical decisions has a bearing on the decision-making process. The smaller the group, organization, or society that is involved in the decision making, the easier the process of arriving at an acceptable alternative. Many of our ethical considerations now involve our society as a whole or, in some cases, the world; therefore, solutions are difficult. For example, an individual couple may choose rhythm and abstinence as their family planning method. If it is not successful for them they must cope with the consequences of having a child. If we mandate this as the only acceptable family planning method for a nation, then there will be thousands of unplanned children and the society will have obligations for support. Thus the issue becomes much more complex applied to wider society.

The value a society places on the individual or the family directly impacts on the standard of care. In Western society we believe in each person's right to exercise choice based on individual beliefs and conscience. We also place high value on preserving individual life. Therefore we often use tremendous resources to try to achieve additional years, months, or even days of life for a person who chooses that care. Another society that places greater emphasis on the community good than on the individual may not choose to use resources in that way. The standard of care might reflect comfort without use of expensive treatment modalities.

A culture's religious values and belief in an afterlife directly affect ethical issues. The Hindu belief in rebirth after death and the immutability of fate affects decisions about using health care resources. Those who believe that the outcome is predetermined by fate will not choose to commit major resources and efforts toward altering that outcome.

The population, or, more accurately, the overpopulation, of a country relative to its resources may also have a direct bearing on the value placed on life. The material resources to provide many health services may not be available. Thus decisions may be made to eliminate certain very costly health care procedures even though they are known to be effective and desired by individuals.

Science and Technology

Scientific advancement and technology have left us wrestling with concerns that would have been considered science fiction 50 years ago. Before the development of kidney dialysis, we accepted the fact that people with nonfunctioning kidneys would soon die. After machines that would filter body wastes became available, a genuine dilemma arose over which of the many candidates would have dialysis and which would not and would consequently die. More people needed treatment than there were equipment, time, and personnel to treat them. As the technology became available the ethical questions arose not over beginning treatment but over decisions to end treatment.

Other technology has had similar effects. The advent of machines that could artificially breathe for someone challenged the medical and legal professions to examine their definitions of life and brought into focus problems of whether and when to turn off a ventilator. Heart and lung machines that could adequately perfuse the body while the heart was stopped for surgical procedures enabled operations to be performed that were unheard of 50 years before. Fetal monitors, which can be attached to mothers-to-be while they are in labor, provide a continuous readout of the status of the fetus. Such monitoring has resulted in an increase in the number of infants delivered by cesarean section. The implantation of an artificial heart in a human subject received worldwide attention. This technology is very costly, and the survival of patients after implantation has been limited, leading to many ethical discussions regarding the appropriateness of using artificial hearts or funding further research. Those individuals with the acquired immunodeficiency syndrome have a limited life expectancy even with the best of health care. Should they be encouraged to participate in sometimes risky research to advance scientific knowledge and the possibility of future benefit to others? Thus scientific and technological advances continue to present ethical questions for which there are often no readily apparent answers.

Legislation

Social change and legislation are constantly in interaction. Legislation may follow changes in society's attitudes, converting new ideas into law.

For example, the social change of increased acceptance of infants born of single mothers resulted finally in legislation that changed the wording of birth certificates and dropped the word "illegitimate."

When social change is desired, legislation may be actively sought to require people to behave in new ways. This was true for much of the civil rights legislation. A change in society was desired, and supporters of civil rights sought legislation as one step in the change. Recent legislative action that speaks to the needs and opportunities available to the disabled has brought about changes in policies, procedures, and even architecture. It has opened many peoples' eyes to the ethics of how the disabled are treated.

Judicial Decisions

The judicial system also provides a major avenue for debating and trying to solve ethical problems. We find that more and more issues are taken to court and judicial decisions are used as the basis for determining the appropriate action. As you continue to study this topic, note that we have often cited a landmark decision in regard to an ethical issue. The process does not stop there, however. Some people may disagree with a judicial decision and continue to oppose it. Judicial decisions may also be overturned by higher courts. Meanwhile, the questions regarding the individual person's role in carrying out a judicial decision remain. For example, although the law in the past forbade abortions, some physicians believed so strongly in the right of the individual to have the procedure done and were so upset by the results of nonprofessional abortions that they were willing to perform them in spite of the law prohibiting them. These physicians were, of course, liable to prosecution if they were caught, and some were prosecuted for performing illegal abortions. Now that abortion is legal in many instances decisions must be made by individuals about participating in care and by the society about funding.

Funding

The financing of health care represents a major area of conflict that has ethical dimensions. The government has become more and more involved in providing funds for health care. Some people are asking how much time, money, and energy we should allocate to health care and how that money should be divided. How obligated are we as a society to make some form of health care available to all? What is it that health care can and cannot provide? Which is more important, prevention or cure? Health care includes controversial procedures, such as abortions and sterilization. Some taxpayers do not ethically sanction these procedures and do not want their tax dollars used to fund them. Thus decisions about funding challenge basic values.

OCCUPATIONAL FACTORS THAT INFLUENCE DECISION MAKING

By virtue of the positions they hold in the health care system, nurses have special forces acting on them as they try to make decisions. An awareness of these factors may help you as you struggle with personal problems in decision making.

Status as an Employee

Most nurses are not in independent practice, but are employed by hospitals, other institutions, or physicians. Thus there are pressures that divide the nurse's loyalty among patient, employer, and self. You will notice that codes do not speak of responsibilities to the employer, yet certainly there are responsibilities to the one who pays the salary and makes decisions in regard to your work. It is not unusual for an ethical decision to involve conflict between the best interests of the employer and the patient.

When discussing ethical decisions in the abstract, most people say that, of course, the patient's best interest should be the only priority. In real situations, however, the issues often are not so clear-cut. If a nurse's decision affects the employer adversely, the result may be job loss, poor references, and severely curtailed economic and career future. As an example, one physician was known to routinely require his patients to sign blank surgical permits on admission to the hospital. One of the staff nurses became upset with this procedure after learning that the patients often did not understand what was being planned. Eventually she discussed the matter with the physician, pointing out that she did not believe that it was ethical to require the patients to sign the blank documents, especially since they were not informed of alternative methods of treatment. The physician became angry and complained to the hospital administration, threatening to take his surgeries elsewhere. This would have created a considerable economic loss for the hospital and, depending on the action of the administrator, the nurse might have been labeled a troublemaker and even discharged to placate the physician.

Collective Bargaining Contracts

Collective bargaining contracts can protect nurses in making ethical decisions. By formalizing reasons and procedures for termination of employment and outlining grievance measures so that individual nurses have a mechanism for protecting themselves, the contract may provide greater freedom. (See Chapter 9 for more discussion of collective bargaining and grievance measures.)

Some people believe that contracts hamper individual freedom. The supervisor who believes that an employee does not deliver optimal care may feel unable to do anything about the situation because the correction and termination processes under a contract are so complex. Often many specific steps related to notifying the employee of unsatisfactory work and providing assistance for employee improvement are required before a person can be discharged.

Collegial Relationships

Relationships among nurses who work together (colleagues) in which they support one another, share in decision making, and present a unified approach to others can provide an excellent climate for ethical decision making. All too often such relationships are lacking in hospitals. Nurses feel alone and are not experienced in seeking out and supporting one another. Greater effort on their part in this area might be rewarding.

Authoritarian and Paternalistic Backgrounds

The historically authoritarian and paternalistic attitudes of physicians and hospitals often have relegated nurses, most of whom are women, to dependent and subservient roles. These role differentiations have in the past inhibited nurses from taking independent stands on issues, and they continue to affect relationships in the health care field. Some physicians have been heard to comment that all ethical decisions rest on the physician's shoulders, and that once the physician has made a decision, all other members of the health care team are obligated to acquiesce. This attitude results in people absolving themselves of moral responsibility by simply following orders. An example of a unilateral decision by a physician would be in the case of a patient suffering from terminal cancer. The physician determines that pain relief is the most important goal and orders that a narcotic be given every half hour through an intravenous line. The cumulative effect of the narcotic will seriously compromise the patient's respirations, perhaps to the point of stopping them. The physician in this situation would expect the nurse simply to carry out the order without participating in the decision-making process that resulted in the narcotic order.

Today's nurses increasingly are speaking out against such an approach, which leaves them out of the decision-making process. In the case just mentioned, nurses of today might expect the physician to discuss the situation with the patient, the family, and the nursing staff. The patient would be encouraged to express his or her needs, and the nurses' input would be part of the decision-making process. The result might be orders that provided broad guidelines as to amount and frequency for the narcotic. The nurses would be expected to make careful assessments and to provide pain medications in light of the overall decisions made at the conference.

Consumer Involvement in Health Care

The widespread consumer movement has become a significant factor in health care. Consumers are demanding a greater voice in all aspects of their own health care delivery. Part of this involvement is at the decision-making level.

Many hospitals have had ethics committees for years. Such committees were traditionally composed of physicians and were for the purpose of monitoring the behavior of physicians. They were called on to act when a physician's inappropriate behavior, such as arriving at the hospital intoxicated, was reported to them. Today the scope of ethics committees has enlarged considerably. They may consider the appropriateness of procedures to be done, which patient should receive treatment, and when treatment should be withdrawn. Membership has grown, and, increasingly, members of the hospital administration, the community, and other health care disciplines are being represented. An ethicist may serve as a consultant or as a member of the committee. If nurses participate, they then have a formal mechanism to share in ethical decision making.

If a nurse makes an ethical decision on the basis of the patient's best interest but contrary to the physician's or hospital's interest, public support may be forthcoming. The public increasingly sees health care as big business and tends to support those who champion consumer interests that conflict with the institution's interests. This support may be short-lived and therefore should not be relied on for protection against the adverse consequences of an ethical decision.

With consumers involved in decision making, nurses again may face a situation in which they are expected to take action or no action based on the conclusions of others. Modern-day nurses may find this as problematic as action based on a physician's decision. For example, an obstetrical patient who has hemorrhaged severely may refuse blood transfusions because of religious beliefs. The nurse, recognizing the benefit of the transfusion, may have difficulty maintaining effective communication and rapport with the patient and family because of her own convictions that a transfusion is the best treatment.

A FRAMEWORK FOR ETHICAL DECISION MAKING

When faced with ethical decisions, most of us hope to find the "right" answer. Unfortunately, there often is no right answer for everyone or every situation. The answer must often be that humans do the best they can in the situation in which they find themselves and continue to struggle with feelings of inadequacy, guilt, anger, and doubt. However, you can proceed from a basic framework that encourages you to look beyond your first thoughts or feelings to basic issues. Andrew Jameton of the Institute for Health Policy Studies at the University of California, San Francisco, presented the following process you can use to help guide you in this task (Jameton, 1984).

Identify The Ethical Problem

In identifying the ethical problem, you will first determine what decision must be made. Then examine that decision. Consider what ethical principles might be involved. Are those principles in conflict? Who are the relevant parties to this decision? Ask yourself what your role and relationship to the problem is. Is this really someone else's decision that you should not assume, or is it one in which a collaborative decision must be made? What are the time boundaries for making this decision?

Gather Data

It is important to have as much information about the unique situation as possible. The facts of the situation will make a difference in what the possible options are. However, remember that most situations do not have some magic pattern of true facts. The facts are always screened through each person's background and experience. What clearly appears to be a "true fact" to one person may seem to be "opinion" to another. Therefore, seeking other viewpoints may help you to see the situation more clearly. You need to understand the relevant people in the situation and their concerns and perspectives as much as possible. Consider whether there are legal cases that might affect decision making in this case.

Identify Options

Most ethical problems do not have only one possible solution. If there were only one solution, there would be no ethical dilemma because there would be no choice. There are usually many options. In some cases more than one may be satisfactory; in others, none of the options will seem satisfactory. The more options you can identify, the more likely you are to find one you can support.

Think the Ethical Problem Through

For each option consider its impact on each person involved. Also think about the impact on society as a whole if this option were to be chosen. Consider the ethical theories presented and ask yourself how each particular option compares with the basic principles of that theory. In this way you might determine that one option is basically a utilitarian approach (seeking the greatest good for the greatest number) while another is clearly supporting a deontological position of doing one's duty.

At this point in some major health care ethical problems, an ethics committee is consulted to assist with analysis. Bringing a wide variety of expertise and experience, the members of the committee may help individuals who must make an ethical decision to identify whether they have all the relevant information, help them to determine other options they have not considered, and provide assistance in comparing the situation with basic ethical principles and theories. Ethics committees may also help institutions establish policies in regard to ethical concerns that tend to recur in that setting.

Make a Decision

At some time you will have to make a decision. This is often difficult and in some instances painful. However, refusing to make a decision that is yours is not a responsible position. There will never be enough time, enough data, or enough alternatives in some situations. No matter how thorough your analysis or how carefully you weighed all competing claims, you may still be left with uncomfortable feelings.

Act and Assess

Once you have chosen a course of action, then you must carry out your decision. This may involve working with others or carrying out plans yourself. Assess the outcomes as you proceed. Unforeseen outcomes are common in ethical situations. Share your thoughts and concerns with others as your proceed and continue to seek new insights into the situation. As you assess the outcome in this particular situation, consider its relevance for a wider range of situations and concerns. Use this situation as a foundation from which to grow and develop.

SPECIFIC ETHICAL ISSUES RELATED
TO THE PROFESSION OF NURSING

Some of the ethical issues that are of concern to nurses relate specifically to the nursing profession, others relate to bioethical issues confronting all of society. In this section we will discuss the areas facing nursing through commitment to the patient, commitment to personal excellence, and commitment to the nursing profession as a whole. Bioethical issues that relate to the whole society are discussed in Chapter 7. We present a definite viewpoint regarding ethics in the nursing profession. We feel strongly about the individual's responsibility for nursing practice and place high value on personal integrity in professional relationships.

Commitment to the Patient/Client

Nursing has a strong history of being committed to the well-being of the patients and clients who need care. Both the ANA Code for Nurses and the International Code for Nurses clearly point out the obligation that the nurse has in fulfilling this commitment. This obligation has been used to try to persuade nurses that they must not be concerned for self, working conditions, salaries, or other aspects of the employment situation. This is not realistic and may even be counterproductive to the development of effective autonomous nurses. However, rejection of a handmaiden philosophy does not require rejection of a basic philosophy that identifies nursing as a profession focused on providing patients and their families with support for growth to maximum health and well-being. Patients/clients can never become objects for nursing but must be approached as unique individuals who deserve concern, respect, and the best we have to offer.

Recommending a Care Provider

Clients and other people of your acquaintance may ask you to recommend a physician or other type of care provider because they believe that, as a nurse, you have special expertise in such matters. In the past, nurses were admonished not to express opinions about care providers and were simply to direct clients to the yellow pages, directories, or hospitals that referred patients to staff physicians on a rotating basis. If you indeed have no personal knowledge about the requested information, then this would be a reasonable approach. But if you do have knowledge, it seems inappropriate to sidestep the issue. You could recommend several competent persons, pointing out characteristics of each that might be factors in personal choice. For example, if asked to recommend an obstetrician, you might recommend three. You could then further state that Drs. A., B., and C. are all board-certified specialists in obstetrics. You might add some information about their practices: Dr. A. is an older physician with a more traditional approach to childbirth; Dr. B. is a young and innovative physician who strongly advocates father participation and the Lamaze natural childbirth method; Dr. C. is new in the community but appears to allow patients a great deal of choice in their approach to childbirth. The client can further research these physicians and make a personal choice.

If you are specifically asked about a physician whose care you believe to be less than satisfactory, you are faced with a different dilemma. Making severely critical statements might leave you open to a legal charge of slander by the physician (see Chapter 5). However, to say nothing is ethically a problem because you are not acting to protect the client. A safe approach is to state, "I personally would not choose Dr. X. as my physician. Instead I would prefer to see Dr. N. or Dr. O." If pressed to give reasons, you are legally more secure if you indicate that you would prefer not to discuss specifics.

You do need to be careful that any recommendations are not based on hearsay or gossip. If you do not have solid information on which to base a referral, do not be drawn into making one. Being a nurse does not obligate you to be an expert on all health care questions.

Confronting Substandard Care

The day has passed when nurses could be expected to provide unwavering support of all members of the health care team, whatever their actions or the outcomes for the patient. Concern for the welfare of patients requires that nurses acknowledge the existence of substandard care and work toward change. We see the issue in terms of the form and extent the involvement should take, rather than whether the nurse should become involved.

A Basic Pattern for Action

The first step in any situation in which you believe substandard care exists is to collect adequate, valid information. Do not make decisions based on gossip, hearsay, or a single isolated instance. If you do, you may create problems for yourself rather than solving problems for the patient. Sometimes a single incident is serious enough that you want to act, but before taking action be sure of your facts.

Your second step is to be certain you understand both the official and the unofficial systems of authority and responsibility within your facility. You need to know which people have the authority to make decisions and changes, what the official prescribed route of change is, and what the hidden priorities of the institution might be. For example, the official lines of authority may provide the physician who has been elected chief of staff with authority within the medical group. Your knowledge of the informal system may reveal that a certain respected physician who does not have an official position actually is able to exert more influence for change. Within the nursing chain of responsibility, you may be aware that the head nurse of your unit, although officially having authority, in reality refers all decision making to the supervisor.

The most commonly recommended initial action is that you take your concerns to your immediate supervisor. If you do this, your legal responsibility, if there is one, usually is satisfied. However, in some states, laws exist that require that poor practice be reported directly to the relevant licensing board. Many people believe that reporting to a supervisor fulfills your ethical responsibility as well as your legal responsibility. If the system always worked effectively, your supervisor would carry the concern onward within the organizational structure, and each person contacted would forward the concern to the next appropriate person until it reached the individual or committee with the authority and duty to act.

Alternative Approaches for Action

However, the system does not always work. Your concern may be dropped or ignored at any one of many points. You may never learn what was done even when positive action has been taken because of the constraints of confidentiality. Occasionally results are identified only much later, when a change in procedure and policy occurs.

Sometimes an alternative initial approach is more appropriate to the situation. You may volunteer to serve on committees such as those that deal with peer review. If there are no such committees, you may work to have them established, perhaps through a bargaining unit. This route of action will require a considerable investment of your own time and effort. The cry of "Why doesn't somebody do something?" may often be answered "Because nobody takes the time." This is a very real constraint on action.

Another initial approach is to use the informal system within the facility. You may discuss your concern with a trusted person who has influence within the system. You may learn that you are not alone in your concerns, that efforts toward change are being made, and that your input of data is welcomed. Be careful when using informal systems; they can backfire. If your immediate superior learns that you went over his or her head with your concerns, he or she may direct anger at you.

If your initial approach is not effective, one formal route for seeking further change would lead you through the official lines of authority within your facility. After discussing your concern with your immediate supervisor and receiving no satisfactory response, you would tell the supervisor formally that you intend to carry your concern to the next higher authority. Technically you could proceed in this manner until you reached the administrator or even the board of directors.

Another formal route for seeking further change is through designated committees or procedures within your facility. This might require a carefully written documented report explaining your concern. You might then be called to answer questions that the committee has.

You might also decide to return to the unofficial power system within the facility. You might seek out other health care professionals whom you believe would be interested and secure support for change in this way.

A final alternative to a problem in your work setting is to offer your resignation if the change is not made. Continuing to exist in an environment in which poor practice exists may place you in conflict with your ethical standards and values. If you find it necessary to do this, be careful that you do not jeopardize your own future with angry letters or intemperate remarks. Render your resignation in polite and professional manner even when expressing dissatisfaction with the system.

Reporting directly to a state licensing board or professional organization's disciplinary committee is an avenue of action outside of the employment setting. These organizations and agencies usually deal with serious problems that represent a breach of the public trust or serious harm. They may not have the capacity or desire to pursue minor though still important problems. The same constraints apply when reporting to these organizations. Remember that their investigation and decisions may be done in a judicial or legal manner. This may involve the requirement that you provide legal testimony in regard to your complaints.

Personal Risks In Reporting

If you decide to pursue any of these routes, you need to be fully aware of the possible consequences. You may be labeled a troublemaker, or worse. You may lose the opportunity to be promoted because you are seen as being antagonistic to the system. It is even possible that you could lose your job for creating too many waves. Officially this should not happen, but in reality it can and does. We do not mean to be unduly discouraging, but we want to warn you that the role of change agent is not easy, and you should be aware of and weigh the consequences before you decide to act.

Commitment to Personal Excellence

In order to meet the commitment to the patient/client, each individual nurse must be committed to personal excellence. Basic to moving toward personal excellence is a willingness to engage in self-evaluation and assume responsibility in the work setting.

Self-Evaluation

Self-evaluation is discussed throughout this text in relationship to personal career goals, legal concerns, and continuing education. There also exists a strong ethical responsibility for the health care professional to practice self-evaluation. You are the one who is best able to identify your weaknesses and practice deficits as well as your strengths. Your careful self-evaluation is the patient's best protection against poor or inadequate care.

Self-evaluation is not always an easy or pleasant task. If we are truly honest with ourselves, we will be likely to uncover areas we wish were not there. Remember, done informally, these do not have to be shared with anyone; that is one of the beauties of self-evaluation. On the other hand, do not hesitate to ask for assistance if you think you need it. One is seldom criticized for trying to do a better job. Many institutions are now including self-evaluation in the formal evaluation of employees. If this is the case, you may be asked to prepare a written self-evaluation that will be shared with at least your immediate supervisor.

One avenue of approach to self-evaluation is the use of the nursing process format. Begin by a thorough personal assessment (Fig. 6-7). To do this you will have to gather data about your own performance. This requires a level of objectivity that is not easy. You might outline areas in which you want to gather data and actually keep notes on yourself.

After data have been collected, you will need to give yourself time to reflect on it and analyze it thoroughly. The self-assessment outline includes questions you would ask yourself; however, the criteria that you use to determine whether your answers reflect the quality of performance you want to attain are not included. Those specific criteria must be individualized to the setting in which you work and the nature of your role in that setting. The breadth of data that represent excellent practice for the nurse in the emergency department differs from what would represent excellence for the nurse working in a rehabilitation setting.

Figure 6–6. One of the advantages of self-evaluation is that it does not have to be shared.

The amount of decision making in which the patient participates differs between the recovery room and the outpatient clinic.

Your analysis can reveal strengths, weaknesses, and areas for growth or improvement. Congratulate yourself on the strengths identified and then clearly identify those areas in which you want to change. As in nursing care planning, clearly identifying and stating the problems or growth needed helps you to plan more effectively.

After you have identified your problems, it is appropriate to establish a plan of action. The plan is more helpful to you if it contains clearly defined goals. What is a realistic expectation for yourself? When is an appropriate time to reach that expectation? As part of realizing these goals, you might find it helpful to establish criteria you will use to identify your progress. Once the goals are set, you are better able to plan appropriate action to meet them. You might consider such things as requesting in-service education, taking continuing education courses, consulting with colleagues, and doing independent reading and study. Some plans would need to include specific things that you will be doing in your daily nursing care for improvement. To do this you may want to request assignments that will provide opportunities for practice of skills.

All this planning must not go to waste. Implementing this plan will require you to remain focused on what you are trying to accomplish. Keeping records on yourself is often helpful.

Periodic evaluation of your progress is necessary so that you do not become discouraged. Any records you have kept will be valuable for this purpose. Sometimes it is hard to identify gradual change. You might even plan rewards for yourself for improvement that occurs. Try not to become discouraged if you do not see the improvement you desire. Remember that just as in patient-care planning, a reassessment and a new or revised plan are often necessary, so may it be in the self-evaluation process. Keep in mind that your overall goal is personal excellence in nursing practice.

Responsibility for Supplies

Pilfering is stealing in small amounts or stealing objects of little value. In fact, many people who are otherwise scrupulously honest do not recognize that taking small items from a place of employment is indeed theft. Hospital employees often take home a thermometer, adhesive bandage strips, and other such objects so routinely that they do not even consider whether this is right or wrong. With the large number

---

SELF-EVALUATION PLAN

Assessment of Patients

1. Do I gather enough breadth of data about patients and families, including both strengths and deficits?
2. Do I gather data in great enough depth?
3. Do I listen closely to the patient and attend to what is being said?
4. Do I regularly use all available sources for information about my patients? (patient, family, other staff, chart, Kardex, and so forth.)
5. Have I recognized problems quickly so that they did not become worse through inattention?
6. Do I recognize physiological, social, and psychological problems?

(continued)

Figure 6–7. Self-evaluation plan.

SELF-EVALUATION PLAN *(continued)*

Planning for Patient Care

1. Do I routinely seek more information on which to base decisions about patient care?
2. Do I include the patient in decision-making whenever possible?
3. Do I consult with others on the health care team when planning?
4. Are my written plans clear, concise, and reasonable to carry out?
5. Do I take into account the realities of the situation when planning care?
6. Are my plans for care sound and appropriate to the individual patient?
7. Do I employ principles from the biological and social sciences in planning?

Intervention

1. Is my work organized and finished on time?
2. Do I maintain optimum safe working habits?
3. Do I perform technical skills in an efficient and safe manner?
4. Do I communicate clearly and effectively with patients, family, and staff?
5. Do I use therapeutic communication techniques appropriately and effectively?
6. Do I use teaching approaches appropriate to the individual patient and family?
7. Do I keep accurate and complete written records?
8. Do I understand and perform any administrative tasks which are my responsibility? (ordering supplies, planning for laboratory tests, and so on.)
9. Do I make the effort to learn about new techniques and procedures?

Evaluation

1. Do I routinely evaluate the effectiveness of the nursing care I give?
2. Do I effectively assist in evaluation of the patient's response to medical care and to ordered therapies?
3. Do I encourage the patient to participate in evaluating both the process and the outcomes of care?
4. Is self-evaluation a planned part of my activities?
5. Do I use data collected during evaluation for the improvement of my own functioning and patient care?

Personal Growth and Relationships

1. Have I established a sound trust and working relationship with co-workers?
2. Do I support and assist my co-workers when possible?
3. Do I communicate effectively with others on the health care team?
4. Have I sought opportunities for learning and personal growth?
5. Is my attitude helpful and productive?
6. Do I have sound working habits? (appearing on time, limiting coffee and lunch breaks to the correct time, and so forth)
7. Is my appearance appropriate to the working environment?
8. Do I use appropriate channels of communication within the institution correctly?
9. Do I handle criticism constructively?
10. Am I doing my share in overall professional activities such as serving on committees or assisting with development projects?
11. Am I honest with myself, being neither too harsh nor too easy going?

Figure 6–7. *(Continued)*

of employees in a modern hospital, this constant petty theft may total thousands of dollars. The cost of this must be passed on to those who pay the bills—the patients. As a leader in the care setting, the registered nurse is often in a position to clearly communicate to all employees that pilfering is unacceptable and to serve as an example of careful steward-ship of the hospital supplies.

Sometimes removing supplies is an oversight rather than a planned action. In order to make efficient use of time, nurses commonly place many small items such as alcohol wipes, extra needles, and pens in their pockets. One hospital unit found that their yearly supply budget for black pens was almost exhausted in the first 6 months of the year. The simple action of placing a basket in the lounge into which nurses dropped everything from their pockets before leaving cut the pen costs dramat-

Figure 6–8. Many people who are otherwise scrupulously honest do not recognize that taking small items from a place of employment is theft.

ically. Perhaps you can be equally creative in helping to solve such problems in your work setting.

Commitment to the Nursing Profession

Commitment to the nursing profession requires that each individual nurse be concerned not only about personal performance but also about how nursing is practiced. This involves participation in peer evaluation, formal evaluation of nursing care, dealing with poor care, and identifying the impaired nurse.

Evaluating Peer Performance

Nurses always have evaluated one another in both formal and informal ways. Some people think that evaluation implies noting error or deficiency. Good evaluation is much broader than this. The main purpose of peer evaluation is to maintain consistent high-quality nursing care. This is an ethical, professional obligation.

Informal Evaluation

The methods of evaluation vary. An important component of peer evaluation is actual observation of the performance of others. Often coworkers are the ones who are best able to observe a nurse's performance. Watching other nurses will also help you to grow in your own practice. When you observe coworkers, you need to strive for objectivity. A common mistake is to let personal feelings, likes, and dislikes influence our observations so that we see only what we want to see. We may view a close friend only in a positive light, whereas we see only the negative aspects of a nurse with whom we have a poor personal relationship.

Another important aspect of evaluation is examining results or outcomes of care. Two nurses may use different approaches or techniques in similar situations, but both may achieve positive results.

Evaluation is not negative. As you observe behavior and outcomes in nursing practice, you will most often see good nursing care. Do not hesitate to commend others and share your positive feelings. Everyone benefits from positive reinforcement of skill. Doing this would help nurses to create a good climate for personal growth and sharing.

An ethical dilemma arises when you observe a colleague practicing what you think is poor patient care, such as poor sterile technique. A variety of avenues of actions are available to you. What you choose to do depends on the seriousness of the situation you have observed. We suggest the following pattern for action as one that may assist in correcting a problem and at the same time maintaining positive working relationships.

Usually the simplest and most effective answer to any problem is to go directly to the person involved and state: "I observed this specific incident and it seemed to me that it was not in the best interest of the patient because. . .How do you feel about it?" This does not level accusations of good and bad nursing and does allow the nurse to give rationale for the action taken. When you understand the situation more fully, you may have a different point of view also. If you disagree and the situation is not critical, you might want to simply state that you do differ. Sometimes just calling an incident to the attention of the person will result in a change in behavior, even if there is no open agreement that a change is needed.

If you observe poor care another time, you might again approach the person. State what you have seen, and note that it is the second time. If the person still disagrees that a problem exists, state that you feel obligated to discuss this with your immediate superior because it is not in the best interest of the patient. You should then follow through on this.

When you approach a supervisor, you need to give specific information with dates, situations, and the action you took. You should not indulge in generalities or sweeping statements but should stick to specific observed instances. Let the supervisor know that you have talked with the person under discussion and have informed the person that you would speak with the supervisor. It is important to specify the action you would like to see occur. You might ask the supervisor to discuss the matter with both of you to clarify the correct nursing procedure. Or you might ask that the supervisor talk about the matter with the other nurse or observe the nurse. A vague declaration of "You should do something about this!" is not helpful.

If your focus has been on enhancing the welfare of patients and you have been quick to praise the good care provided by others, your action in response to poor care will be more readily accepted. Remember that your attitude when approaching another nurse is crucial. Facial expressions and tone of voice as well as words need to be considered. If you are perceived as friendly and caring, your comments probably will be accepted in a far different manner than if you are seen as being negative and critical.

But you cannot always count on this. Many nurses feel threatened by the idea of evaluation or have had bad experiences in which evaluation only involved pointing out deficiencies. These nurses may be angry and upset with any colleague who deems evaluation to be part of the colleague role. There is a great deal of pressure in these situations to close your eyes to what is happening around you and concentrate only on your own care.

If you observe an incident that has the potential for serious danger to the patient (such as an unreported medication error) or one that has legal ramifications (such as falsifying narcotic records), you would have a legal as well as an ethical responsibility to go immediately to a supervisor with your information. In a situation that has the potential for legal involvement, it is prudent to keep an exact personal record of your observations and actions. Your record should include times and dates of the incident and of your reporting efforts (see Chapter 5).

Formal Evaluation

Formal evaluation of nursing is occurring in most settings under the title of quality assurance. Quality assurance is a planned program of evaluation that includes ongoing monitoring of the care given and of outcomes of care. It includes a mechanism for instituting change when problems or opportunities for improvement are identified. Quality assurance programs are required by the Joint Commission on the Accreditation of Health Care Organizations and by Medicare.

The first aspect of nursing care that is usually evaluated is whether the nursing actions taken were complete and appropriate for the situations. Criteria developed to evaluate this aspect are called process criteria. One basis for developing process criteria is the *Standards for Nursing Practice* developed by the ANA (American Nurses' Association, 1973). There are general standards that refer to all settings and more specific ones for gerontological, maternal-child, community health, psychiatric-mental health, and other specialty areas of nursing. Some specialty organizations such as the Intravenous Nurses' Society have also published standards that refer to their specific specialty.

Another basis for formal evaluation is the use of outcome criteria for patient care. Outcome criteria are specific, observable patient behaviors or clinical manifestations that are the desired result of care. They usually are established by nurses working in groups. Nursing literature is consulted so that appropriate criteria are established.

A number of methods have been used to evaluate both the process and the outcomes of nursing care. Conferences designed to discuss the matter to be evaluated are personal and flexible but may lack objectivity. Simple interviews with either patients or staff also lack objectivity, although valuable insight and direction may be gained from them. Direct observation of patients provides an excellent means of evaluation if specific criteria are set up before the observation, but it is time consuming. The method that is gaining wider acceptance in nursing is the audit based on review of the patient's record. If information does not appear in the record, then, for the purposes of the audit, the observations were not done or the action was not taken. This may come as a shock to nurses who reply, "But we always do that!"

All types of evaluation first call for establishing specific criteria to be used in the evaluation. These criteria may refer to process, to outcome, or to both. The creation of the criteria is a professional nursing responsibility. The chart review involves comparing the patient record with the criteria. Often medical records personnel may do this. The accuracy of the review depends on the adequacy of the charting. This is just one of the reasons why you must recognize the importance of your charting and make sure that you maintain a high standard in written records. If audits are being done at your institution, you should become familiar with the criteria being used. These criteria can serve as guidelines for you in evaluating your own care and in record keeping.

This kind of review has raised some serious concern and often results in increased attention to charting and even revision of charting systems in some areas. Once the information has been gathered, nurses again take the initiative in determining the meaning of the data and what the next step should be. Because the goal is improvement of patient care, it is hoped that the audit will result in plans to enhance patient well-being. Changes in policies and procedures and in-service education classes are some of the approaches that have been used. Once remedial action has been taken, reevaluation is done to determine its effectiveness. Formal evaluation of nursing care is successful only if all nurses recognize their individual responsibility and accountability for practice and are willing to learn and grow in order to enhance patient care.

The Chemically Impaired Nurse

The *chemically impaired nurse* is a term used to describe that person whose practice has deteriorated because of chemical abuse, specifically the use of alcohol and drugs. There is a strong possibility that each of you, if you remain active in the profession, will at some time find yourself working with a chemically impaired colleague.

One would like to believe that nurses, who have studied the physiological effects of alcohol and drugs on the system, would avoid the chances of such abuse. This is not the case. Statistics regarding chemical dependency in nurses are flawed owing to the social stigma and the subsequent efforts to protect the individuals involved (Sullivan, Bissell, and Williams, 1988). From September 1980 to August 1981 the National Council of State Boards of Nursing collected data on disciplinary actions from its member state boards. Of the cases reported during that period, it was determined that 67% of the disciplinary proceedings involving nurses were related to some form of chemical abuse (Sullivan, Bissell, and Williams, 1988). The state boards have not published data since that time. Several studies of alcoholic physicians and nurses have revealed that only a small percentage were ever reported to their respective state boards (Bissell and Haberman, 1984; Bissell and Skorina, 1987). In their discussion of chemical dependency in nursing, Sullivan, Bissell, and Williams (1988) estimated the numbers of chemically dependent nurses based on statistics for the general population and the numbers in treatment. Although both physicians and nurses are overrepresented among those in chemical dependency treatment programs, it may be that they are more predisposed to enter treatment than is the population at large. They conclude that the percentage of chemically dependent nurses is as at least as great as the percentage of chemically dependent people in the general population, and it may be that there is a greater percentage in the nursing population based on accessibility of drugs.

Why are nurses affected by this problem? Factors that lead to chemical dependency include the stress that one encounters in the nursing profession, particularly in intensive care units and emergency departments. Frequent shift changes and staffing shortages add to the situation. Unrealistic personal expectations, frustration, anxiety, and depression contribute to the problem. Once the problem exists, denial is a big part of the disease.

Jefferson and Ensor (1982) provide the following information about addiction:

> Addiction is an insidious process that occurs as the result of a) prolonged intake of a chemical, b) processes going on within the individual (including genetic, psychological, and chemical), and c) processes external to the individual (that is, the actions and reactions of family, friends, co-workers, supervisors, and society). . . .Addiction is present any time a chemical interferes with any aspect of a person's life and that person keeps using the chemical.

In 1981 the ANA appointed a Nursing Task Force on Addiction and Psychological Disturbance to develop guidelines for treatment and assistance for nurses whose practice was impaired by alcoholism, drug abuse, or psychological dysfunction. The guidelines were designed for use by state nurses' associations.

The concerns for the chemically impaired nurse are twofold. The first is on a personal level for the nurse who is afflicted: the illness may go undetected and untreated for years. The second concern is for the patient, whose care is jeopardized by the nurse whose judgment and skills are weakened.

Because nurses, by virtue of their education, are socialized into caring roles, they have not always dealt with the problem in a straightforward fashion. The impaired nurse was often protected, transferred, ignored, and, in some instances, promoted. None of these actions helped the problem.

What are some of the behaviors you will notice in a chemically impaired colleague? Some similar behaviors will be seen in the nurse impaired by either alcohol or drugs. They include the following:

- Increased absenteeism
- Inability to meet schedules
- Tendency to shrink from new and challenging assignments
- Changes in personality and mental status, mood swings
- Changes in behavior
- Illogical and sloppy charting
- Excessive errors
- Unkempt appearance
- Decreased ability to concentrate
- Poor to inaccurate recall
- Medication "errors" that require many changes in charting
- Arriving on duty early or staying late for no valid reasons

In addition, the nurse who is consuming alcohol while working may have alcohol on the breath, have slurred speech and an unsteady gait, and have a flushed face (Jefferson and Ensor, 1982).

Problems related to drug abuse are complicated by the fact that the nurse usually is obtaining drugs from the supply available on the hospital unit and is therefore in violation of the Controlled Substances Act. Some additional factors that may indicate a problem with a drug abuse include increased incidents of dropped or wasted medication when that nurse is on duty and complaints of little or no relief from pain medication from patients assigned to that nurse. (This may occur because the nurse takes all or part of the medication prescribed for the patient and gives the patient distilled water, saline, or diluted narcotic.) Eventually you may notice that the nurse in question makes frequent use of the bathroom, and you may find used syringes and bloody cotton balls left there.

Nurses who abuse narcotics usually prefer to work alone, may express a desire to work on a night shift (where there is less contact with others), or may express a preference for areas of the hospital where many narcotics may be given with less surveillance because of patient short-stay (e.g., emergency departments or delivery rooms).

What should you do if you suspect that a colleague has a chemical dependency problem? First of all, you need to know what the law in your state requires of you. In many states any professional is legally obligated to report such a chemically dependent health care professional. This reporting most commonly is done through channels at the place of employment but may also be done directly to the state board of nursing. If you do not know the requirements, you should immediately check them out. In some states failure to report can result in disciplinary action toward you.

When planning to report you do not have to be sure beyond any doubt that a problem exists. You need to have enough data to represent a reasonable concern. The investigation to clearly establish the problem is the responsibility of the employing agency and/or the state board.

To establish reasonable concern, collect data and document it, including dates and times that support your concern. Do not confront or accuse the person whom you suspect. There are at least several good reasons you should not confront the person whom you suspect at this time.

First, the person may become more secretive about the behavior because of the danger of being caught. This will make collection of data more difficult, if not impossible. Personal defenses and denial may become stronger. The suspected person may ask for a transfer to another shift or to a different part of the hospital, or, if truly threatened, may seek employment in another hospital.

Second, the person may feel attacked and rejected. A confrontation needs the support of a knowledgeable professional in order not to end in disaster. Through the support of the appropriate health care person, the individual may be be guided into appropriate choices for treatment and rehabilitation.

We have already alluded to another reason you should not confront the suspected person at this time. You are still collecting data and documenting it. You cannot be sure from a single observation that a problem exists. There are often reasons why things are not the way we initially perceived them.

Once you feel you have data to support a realistic concern, you should report it to a supervisor to validate your observations. Usually once you have notified your supervisor, he or she will assume responsibility for the problem but may ask for your continued assistance with data collection or with confrontation.

Once adequate information has been gathered, hospital administrative personnel will notify the state board of nursing. In addition they usually must notify the state board of pharmacy if drugs are involved. More investigation will be carried out; records will be examined. If a problem exists, actions appropriate to the situation will be taken. These usually include a carefully planned confrontation by an intervention team, a requirement that treatment be sought, and a presentation of the consequences of not seeking treatment.

The worst thing you can do if you suspect a problem is to ignore it or help a colleague "cover" for inadequacies. The problem will not get better if it is not recognized and treated. The longer the delay, the greater the chance that an innocent patient will be placed in jeopardy.

Fortunately help and rehabilitation are being made available to those who need it. Many states now have programs to provide support for treatment of health care professionals with chemical dependency. The board of nursing may suspend a license and provide monitoring and supervision as the individual seeks treatment. When treatment is completed, the board may reinstate the license with temporary limitations and continued monitoring and support. The goal is the eventual full rehabilitation of the health care professional to the service of the community. Therefore, reporting a chemically dependent colleague may be the most caring action you can take.

CONCLUSION

Understanding the basic concepts related to ethics sets the stage for approaching a wide variety of concerns in the nursing profession specifically and in society as a whole. Here we have tried to help you understand the many forces that impact an ethical decision maker and the factors that make each situation so complex. We believe that nurses have a special obligation to the patient/client, to personal excellence, and to the profession of nursing as a whole. We encourage each prospective nurse to examine these issues and his or her own responses to them.

REFERENCES

American Nurses' Association. Standards for Nursing Practice. Kansas City, MO, American Nurses' Association, 1973

Bissell L, Haberman PW: Alcoholism in the Professions. New York, Oxford University Press, 1984
Bissell L, Skorina J: 100 alcoholic women in medicine. JAMA 257:2939–2944, 1987
Bok S: Lying: Moral Choice in Public and Private Life. New York, Pantheon Books, 1978
Cohen MM, Cohen EN, Thomasma DC: Making treatment decisions for permanently unconscious patients. *In* Monagle JF, Thomasma DC: Medical Ethics: A Guide For Health Professionals. Rockville, MD, Aspen Publishers, 1988
Help for the helper. Am J Nurs 82(4):572, 1982
Jameton A: Nursing Practice: The Ethical Issues. Englewood Cliffs, NJ, Prentice-Hall, 1984
Jefferson LV, Ensor BE: Confronting a chemically impaired colleague. Am J Nurs 82(4):574, 1982
Kroeger-Mappes EJ: Ethical dilemmas for nurses: Physicians' orders versus patient's rights. *In* Mappes TA, Zembaty JS: Biomedical Ethics, 2nd ed, p 127. New York, McGraw-Hill Book Company, 1986
New encyclopedia of bioethics includes A.N.A. code. Am J Nurs 77(8):872, 1977
Sullivan E, Bissell L, Williams E: Chemical Dependency in Nursing: The Deadly Diversion. Menlo Park, CA, Addison-Wesley Publishing Co, 1988

FURTHER READINGS

Bagwood T: Substance abuse and obligations to colleagues. Nurs Manage 21(8):40–41, 1990
Czerwinski BS: An autopsy of an ethical dilemma. J Nurs Admin 20(6):25–29, 1990
Dilday RC: What the SNA's are doing: In Georgia. Am J Nurs 82(4):582–583, 1982
Ecklund V: Is there a chemically dependent nurse on your staff? Prof Nurs Q 1(1):22, 1986
Ensor BE: What the SNA's are doing: In Maryland. Am J Nurs 82(4):581–582, 1982
Gilfand G, Long P, McGill D, Sheerin C: Prevention of chemically impaired nursing practice. Nurs Manage 21(7):76–78, 1990
Harakul BM: What the SNA's are doing: In Ohio. Am J Nurs 82(4):583–584, 1982
Heins M, Bowman RA: What the SNA's are doing: In Tennessee. Am J Nurs 82(4):581–584, 1982
Holder AR, Lewis JW: Informed consent and the nurse. Nurs Law Ethics 2(2):2–8, 1981
Lachman VD: Why we must take care of our own—drug and alcohol abusers in our own profession. Nursing 86(5):41, 1986

Naegle MA: Educational and clinical perspective in alcoholism. *In* Perspective in Nursing 1985–87, pp 124–129. Based on Presentations at the 17th NLN Biennial Convention. Publication No. 41-1985. New York, National League for Nursing, 1985.

New ANA Task Force will seek answers for impaired RNs. Am J Nurs 82(2):242, 1982

Sherry D: Autonomy vs. beneficence. Home Healthcare Nurse 8(6):13–15, 1990

Supples JM: My colleague, my friend: The impaired nurse. Nurs Manage 21(8): 48I–48P, 1990

7

Bioethical Issues in Health Care

Objectives

After completing this chapter, you should be able to

1. *Define bioethics.*

2. *Discuss the history of family planning practices in the United States.*

3. *Discuss at least three positions people take related to family planning practices.*

4. *Outline the major arguments for and against abortion.*

5. *Discuss the arguments some people have against genetic screening and sterilization.*

6. *List some of the possible ethical and legal problems associated with the practice of employing a surrogate mother.*

7. *Discuss the problems associated with determining when death has occurred.*

8. *Review and examine right-to-die issues.*

9. *Differentiate between active euthanasia and passive euthanasia.*

10. *Discuss the major issues related to withholding or withdrawing treatment.*

11. *Identify at least three patients' rights with regard to informed consent and treatment.*

12. *Identify major concerns associated with organ transplantation.*

13. *Discuss reasons we have difficulty establishing firm rules regarding the treatment of the mentally ill.*

14. *Outline concerns related to the rationing of care.*

Bioethics is the study of ethical issues that result from technological and scientific advances, especially in biology and medicine. This area of study may also be called biomedical ethics because of its association with medical practices. It is a subdiscipline within the larger discipline of ethics, which, as discussed in Chapter 6, is the philosophical study of morality or what is right and what is wrong. This chapter should be read, studied, and discussed within the framework of the information concerning ethical decision making that was provided earlier. Perhaps even more than before you will be looking to judicial rulings, legal mandates, and social standards to assist in resolving some of the concerns with which you will be faced. You have had some exercise in looking at what is right or wrong with regard to your personal professional practice. This chapter examines more specifically those issues that apply to the bioethics of patient care.

MAJOR AREAS OF BIOETHICAL CONCERN

The bioethical issues surrounding the delivery of health care are numerous and multifaceted. They are also always changing. At an earlier point in time most of the truly serious debates related to birth, death, or the processes that bring a person to either point. Today that represents just the "tip of the iceberg" as we explore such concerns as access to health care, rationing of health care, where and how federal dollars should be spent with regard to the nation's health, and the obligation of others to assist the homeless.

These concerns confront us because as a nation our population is getting older and living longer. More people who in earlier days would have died now grow old and infirm. Diseases such as Alzheimer's, for which no effective treatment exists, increase in prevalence. New technologies result in treatments that were not available 15 years ago. Many of the technologies are so expensive that they are priced beyond what an individual or family can afford without help from third-party payers. New diseases such as the acquired immunodeficiency syndrome challenge us to find methods of prevention and treatment.

Entire textbooks have been devoted to bioethical considerations. Initially most of these were written for medical students, but now just as many are written for nursing students. Centers for research in bioethics have emerged, most notably the Institute of Society, Ethics, and the Life Sciences, located in Hastings-on-Hudson, New York (often called The Hastings Center), and the Kennedy Institute Center for Bioethics, located at Georgetown University in Washington, D.C. Journals such as the *Hastings Center Report* and the *Journal of Medicine and Philosophy* have come into being and an encyclopedia, *The Encyclopedia of Bioethics,* has been published.

Most of the bioethical issues with which we wrestle were not a concern 20 or even 10 years ago. They are a product of the technological advances that have occurred in medical practice and research. Twenty years ago heart-lung and other organ transplantations were not being done. Therefore, there was no need for donor organs or critical decisions with regard to the life status of the possible donor. We were not able to fertilize ova outside the human body and reimplant fertilized eggs in a woman's uterus. Lifesaving machines, such as respirators, and miracle drugs, such as some of the chemotherapeutic agents used today, were not available to offer extension of life. Technologies that allow for early diagnosis were not available. Concerns related to the quality of life were often more clear-cut. As advances occur in medical practice, so must we challenge ourselves to think through our own beliefs and feelings with regard to these practices.

It is our intent in this short section to share with you some of the major bioethical issues confronting the new graduate today. Through exposure you will have opportunity to gain information, explore philosophical and religious issues, and integrate your own beliefs into your concept of the nurse's role.

BIOETHICAL ISSUES CONCERNING THE BEGINNING OF LIFE

A number of the bioethical issues with which we wrestle are focused on the process by which conception occurs, the products of conception, and the beginning of life, including whether it should occur. Much of the early debate related to family planning.

Family Planning

The modern population control movement probably can trace its beginnings to the writing of a minister in the Church of England. In

1798 Thomas Malthus, in an essay titled "On Population," expressed deep concern about a population that was growing faster than were the resources to support it. To offset this problem he advocated late marriage, no marriage, or abstinence in marriage. No forms of contraception as we know them today were available, although women may have had homemade devices that they developed in an effort to prevent pregnancy. Most commonly these devices were sponges dipped in various herbs and other substances that, when inserted in the vagina, soaked up semen.

Those starting life in the United States during its early development were no more enlightened. Some of the controversy related to the issue of birth control has its roots in early legislation that was passed in the United States. In 1873 Congress passed the Comstock Act prohibiting the sale, mailing, or importing of any drug or article that prevented conception. This resulted in the illegal importation and distribution of contraceptive devices. You may have read about Margaret Sanger in some of your other studies. She championed for contraceptive practices at a time when such activities and viewpoints were extremely unpopular.

It was not until 1965 that a clear, legal concept of planned parenthood was developed, when the Supreme Court of the United States established the right of the individual to obtain medical contraceptive advice and counseling in the case of *Griswold and Buxton v. the State of Connecticut* (Hayt, 1977).

Additional controversy over birth control is related to theological teachings of some religious groups. According to their beliefs, interference with procreative powers is wrong. Orthodox Judaism has specific rules about when sexual intercourse may or may not occur; these rules are geared toward increasing the Jewish population. The Orthodox Jewish population is so small, proportionately, to other groups that the impact is not significant. Encyclicals from popes of the Roman Catholic Church from early time to the present have forbidden the use of artificial birth control. The Catholic Church believes strongly that the natural use of reproductive powers assures the propagation of the human race and that anything that impedes attainment of the purpose for which these organs were created (i.e., reproduction) is immoral. We see high birth rates in countries that are predominantly Catholic. The members of the Church of Jesus Christ of Latter-Day Saints (Mormons), although less adamant in their teachings, also discourage the use of artificial birth control under normal circumstances.

When working with patients whose personal beliefs prohibit the use of artificial birth control, you must be knowledgeable about natural methods of family spacing that will meet the patient's need. Your personal views regarding contraception must be set aside as you focus on meeting the patient's needs.

Of the methods of birth control available to those who have no religious sanction against their use, not all methods are acceptable to all people. For example, some find the intrauterine device unacceptable because they believe that interfering with a fertilized egg should be viewed as abortion. (Researchers are not entirely sure how the intrauterine device works but believe that it prevents the fertilized egg from implanting in the wall of the uterus.) The other extreme is represented by those who find abortion an acceptable method of family spacing.

Central to all discussions of contraception is the issue of freedom to control one's body. This immediately raises a second question: who has that right? Is it the woman's right because it is her body? Avid feminists would answer with a resounding "yes." What if the partners disagree about family planning practices? Does one have more say than the other? What if one partner wants to have a family and the other does not? It is not within the scope of this chapter to explore the ramifications of all these concerns, but nurses working in this area need to be aware of the many issues that are present.

Largely because of personal values, there is disagreement over how contraception should be practiced, by whom, and at what age. In general, it is assumed that adults are capable of giving free and informed consent. The ability to procreate precedes what is generally considered legal age, however, and we find ourselves grappling with problems related to age of consent and its definition.

Problems of Consent and Family Planning

In legal terms, the *age of consent* is "the age at which one is capable of giving deliberate and voluntary agreement, especially to marriage or to unlawful sexual intercourse" (Thomas, 1989). Implied in this is physical and mental ability and the freedom to act and make decisions. Before reaching the age of consent, parents are required to give consent for care of their children. Implicit in this is the assumption that the parents have the best interests of the child at heart and that they are better qualified than the child to make decisions in the child's best interest. The authority to give consent goes along with the understanding that the parents are responsible for the care and education of the minor, including medical costs. However, trends of today cloud the issue, and legislators and concerned citizens continue to struggle with legislating "rights" through arbitrary points such as age. In former times the age of 7 was believed to be a sufficient age at which to give consent because by age 7 children were expected to know right from wrong and to have reached the age of reason. Although few of us would think that this is an age at which a child should be responsible to give consent for medical treatment, guidelines of the Department of Health and Human Services have allowed that it is sufficient to refuse consent, despite parental opinion (Hellegers, 1975).

The trend recently has been toward the concept of the "emancipated minor." Although *emancipation of a minor* legally means "the entire surrender by the parents of the right to care, custody, and earnings of such a child as well as renunciation of parental duties," it is done with the agreement of the parents. Both parents and child agree that the child is able to care for self, may leave home, may earn a living, and may pay for cost of health care. This usually does not take place before the age of 16, but it may. Most states recognize some form of emancipation of minors (Mancini, 1978).

Another term we often hear is *mature minor,* a relatively new concept. This term is applied to "youths who are sufficiently mature and intelligent to understand the nature and consequences of a treatment that is for their benefit" (Mancini, 1978, p 126). Under this definition, a minor who wants birth control devices because he or she is sexually active demonstrates ability to make a mature decision, although the parents may not agree with the decision. This definition also allows minors to consent to therapy for venereal disease and drug abuse as well as pregnancy care.

Health care workers have no legal obligation to inform parents of this treatment. The most liberal legislation applies to the treatment of venereal disease and is endorsed by most states. Minors of any age can consent to diagnosis and care for venereal disease.

Many parents strongly oppose this position. They believe that this undermines their parental role and sanctions sexual activity between young people. To illustrate this viewpoint let us consider the case of an 11-year-old girl who sought treatment for gonorrhea. At her insistence the physician promised to honor her legal right to confidential health care and not to inform her parents. Later a public health nurse who was working with the girl learned that the child was being repeatedly sexually assaulted after school by a 16-year-old neighbor while her parents were still at work. The nurse also felt bound to a pledge of confidentiality but was able, with modest encouragement, to get the child to discuss this with her parents and enlist their support. In this instance the statute that protected the "rights" of the child may have led health care professionals to become involved in activities that did not serve the best interests of the child.

In 1973 the American Academy of Pediatrics developed the Model Act, which addresses the issue of consent of minors for health care. This act recommends that minors be allowed to give consent for health services when they are pregnant or afflicted with reportable communicable disease, including venereal diseases, or drug and substance abuse, including alcohol and nicotine. It is generally accepted that the age of the patient is not to be considered for some treatments, but that parental consent is automatically required for other treatments if the patient is younger than 18. Certainly there will be times when physicians' ethical and moral convictions will prevent them from complying with adolescents' requests for care. This occurs most commonly with requests for contraceptive pills and abortions. In such cases physicians often discuss their beliefs with the adolescent and frequently refer the patient to a medical colleague for assistance.

A major controversy exists around the role of the school in the sex education of high school students and the dispensing of contraceptives. Those who are concerned about the rising incidence of teenage pregnancies and sexually transmitted diseases argue that the information must be disseminated, regardless of who does it. Conservatives think that this is an erosion of the role of the family, and worry that the indiscriminate dispensing of contraceptives encourages promiscuity among teenagers. Concern about the spread of the acquired immunodeficiency syndrome has done much to liberalize thinking regarding the dispensing of condoms in particular.

Abortion

What has been said about contraception becomes an even greater issue when related to abortion. In medical terms, abortion is the termination of the pregnancy before viability of the fetus, that is, any time before the end of the sixth month of gestation. An abortion may occur spontaneously as a result of natural causes (*spontaneous abortion*). The pregnancy may be interrupted deliberately for medical reasons (*therapeutic abortion*), or for personal reasons (*elective abortion*). It is these last two classifications, especially the latter, that induce bioethical debate. Ethically, the entire debate revolves around the definition of human life and when the fetus should be considered a human being. There exist two schools of thought about the nature of the fetus. One believes that new life occurs at the moment of conception. The other contends that human life does not exist until the fetus is sufficiently developed biologically to sustain itself outside the uterus.

The legal aspects of abortion were clarified on January 22, 1973, when the U.S. Supreme Court ruled that any state laws that prohibited or restricted a woman's right to obtain an abortion during the first 3 months of pregnancy were unconstitutional. In the case of *Roe v. Wade* the Supreme Court recognized that during the first trimester of pregnancy a privacy right exists that allows the individual to make the final decision with regard to what happens to her own body (*Roe v. Wade,* 1973). "Jane Roe" was the fictitious name Norma McCorvey used when two young attorneys, both female, filed her lawsuit. A pregnant, divorced waitress, a victim of a gang rape and beating, Jane Roe sued the state of Texas because she could not obtain a legal abortion in that state and was too poor to travel to New York or California where abortion was legal. Without access to abortion, she had the baby, whom she placed for adoption. Four years later the Supreme Court struck down the laws that prevented her seeking abortion. It was also determined that some time limitations as to when an abortion can be performed were necessary because of the states's interest in protecting potential life. At the period of viability the state's interest took precedence over the mother's desire for an abortion. Supreme Court Justice Blackmun, in writing an opinion that met with agreement from six other justices, decided that a woman's decision to terminate a pregnancy was encompassed by the right to privacy, up to a certain point in the development of the fetus (Blackmun, 1981). It was established that this lasted until the end of the first trimester. Thus, the courts ruled that the state could not prevent abortions during the first trimester but could regulate abortions in the second and third trimesters of pregnancy, at which point the interests of the fetus took precedence over those of the mother.

Despite these rulings the issue of abortion versus right to life continues to surface with new legislation and rulings being considered each year. The legal positions also do little to help us deal with the bioethical concerns. Many people view termination of life at any point after conception as murder. The position of the Roman Catholic Church remains firm on the church's position on abortion.

Others believe that although abortion is usually an unpleasant procedure, there may be certain circumstances that would make it justifiable, for example, in the cases of rape or incest or in instances where amniocentesis indicates that a fetus would be born retarded or genetically defective. Still others think that early termination of the pregnancy could be acceptable but any termination after the fourth month would not be desirable.

Those supporting abortion without restriction usually do so because they believe that women should have control over their own bodies. They further argue that the quality of life of a child who will be born as "unwanted" or with a deformity or genetic defect may be minimal. Interesting and challenging cases have emerged with respect to this concept. These are generally known as "wrongful birth" cases and are based on the principle that it is wrong to give birth to a child whose life will not have the same quality as that of other children, as in the case of children with birth defects or limitations that can be diagnosed or anticipated before birth.

As a nurse, these issues may present some difficult questions you will need to answer. To what extent do you believe you can personally participate in the abortion procedure? You may find it easier to assist with an abortion done as a dilation and curettage at 10 weeks' gestation in a doctor's office or clinic than to assist with a saline abortion carried out at 5½ months' gestation in a hospital labor room. The products of conception aborted at 10 weeks have little that is lifelike in their appearance. The fetus aborted at 5½ months appears much like a premature infant. Certainly, as a nurse, you have the right to refuse to be involved in abortive procedures or the care of patients seeking abortion. However, employment in a given area, for example, labor and delivery room, may rest on the nurse's willingness and ability to assist with abortions and to give conscientious care to the patient who has had the abortion. Some religiously affiliated hospitals have elected to close their labor and delivery suites rather than perform abortions.

Attention has been focused on events in which an abortion was attempted toward the end of the fifth or sixth month of gestation and the fetus was born showing signs of life. Is the doctor or nurse obligated to try to keep the infant alive? Is the doctor or nurse guilty of malpractice, or even murder, if he or she does anything to hasten the infant's death? Should this infant be considered a human being? Does the infant have "rights"? Does the mother have legal possession of and responsibility for the child if, in fact, she attempted to abort the fetus? This issue, like so many others, probably will be settled in a court of law while we continue to debate it ethically.

The abortion issue is also complicated by consent problems. Many states have recognized the special problems related to parental consent and to health care involving pregnancy and have legislated special exceptions.

As a society it seems likely that we will continue to debate the issue of abortion. Ultimately the decision rests with the individual who is having to make the choice. Certainly the legal entanglements become more complex with each court ruling and seem to be limited only by someone's willingness to challenge another aspect of the question.

Recently the abortion issue has been made more complex by research that would use the fetal tissue wasted by the abortion for therapeutic purposes. Research has suggested that implantation of fetal brain tissue recovered at the time of abortion may be helpful in the treatment of

Parkinson's disease if implanted in the brain of the patient with that diagnosis. The ramifications of this type of research and treatment are so great that a special committee has been appointed to develop guidelines to govern future research and treatment activities.

Amniocentesis, Prenatal Diagnosis, and Genetic Screening

A major breakthrough in our ability to detect genetic abnormalities before birth occurred in the 1970s with the development of techniques to carry out amniocentesis. An amniocentesis is done between 14 and 20 weeks after the last menstrual period. With this test, a 4-inch needle is inserted through the pregnant woman's abdomen and uterus, and about 20 mL of amniotic fluid are removed and analyzed. From these cells a number of genetic problems can be diagnosed prenatally, among them such conditions as Down's syndrome, hemophilia, Duchenne's muscular dystrophy, Tay-Sachs disease, and problems related to the brain and spinal column (e.g., anencephaly and spina bifida). Down's syndrome, a condition occurring with predictable frequency in mothers in their early 40s and older, is the most common reason for seeking amniocentesis. The obvious alternative for the mother is that when genetic screening reveals a genetic disease she will often choose to have an abortion. Rothstein (1989, p 39) reports that "termination rates for muscular dystrophy, cystic fibrosis, and alpha and beta thalassemia are nearly 100%; they are 60% for hemophilia; and 50% for sickle cell anemia." Some couples request amniocentesis if they are in an "at-risk" group but state that under no circumstances would they abort the fetus. They believe that the additional 5 months will give them time to adjust to the fact before the baby is born. Usually doctors are reluctant to do an amniocentesis under these circumstances because the risk, although small, does not seem justified.

Some people are concerned about this procedure because of where it might end. Is mass genetic screening a possibility? Ethicists have expressed concern about the government's making diagnostic amniocentesis and abortion of all defective fetuses mandatory. Still others argue against genetic counseling and amniocentesis because of the stress it places on the marriage of the couple and, in cases in which it can be determined, the guilt that is placed on the partner carrying the defective gene. Their argument is that there are some things we are better off not knowing. Genetic screening also may result in at least one of the partners, often the carrier, seeking voluntary sterilization to prevent pregnancies with less than favorable outcomes.

There are some positive aspects of amniocentesis. Prenatal diagnosis, for example, may save more fetal lives than it terminates. Many women carrying fetuses at high genetic risk might resort to abortion if the diagnostic techniques were not available. Such women, unwilling to take a chance, would rather abort a healthy fetus than risk bearing a defective one.

The advent of amniocentesis has heralded the development of yet another medical specialty, that of prenatal surgery. Although the specialty is still new, some corrective surgery is being done on infants while they are in their intrauterine environment.

As a nurse you may care for patients with any one of many viewpoints regarding amniocentesis and abortion and you will also have your own values to consider. Will your values conflict with those of your patient? Are you obligated to advocate for the patient if the patient's request is squarely in opposition to what you believe to be right? Should you try to sway a woman who is indecisive toward either decision?

Sterilization

For years surgical operations that have resulted in permanent sterilization of the patient have been performed for purposes of therapy. Examples of this could include removal of reproductive organs to halt the spread of cancer or other pathological processes. Although problems may arise for the patient and his or her family as a result of such surgeries, usually they are resolved without serious ethical debate, depending on the family's religious values, the patient's body concept, family plans, and personal values.

With increasing frequency, voluntary sterilizations have been requested by couples for purposes of terminating reproductive ability. These surgical procedures, performed on either the man or the woman, should, for all intents and purposes, be considered permanent and irreversible. For those who have the number of children they desire, sterilization may pose few problems. In most cases, full and informed consent generally is obtained from both husband and wife, and the surgery is performed. (Questions have been raised whether the husband or wife is free to make an independent decision regarding sterilization without consultation with their partner.) Although many people see this as the prerogative of the couple, others find any type of sterilization in conflict with their religious and moral beliefs. A few states still have laws forbidding voluntary sterilization for contraceptive purposes, although in fact these laws may not be enforced.

Eugenics

Of greatest controversy is any type of sterilization performed for eugenic purposes, especially if there is any question about the procedure being voluntary. Eugenics is the movement devoted to improving the human species through genetic control. The practice of eugenics is not new. The idea of improving the quality of the human race is at least as old as Plato, who wrote on the topic in his *Republic.* The modern eugenic movement is thought to have started in the 19th century. Charles Darwin's theory of evolution was advanced by his cousin Francis Galton, who created the term *eugenics.* Keyed to this were philosophical beliefs of certain 18th-century thinkers about the notion of human perfectibility. When Mendel's law provided an explanatory framework about the transmission and distribution of traits from one generation to another, the eugenics movement took hold. Organizations focusing on eugenics were created around the world.

The center of the eugenics movement in the United States was the Eugenics Record Office at Cold Spring Harbor, New York, and its leader was geneticist Charles Davenport. Up to the early 1930s the eugenic movement grew. Eugenicists presented a two-part policy. Negative eugenics advocated the elimination of unwanted characteristics from the nation by discouraging "unworthy" parents. This movement included a variety of approaches such as marriage restriction, sterilization, and permanent custody of "defectives." Many eugenicists were actively involved in other issues of the day including such timely causes as prohibition, birth control, and legislation that would outlaw miscegenation (marriage between two persons of different races, especially between white and black in the United States). During this time states passed compulsory sterilization bills.

Also passed at this time was the Immigration Restriction Act of 1924. This bill dramatically limited the immigration of people from southern and eastern Europe on the grounds that they were "biologically inferior."

Positive eugenics encouraged the increase of desirable traits in the population by urging "worthy" parents. "Superior" couples were encouraged to have more children.

The eugenics movement grew in Germany as well as in the United States. In 1933 Hitler sanctioned as law the Hereditary Health Law, or the Eugenic Sterilization Law, which assured that the "less worthy" members of the Third Reich did not pass on their genes. It also provided for the mass murder of millions of others considered "undesirable."

By the late 1930s eugenics in the United States began a tremendous decline. Americans became concerned about the concept of a "master race." At the same time psychologists and anthropologists were conducting research that indicated that culture and environment also had great influence over human development.

When the eugenic movement was rekindled in the 1960s, it had a different focus—one related to genetic counseling and genetic research. Today a couple who gives birth to a defective child or who realizes that one of them is carrying a genetic trait that could result in a defect in the child might voluntarily seek genetic counseling and possibly opt for sterilization of one of the partners. Again, this approach may offend the religious and moral values of some, but generally it is viewed as the couple's prerogative.

Problems are created when the concept of eugenics is applied to minors or to institutionalized people. Problems also arise in the language of laws in certain states that would include "epileptics, habitual criminals, and moral degenerates" among those eligible for compulsory sterilization. Some states have expanded compulsory sterilization to include those who might become wards of the state (Hayt, 1977). In the case of epileptics, modern medical advances have changed our understanding of the role of heredity in disease and our attitudes toward people who are affected. The trend in recent years has been for states to either modify or repeal their eugenic sterilization laws.

In states that still permit compulsory eugenic sterilization, questions can be raised as to who would request the sterilization, who would sign the consent, and who would fund the procedure. As the result of a court decision, federal monies may not be used for this purpose (Hellegers, 1975). However, the taxpayer contributes to the costs of institutionalization for people who are not capable of existing independently in today's society and for the care of those with severe illnesses and disabilities. Therefore, it is not only a personal concern but also society's concern.

In Vitro Fertilization

Another interesting bioethical issue relates to the creation of life or, more correctly, the conditions under which it may occur. In 1978 in England, attention was directed at the birth of a child who was conceived in a test tube, a process we refer to as *in vitro fertilization*. Owing to a blockage in the mother's fallopian tubes, conception in her tubes was impossible. The ovum was removed from the mother, united with the father's sperm in a laboratory test tube, and then implanted into the mother's uterus, where it grew to term and was delivered by cesarean section.

Figure 7-1. Another interesting issue involves the creation of life or, more correctly, the circumstances under which it may occur.

Many heralded this as one of medical science's great advances. Others thought that this was going too far, that there are already too many risks involved in the birth process, and that we are only asking for more complications. Others expressed concern about the ethics of using tax dollars to fund this type of research.

Despite the objections that have been raised against in vitro fertilization, it is now recognized as a viable alternative for many couples who would otherwise be childless (at least as far as natural parenting is concerned). Reproductive problems often stem from blocked fallopian tubes in the female. By means of a laparoscope, mature eggs are obtained from the female. These are then fertilized with the husband's sperm. A number of fertilized ova are then allowed to develop. Three to five of the fertilized ova are then implanted in the woman's uterus in the hope that at least one will survive the procedure (a process that has resulted in some multiple births). The remainder of the fertilized ova are discarded. In some instances when more of the implanted fertilized ova continue to develop within the uterus than was anticipated, several of the embryos will be aborted to allow one or two the opportunity to reach viability. Once again a serious bioethical concern is raised if one believes that life begins at conception.

In 1990 British researchers announced that they had identified the sex of human embryos just three days after they were conceived through in vitro fertilization. This medical discovery would allow a mother to be implanted with only female embryos and could be used to prevent the birth of boys in situations where the mother was at risk of passing on a severe genetic disease that occurs only in males (there are about 200 known sex-linked genetic diseases). It also provides the opportunity to identify severe genetic problems from a single cell and raises the question of whether couples would seek the "test tube baby" procedure to be assured of genetically perfect children, or even to select a child's sex.

Artificial Insemination

Other discussions revolve around the topic of artificial insemination, which is the planting of sperm in the woman's body to facilitate conception. Although we tend to think of this as a fairly new procedure, the first time artificial insemination is said to have been used was in Philadelphia in 1884 (Fromer, 1981). There are two different kinds of artificial insemination: homologous, in which the husband's sperm is used; and heterologous, in which a donor's sperm is used. Using the husband's sperm is by far the most common and creates the fewest problems legally, ethically, and morally. In some instances the sperm from the husband and the sperm from a donor with similar physical characteristics are mixed together.

Although some religious groups may have objections, few concerns arise if the husband's sperm is used. That is not true with a donor sperm. If the wife is artificially inseminated with donor sperm without the knowledge and consent of her husband, the problems are multiplied. One of the major questions that is raised is that of adultery, which is considered a criminal act in most states. If conception occurs and the child is not biologically that of the husband, can one say that adultery has occurred? In at least one instance the wife was found guilty of adultery after being artificially inseminated with donor sperm (Hayt, 1977). Others question whether the child should be legally adopted by the husband, an act that, to some extent, helps to clarify issues of inheritance, child support (if the couple should later divorce), and the legitimacy of the child.

Surrogate Mothers

Unique problems arise with surrogate mothers, a practice by which a woman agrees to bear a child conceived through artificial insemination and to relinquish the baby at birth to others for rearing. This practice has occurred with increasing frequency and in a variety of relationships.

In one instance a 47-year-old grandmother agreed to serve as gestational surrogate for her own daughter whose uterus had been removed. The daughter's eggs were inseminated with her husband's sperm and the embryos were then implanted in the grandmother who gave birth to triplets when she was 48. Thus this woman became the gestational mother and the genetic grandmother to triplets.

What happens if the child is born defective, as occurred with a New York couple in 1982? The man who paid a woman to be artificially inseminated with his sperm and carry his child rejected the infant, who

Figure 7–2. Complexities arise when surrogate mothers are unwilling to relinquish the infant after birth.

was born with microcephaly, stating that he could not be the father. The surrogate mother and her husband also did not want to accept the responsibility for parenting the child. How are these dilemmas to be solved? What will eventually become of the child?

More recently problems associated with surrogate mothering have centered around the surrogate mother's unwillingness to give up the child after birth, as in the case of "Baby M," as the court calls her. This baby was born to a surrogate mother after she was impregnated with the sperm of a man for whom she agreed to bear the child. This man's wife, a pediatrician, believed that she could not bear a child because she had multiple sclerosis. Although signed agreements existed, the surrogate mother broke the contract within days of the baby's birth and asked for custody of the child.

These artificial means of reproduction have complicated even the language that we are accustomed to using. The term *biological* is no longer adequate for making some critical conceptual distinctions. Macklin (1991, p 6) states, "The techniques of egg retrieval, in vitro fertilization (IVF), and gamete intrafallopian transfer (GIFT), now make it possible for two different women to make a biological contribution to the creation of a new life." Macklin further believes that the woman who contributes her womb during gestation is also a biological mother. We find terms such as *genetic mother* used to refer to the individual contributing the ovum and the term *gestational mother* being used to refer to the individual who provides the uterus in which the child developed. In some instances the surrogate mother is both.

Single Parents

Another ethical issue has arisen as our society has granted greater acceptance to single-parent families. More single women are trying to adopt children, and some see artificial insemination as a logical solution. In some instances these women have also professed to being lesbians. One of the couple will seek artificial insemination with a donor sperm. The child is then raised as family in the lesbian relationship. Providing a parenting option to lesbians is totally unacceptable to many people. Aside from the additional emotion that the issue of a lesbian life-style may introduce, there is the argument against artificial insemination of any single woman on the basis that the traditional two-parent family composed of a male and female is in the best interest of all children.

Sperm Banks

Another aspect of the artificial insemination issue is the issue of sperm banks. Sperm banks have been established in different parts of the United States for various reasons. Men who want to have a vasectomy may contribute to a sperm bank "just in case" they change their minds at some future time. Men who are to be exposed to high levels of radiation or other harmful substances that might result in sterility or mutation of genes also have had sperm stored. In most cases the sperm banks are established by the medical community so that sperm is available for artificial inseminations. In California a sperm bank was started that contains sperm of only outstanding and brilliant men. The idea was to create children with this sperm who will be genetically endowed with greater intelligence and creativity. Many find this unacceptable because it brings up the issue of creating a super race.

The Right to Genetic Information

All the issues of artificial insemination with donor sperm, surrogate mothering, single parenting, and sperm banks are further complicated by a recent trend toward providing individuals with information regarding their genetic background, make-up, and history. You can readily anticipate the problems that would be created if a donor sperm were used for insemination. In some instances no record has been maintained with regard to who donated the sperm.

How many individuals would be willing to donate sperm if it were to include a detailed genetic background? What might be the ultimate legal involvement? On the other hand, what are the rights of the child with regard to knowing what genetic factors he or she carries? Whose rights should take precedence?

BIOETHICAL ISSUES CONCERNING DEATH

One of the most important areas of ethical debate involves the topic of death and dying. As mentioned earlier, the advent of lifesaving procedures and mechanical devices has required redefinition of the term *death,* has caused us to examine the meaning of "quality of life," and has created debates about "death with dignity."

Also associated with the issue of death are a number of companion concerns that did not exist before we had some of the technological advances that have occurred within the past 10 years. Some of these concerns relate to euthanasia, the right to refuse treatment, and the right to die. Another set of concerns relate to organs retrieved from the dying because of the scarcity of these medical resources. Generally, there is more demand for donated organs than there are organs to meet the needs. Superimposed on all these issues is that of informed consent.

Death Defined

Until recently the most widely accepted definition of death was from *Black's Law Dictionary*, which defines death as the irreversible cessation of the vital functions of respiration, circulation, and pulsation (Rothman and Rothman, 1977). This traditional view of death served us well until the development of artificial respirators, pacemakers, and other advances in medical science made it possible to sustain these functions indefinitely. We also have learned that various parts of the body die at different times. The central nervous system is one of the most vulnerable areas, and brain cells can be irreversibly damaged if deprived of oxygen, whereas other parts of the body will continue to function.

Newer definitions of death have been built around the concept of human potential, in other words, the potential of the human body to interact with the environment and with other people, to respond to stimuli, and to communicate. When these abilities are lacking, there is said to be no potential. Because this potential is directly related to brain function, the method most generally used to assess capability is electroencephalography. Brain activity, with few exceptions, is said to be nonexistent when flat electroencephalographic tracings are obtained over a given period of time, often 48 hours (Rothman and Rothman, 1977). At this point the person may be considered dead, although machines may be supporting the vital functions of respiration and circulation. Many institutions now accept this definition of cerebral death and use it as a basis for turning off respirators and stopping other treatments.

Euthanasia

Euthanasia, meaning "good death," may be classified as either negative or positive. The word, as it is generally applied, refers to the act or method of causing death painlessly so as to end suffering.

Negative Euthanasia

Negative, or passive, euthanasia refers to a situation in which no extraordinary or heroic measures would be undertaken to sustain life. The concept of negative euthanasia has resulted in what are called "no codes" (also designated as "DNR"—do not resuscitate) in hospital environments, a situation in which hospital personnel do not attempt to revive or bring back to life persons on this status whose vital processes have ceased to function on their own.

This raises the question of consent. Often the person receiving the care is unconscious or unable to give consent. Does the responsibility for action, or the lack of action, then fall to the physician, the family, or the nurse? Would the ethical answer to this question be the same as the legal answer? Who is to decide?

In an attempt to gain greater control over the area of dying, many people are now signing living wills. By signing a living will the person requests that no extraordinary procedures be implemented to sustain life. Although the living will (Figure 7-3) is not necessarily considered legal consent, it does reveal the desires of the person under consideration.

**TO MY FAMILY, MY PHYSICIAN, MY LAWYER, MY CLERGYMAN
TO ANY MEDICAL FACILITY IN WHOSE CARE I HAPPEN TO BE
TO ANY INDIVIDUAL WHO MAY BECOME RESPONSIBLE FOR MY
HEALTH, WELFARE OR AFFAIRS**

Death is as much a reality as birth, growth, maturity and old age—it is the one certainty of life. If the time comes when I, _____
can no longer take part in decisions for my own future, let this statement stand as an expression of my wishes, while I am still of sound mind.

If the situation should arise in which there is no reasonable expectation of my recovery from physical or mental disability, I request that I be allowed to die and not be kept alive by artificial means or "heroic measures". I do not fear death itself as much as the indignities of deterioration, dependence and hopeless pain. I therefore, ask that medication be mercifully administered to me to alleviate suffering even though this may hasten the moment of death.

This request is made after careful consideration. I hope you who care for me will feel morally bound to follow its mandate. I recognize that this appears to place a heavy responsibility upon you, but it is with the intention of relieving you of such responsibility and of placing it upon myself in accordance with my strong convictions, that this statement is made.

Signed _____

Date _____

Witness _____

Witness _____

Copies of this request have been given to _____

Figure 7-3. The Living Will.

Another approach that is being used with increasing frequency is the signing of a durable power of attorney, particularly as it relates to health care decisions. In entering into this type of an agreement an individual (referred to as the "principal") may designate another person who is given the power and authority to make health care decisions for the principal should the principal be unable to make those decision for himself or herself. The durable power of attorney does not go into effect until after the principal is not longer capable of making decisions. Figure 7-4 provides an example of this form. These forms can be purchased in most office supply stores and become effective if signed before a notary public. However, it is best to consult an attorney before entering into such an arrangement.

It is difficult to describe what constitutes extraordinary measures and on whom they should or should not be used. Is it one thing to defibrillate a 39-year-old man who is admitted to an emergency department suffering from an acute heart attack and quite another to defibrillate a 90-year-old man whose body is riddled with terminal cancer and whose heart has stopped? Often people who are involved in giving medical and emergency care develop an almost automatic response to lifesaving procedures and have difficulty accepting dying as an inevitable part of the life process. It is difficult to know when it is permissible to omit certain life-supporting efforts, or which efforts should be omitted. If the 90-year-old man who is dying of terminal cancer were to also develop pneumonia, should the physician prescribe antibiotics? This brings us to a distinction between stopping a particular life-supporting treatment or machine or withdrawing treatment, as discussed earlier in the chapter, and not starting a procedure in the first place, that is, withholding treatment.

Positive Euthanasia

Positive, or active, euthanasia occurs in a situation in which the physician would prescribe, supply, or administer an agent that would result in death. In the case cited later in this chapter in which the parents chose to let a newborn with Down's syndrome and an intestinal blockage die, positive euthanasia would have been used if the doctors had hastened the infant's death with medication. There may well be more instances of positive euthanasia than we know about publicly. In these cases would the doctor be guilty of murder? And what should be decided about the involvement of nurses who carried out the physician's orders?

The issue of positive euthanasia is cloudy. On some occasions the physician will prescribe strong narcotics for a terminally ill patient and

[PLEASE NOTE: This is a standardized legal document that may not be appropriate for a person in your particular situation. You should consult your attorney before signing this or any legal document.]

DURABLE POWER OF ATTORNEY FOR HEALTH CARE DECISIONS

I, _____ as principal, domiciled and residing in the State of Washington, hereby enter into a Durable Power of Attorney to provide informed consent for health care decisions pursuant to the laws of the State of Washington.

1. **Designation.** I designate _____ , if living, able and willing to serve, as my attorney-in-fact. If he or she is not living, able and willing to so serve, then I designate _____ , if living, able and willing to serve, as my attorney-in-fact.

2. **Powers.** The attorney-in-fact, as fiduciary, shall have all powers to provide informed consent for health care decisions on principal's behalf.

3. **Effectiveness.** This power of attorney shall become effective upon the disability or incompetence of the principal. Disability shall include the inability to make health care decisions effectively for reasons such as mental illness, mental deficiency, physical illness or disability, advanced age, chronic use of drugs, chronic intoxication, confinement, detention by a foreign power or disappearance. Disability may be evidenced by a written statement of a qualified physician regularly attending me. Incompetence may be established by a finding of a Court having jurisdiction over me.

4. **Duration.** This power of attorney shall remain in effect to the extent permitted by RCW 11.94 notwithstanding any uncertainty as to whether the principal is dead or alive.

5. **Revocation.** This power of attorney may be revoked in writing by notice mailed or delivered to my attorney-in-fact, and by recording the written instrument of revocation in the office of recorder or auditor of the county of my residence.

6. **Termination.**

   a. By Appointment of Guardian. The appointment of a guardian of the person of the principal terminates this power of attorney. The appointment of a guardian of the property only does not terminate this power of attorney.
   b. By Death of Principal. The death of the principal shall be deemed to revoke this power of attorney upon proof of death being received by the attorney-in-fact.

7. **Reliance.** The designated and acting attorney-in-fact and all persons dealing with the attorney-in-fact shall be entitled to rely upon this power of attorney so long as neither the attorney-in-fact nor person with whom they were dealing at the time of any act taken pursuant to this power of attorney had received actual knowledge or actual notice of the revocation or termination of the power of attorney by death or otherwise, and any action so taken, unless otherwise invalid or unenforceable, shall

Figure 7–4. Durable Power of Attorney.

be binding on the heirs, devisees, legatees, or personal representatives of the principal.

8. Indemnity. The estate of the principal shall hold harmless and indemnify the attorney-in-fact from all liability for acts done in good faith and not in fraud on behalf of the principal.

9. Applicable Law. The laws of the State of Washington shall govern this power of attorney.

10. Execution. This power of attorney is signed on this _____ day of _____, 199 _____ , to become effective as provided in Paragraph 3.

Signature: _____
Print name: _____

STATE OF WASHINGTON)
) ss.
COUNTY OF KING   )

    I certify that I know or have satisfactory evidence that _____ is the person who appeared before me, and said person acknowledged that _____he signed this instrument and acknowledged it to be h_____ free and voluntary act for the uses and purposes mentioned in the instrument.

    DATED: _____

_____
NOTARY PUBLIC in and for the State of Washington residing at _____.
My commission expires: _____

Figure 7–4. *(Continued)*

will request that the medication be given frequently enough to "keep the patient comfortable." Nurses often are reluctant to administer a medication that they realize has a potentially fatal effect when given in that dosage. In such cases the ethical intent of the action is often considered. Medications given for the comfort of the dying patient may be ethically justifiable even if they hasten death to some extent. When nursing staff have difficulty with this issue, a patient conference with an oncology specialist or with a nurse skilled in the area of death and dying will help the staff to clarify values and deal with individual feelings.

Right-to-Die Issues

Much debate currently rages around the issue of maintaining the lives of persons considered to be in a persistent vegetative state. Some of the issues that arise are the patient's rights, the families wishes, and the cost to society. In most cases the problems emerge when the life of a family member is being maintained through support measures that might be considered extraordinary.

In 1991, St. Francis-St. George Hospital in Cincinnati was sued in one of the first cases of its kind. The suit charged that the nurses should not have resuscitated an 82-year-old man when he suffered a heart attack. In so doing they disregarded a "no code" status of the patient ("Hospital Sued," 1991).

Withholding Treatment

Withholding treatment could be considered as negative euthanasia. A historic case occurred in 1963 when a couple on the East Coast gave birth to a premature infant who was diagnosed as having Down's syndrome, with the added complication of an intestinal blockage. The intestinal blockage could be corrected by surgery with minimal risk; without the surgery the child could not be fed and would die. The Down's syndrome, however, would result in some degree of permanent mental retardation. The severity of the retardation could not be determined at birth but would usually run from very low mentality to borderline subnormal intelligence.

The parents (the mother a nurse, the father an attorney) had two normal children at home. They believed that it would be unfair to the other children to raise them with a child with Down's syndrome and refused permission for the corrective operation on the intestinal blockage. Although it was an option, the hospital staff did not seek a court order to override the decision, believing that it was unlikely that the court would sustain an order to operate on the child against the parents' wishes because the child had a known mental handicap and could be a burden to the parents financially and emotionally, and perhaps to society. The child was put in a side room (an interesting action) and was allowed to die, a process that took 11 days. When confronted with the possibility of giving medication to hasten the infant's death, both doctors and nurses were convinced that it was clearly illegal (Gustafson, 1973). Certainly this case represents an extreme of withholding treatment.

The situation above stimulates both ethical and legal questions. Would the approach have been the same if the infant had not been mentally retarded? Would the staff have been guilty of murder if the infant had been given medication to hasten death? If a court decision had been requested and granted to proceed with the surgery, who would have been responsible for the costs incurred? What are the rights of the child? Who advocates for those rights if the child is unable to do so?

On March 22, 1983, federal regulations went into effect that required a sign to be conspicuously posted in nurseries, neonatal intensive care units, and pediatric and maternity wards alerting people to the fact that handicapped infants are accorded protection by the Rehabilitation Act. This act states that no person can be discriminated against on the basis of handicap. Any violation of this act was to be reported to the Department of Health and Human Services (DHHS) for immediate investigation of hospital records. The address and 24-hour hot line telephone number of the DHHS were also to be posted.

The legislation, popularly called the Baby Doe rule, was the result of an Indiana case in which another infant was born afflicted with Down's syndrome and a digestive tract blockage. The parents refused to authorize treatment, although the blockage could have been surgically corrected. Nothing could be done about the Down's syndrome. The hospital sought court guidance. After widespread publicity, President Reagan sent the secretary of the DHHS a memo, reminding him of the Rehabilitation Act. A regulation requiring a posted notice and the establishment of the hot line resulted.

The regulation was challenged by the American Academy of Pediatrics and several other medical groups. Their concern was that the hot line was allowing government agencies to become involved in private medical decisions. After the refusal of a Long Island hospital to allow examination of a baby's medical record and a government suit to obtain the records, a federal judge struck down the regulation. The Ninety-Eighth Congress then attached an amendment to anti–child abuse legislation that required that handicapped infants receive treatment when, in the physician's judgment, such treatment would probably correct or lessen the severity of the child's health problem. It did not require treatment of infants whose condition was irreversible or when care would be futile. Responsibility for monitoring such problems was placed with the state.

Withdrawing Treatment

In some instances the family has sought court orders to have extraordinary life-support measures discontinued. A historic case is that of Karen Quinlan, a young woman left in a vegetative state after suffering severe brain damage as a result of chemical abuse. She was placed on a respirator, and her physicians thought that she would live only a short time if it were to be removed. Her parents requested that the respirator be discontinued, but because she continued to manifest a minor amount of brain activity, their request was refused. After previous petitions to the Supreme Court of New Jersey had been rejected, the courts ruled on March 31, 1976, that her parents could exercise her privacy right on her behalf and the respirator was discontinued. Much to everyone's surprise, Karen continued to live after the respirator was stopped, although she never emerged from her comatose condition; she died in 1986.

A more recent case has attracted equal publicity. In March 1988 Joe and Joyce Cruzan requested through the Jasper County Probate Court they be allowed to remove the gastrostomy tube that kept their daughter Nancy alive. Nancy had been in a persistent vegetative state since an automobile accident in 1983. Although the request was granted, Missouri's attorney general appealed the decision, asking for a clear precedent from a higher court. In June 1990 the U.S. Supreme Court effectively denied the request in asking for "clear and convincing" evidence of the patient's view. In reaching this point, a fine line was drawn between initially withholding medical treatment and later withdrawing it. In Missouri, once the family gives initial consent for treatment they forfeit all power to undo that consent or to stop treatment. No other state has such a law (Colby, 1990). Treatment can be stopped only two ways: if it can be demonstrated that it causes pain or if the patient left behind clear and convincing evidence of his or her wishes prior to incompetency. The first was not an option because of Nancy Cruzan's persistent vegetative state. Therefore, her parents presented a state court with testimony from her physician and three more friends that Nancy would not have wished to continue existing with irreversible brain damage. The circuit court judge ruled that this met the test and Nancy's feeding tube was removed on December 14, 1990. She died on December 26.

Both the Quinlan and the Cruzan cases represent examples of situations in which treatment was withdrawn. Such cases represent hard decisions for all involved and evoke legal, moral, and ethical questions in almost all instances.

Other cases have reached the headlines as individuals and families strive to have more voice in determining issues related to the right to die. In all cases, much conflict exists in the arguments put forth by those supporting the right-to-die and those supporting right-to-life movements. In the fall of 1990, Congress took a major step regarding this issue by passing legislation that requires all Medicare and Medicaid providers to inform patients, on admission, of their right to refuse treatment. The matter is far from settled and will be discussed in greater detail later in this chapter.

Of particular concern to nurses are their own feelings when a decision is reached to remove life-supporting measures, whether they are tube feedings or ventilators. Over the years of caring for the patient, strong emotional attachments often are formed between nurses and patients, even when the patient is in a vegetative state. Nurses who have worked to preserve the patient's dignity have great difficulty "letting go." In some instances, patients have been transferred to other facilities to be allowed to die in an environment where the nurses are not so emotionally involved with the patient.

Positions on Withholding and Withdrawing Treatment

Several organizations or groups have issued guidelines for use of their members and others who would find them useful with regard to the issue of withholding or withdrawing treatment. Key to all of these guidelines is whether the patient is able to make decisions for herself or himself or whether someone else must make those decisions, which is referred to in legal terms as *competent* and *incompetent*.

In 1983, the President's Commission Report, *Deciding To Forego Life-Sustaining Treatment*, focused on the ethical, medical, and legal issues in treatment decisions, especially as applied to individuals who could not make those decisions for themselves. The report distinguished between withholding and withdrawing treatment, referring to "withholding" as not starting treatment, while "withdrawing" meant stopping treatment after it was started. The commission did not make a moral distinction between the two but suggested that more justification may be needed for withholding treatment because the decision would be made without knowledge of the positive effects of treatment. On the other hand, withdrawing treatment is always initiated after it has been determined that the treatment has not helped the patient. The commission concluded that there was not a morally significant difference between decisions to withdraw or withhold treatment (Fry, 1990).

In May 1986 the American Medical Association issued a *Statement on Withholding or Withdrawing Life Prolonging Medical Treatment*. This document stated that life-prolonging medical treatment and artifically or technologically maintained respiration, as well as nutrition and hydration, could be withheld from a patient in an irreversible coma even when death is not imminent.

In 1987 the Office of Technology Assessment of the Congress of the United States issued the results of its study of the use of life-sustaining technologies on elderly persons. This report noted that the most controversial of the technologies was that of nutritional support and pointed out that this issue was emotionally highly charged. They identify that the most troublesome part of nutritional support is whether it is intravenous feeding and hydration or a tube feeding (Fry, 1990).

The Hastings Center issued *Guidelines on the Termination of Life-Sustaining Treatment* in 1987, which provide clear definitions of key terms and a general guideline for making decisions regarding treatment. They view nutrition and hydration as medical interventions that may be foregone in some cases much as other life-sustaining measures (i.e., ventilators) can be foregone in some instances. The *Guidelines* place emphasis on the patient's ability to make decisions and would require careful assessment on a case-by-case basis (Fry, 1990).

In January 1988 the American Nurses' Association issued its *Guidelines on Withdrawing or Withholding Food and Fluid.* In general, these guidelines indicate that there are few instances under which it would be permissible for nurses to withdraw food nor fluid from their patients. Neither the American Nurses' Association or American Medical Association guidelines make a distinction between withholding treatment or withdrawing treatment.

Assisted Death

Much attention has been given to "right to die" issues. The case of an Oregon woman who was said to be suffering from Alzheimer's disease drew national attention. She sought the assistance of a physician in Michigan, who assembled intravenous equipment and medication in the back of his Volkswagen van. The physician then drove the van to a Michigan campground with the woman from Oregon. He set up the medication and started the intravenous solution. She initiated the administration of the solution that would allow her to end her own life. The physician was charged with murder, but when the case came to trial it was thrown out of court because Michigan does not have laws against assisting in a suicide and the Oregon woman's death was a suicide not a murder.

In 1991 the Washington legislature wrestled with a referendum-initiative sponsored by the Washington Citizens for Death with Dignity that would allow patients who are in a medically terminal condition to request and receive "physician aid-in-dying." The initiative permitted a medical procedure to be performed by a physician that would end the life of a "qualified" patient and changed Washington State's Natural Death Act to the Death with Dignity Act. As we go to press the election is yet to be held.

The Right to Refuse Treatment

This issue is very closely aligned to the right to die but carries some special implications that require separate consideration. Although we discussed some of the outer parameters of this issue in the previous section on the right to die, there are some other aspects that can create even bigger problems for the nurse.

The moral, if not legal, precedent for refusing treatment occurred in 1971. Carmen Martinez was dying of hemolytic anemia, a disease that destroys the body's red blood cells. Her life could be maintained by transfusions, but her veins were such that a "cut-down" (a surgical opening made into the vein) was necessary to accomplish the transfusions. Finally Martinez pleaded to have the cut-downs stopped and to be "tortured" no more. The physician, fearful of being charged with aiding in her suicide, asked for a court decision. The court ruled that Martinez was not competent to make such a decision and appointed her daughter as her guardian. When the daughter also asked that no more cut-downs be performed, the compassionate judge honored the daughter's request. He decided that although Martinez did not have the right to commit suicide, she did have the "right not to be tortured." She died the next day (Veatch, 1976).

People working in the health care profession are frequently confronted by such dilemmas. Cases in which a patient refuses to have a leg amputated, although it is evident that not performing the surgery will undoubtedly result in death, frequently make the news. When children are involved, it is even more newsworthy. In such cases the courts usually are involved. A case in Illinois in 1952 is typical. Eight-day-old Cheryl suffered from erythroblastosis fetalis (Rh incompatibility). Her parents, who were Jehovah's Witnesses, refused to authorize the administration of blood that was necessary to save her life. The judge in the case ruled that Cheryl was a neglected dependent and overrode the parent's refusal. In such instances the child is usually made a temporary ward of the court and legal documents are attached to the chart authorizing the needed treatment. Such court decisions usually have been based on the premise that the right to freedom of religion does not give parents the right to risk the lives of their children or to make martyrs of them (Veatch, 1976).

In some cases in which time is not a factor, the court will recommend that treatment be delayed until the child is aged 15 or 16 and can make a decision for himself or herself as an older minor. Other judges will rule just the opposite, deciding that it is cruel to place the burden of the decision on this older minor. Such was the case of Kevin, whose parent's refusal of a blood transfusion made the surgery to correct a deformity of his face and neck too risky to consider. The family court judge ruled against the delay and against letting Kevin participate in the decision on the basis that it would cause him psychological harm if he had to choose between his parents' wishes and his own (Veatch, 1976).

Situations like the above are always difficult for those involved. Because they have the most contact with the patient, nurses in particular must examine their own feelings and attitudes. They must recognize that patients also have the right to attitudes and beliefs. If the nurse decides that his or her own feelings are so strong that they may interfere with the ability to give compassionate care, it would be wise for the nurse to ask to be assigned to other patients.

The right to refuse treatment can take on additional implications when the patient, by refusing one type of treatment, is essentially demanding alternative medical management. Our support of the right to refuse treatment is based on basic beliefs and respect for the autonomy

Figure 7-5. People working in the health care field are frequently confronted with the dilemma of patients who may wish to refuse treatment.

of the patient. When the refusal of medical intervention means that the individual is no longer a patient, it is known as a *negative right simpliciter* by bioethicists. In these cases the patient's physician need only do nothing, as in cases in which the patient discharges himself or herself from the hospital. When the patient refuses treatment but does not withdraw from the role of being patient the matter becomes more complex. An example would be the patient who refuses to have a gangrenous toe surgically removed and demands to have it treated otherwise. Another instance would be a woman with a complete placenta previa who refuses to have a cesarean delivery. These are referred to as positive rights. In the first instance regarding treatment of a gangrenous toe, one form of treatment may be more accepted than the other but both may be successful. In the second instance failure to agree to the cesarean section by a patient with a well-documented placenta previa may virtually doom the interests of both mother and child. Certainly the death of the fetus is highly probable. Should the physician have the right to limit the patients' refusal for treatment when the request for an alternative is unreasonable? The logical approach is informed consent and the sharing of information about the success of various approaches to treatment in the hope that the patient will consider and consent to those with higher success rates. Court intervention would be a less desirable approach.

ADDITIONAL BIOETHICAL CONCERNS

Most of you will probably find the area of bioethics interesting. While many topics are central to the area of bioethics, such as right-to-die, right-to-refuse treatment, and all the issues related to birth, a number of less well-defined concerns are encountered in our health care delivery system. We cannot discuss all of these without creating a separate bioethics textbook; however, several deserve some review.

Organ Transplantation

Developments in the area of organ transplantation have created a number of concerns. In many ways it has necessitated a clearer definition of death. The supply of organs that can be used for transplantation has not been able to keep up with the demand. This is due to the larger number of organs that are being transplanted today. It is also due to the decreased availability of organs as a result of modern technology being used to save more lives.

Concerns About Procurement

Conflicts between the interest of the potential donor and the person receiving the donor organ are easy to anticipate. Certainly no one would want to remove an organ from a donor as long as that person had any potential for recovery. On the other hand, it is imperative that donor organs be removed soon after the death of the host, before the organ to be removed is rendered unusable.

Although there is lack of uniformity in the definition of death throughout the 50 states, it is generally accepted that organs can be removed from donors who have a flat electroencephalogram. This action is based on the 1975 definition of death, which states: "For all legal purposes, a human body with irreversible cessation of total brain function, according to usual and customary standards of medical practice, shall be considered dead" (Capron, 1978, p 300).

The idea of consent again comes into play when we talk about organ transplantation. It is more desirable if the consent can be obtained from the donor. This has been facilitated in many states by the Uniform Anatomical Gift Act, which was drafted by a committee of the National Conference of the Commissions of Uniform State Laws in July 1968 and adopted in all American jurisdictions in 1971 (Hayt, 1977). People who are willing to donate parts of their bodies after death may indicate the desire to do so in a will or other written documents or by carrying a donor's card. Many states now provide a space on driver's licenses where the person can authorize permission for organ donations.

The spouse or the next of kin can also grant permission for the removal of organs after death. However, the time factor is crucial; the deaths are often accidental, and the relatives are often so emotionally distressed at the time that the process of obtaining permission may be difficult. Most medical personnel have at least some initial hesitancy in requesting permission for donor organs at this critical time.

In response to the inadequate supply of organs to meet societal needs—a situation labeled scarce medical resources—some states have passed legislation that requires that donor organs must be requested of the family when it is apparent that the patient has no chance for survival. This brings forth other problems. Who is to be responsible for approaching the family and requesting the organs? Must it be the family's physician? Would critical time be saved if it were the emergency department nurse or hospital social worker? Policymaking groups within the American Hospital Association are currently wrestling with this problem, and protocols are being developed in hospitals. An increasing number of hospitals are designating a nurse as transplantation coordinator to facilitate this process.

Figure 7–6. The need for organs that can be used for transplant has become greater, and obtaining these organs has become more difficult.

An interesting and controversial case occurred in California in 1990. An 18-year-old woman, an only child, was diagnosed as having chronic myelogenous leukemia. Although this form of leukemia responds favorably to bone marrow transplants, no compatible donor could be found after testing the girl's family and contacting the National Marrow Donor Program. In desperation the parents decided to have another child in hopes that the new baby would genetically have matching tissue type. This required that the father have a vasectomy reversed and that the mother, aged 43, go through another pregnancy that terminated in a cesarean section. The baby provided a good match and was able to provide donor tissue for her sister. The case drew considerable attention as medical ethicists voiced concern about creating one child to save another. Citing Immanuel Kant, they argued that the baby was conceived, not as an end in itself, but for utilitarian purposes. Some medical ethicists argue the rights of the individuals involved, saying that it is not the concern of biomedical ethicists to intrude into matters affecting private citizens, especially when that intrusion approaches "intruding into a couple's bedroom." Still others say that striking cases must be brought before the public because an obligation to inform society exists.

The critical need for human organs also causes us to challenge previous decisions. A good example is that raised when considering organs removed from an anencephalic infant. An anencephalic infant is one born with only enough brain to support such vital functions as heartbeat and respiration. It has been estimated that about 60% of these infants are stillborn and of those born alive only about 5% will live more than 3 days (Capron, 1987). Because anencephaly affects only the brain, other organs can be used for transplantation if the infant is kept alive on a respirator until a donor is located. This would challenge our definitions of death. How can current definitions of "brain" death be applied to a condition in which there is no brain as we normally recognize it?

Other problems arise with regard to organ transplantations, especially because there are more people who need organs than there are organs available. The skill of modern technology resulted in the development and implantation of artificial organs such as the heart. Such technological advances were once viewed as science fiction. As a result, historic cases received a great deal of publicity, such as the implantation of an artificial heart in Barney Clark. Over the years the use of artificial organs has not proven effective, and the practice of implanting artificial organs is not common today. This is not true of artificial parts. The use of artificial joints, heart values, and other prostheses continues to grow.

Concerns About Allocation

How will it be determined who will receive a donated organ? Is there any "elitism'" in their distribution, that is, does a white-collar worker have a better chance to receive an organ than does a blue-collar worker? Insurance policies and Medicaid refuse to pay for the cost of many organ transplants, although the cost of corneal transplants and kidney transplants are usually covered by Medicare. Transplants are expensive procedures, often running into several hundreds of thousands of dollars. If money is required "up front," as it sometimes is, where can the needy person procure such funds? Other questions involve both donor and recipient. Should the donor or the donor's family be able to say who will receive the organ? How can one "get in line" for an organ, and how can that need be made known?

In 1982, the father of a child dying because of the need for a liver transplant made national news when he made an impassioned plea before a meeting of the Academy of Pediatrics for them "to keep their eyes and ears open" for a donor for his child. Several days later he received a donation from a family in Salt Lake City, Utah. But his approach has been criticized because his daughter lived while others who needed liver transplants died. Who shall decide?

Much has been written about the problem of selecting recipients for organ transplantation when the number of applicants exceeds the number of available organs. Many criteria have been suggested, and as one might anticipate, these criteria have received arguments both pro and con. The criterion requiring medical acceptability is probably the only exception. Many transplants require that compatibility exist in the tissue and blood type of donor and recipient. It would not be logical to give a much needed organ to a person whose body would automatically reject it.

The criterion of the recipient's social worth is probably one of the hardest to defend, although it was used in the Pacific Northwest in the early 1960s to decide who should be allowed to live by kidney dialysis. Social worth, both of past and future potential, was considered, and even such factors as church membership and participation in community endeavors were considered.

Others suggest some type of random selection once the criterion of medical acceptability has been met. This could be either a natural random selection of the first come, first served variety or an artificial selection process such as a lottery. A criticism of this method is that it removes rational decision making from the process.

We offer no suggestions to solve this problem but merely demonstrate the difficulty it presents. Even the issue of who should serve on the decision-making committee can be touchy. The problem of personal biases is one big concern.

In an effort to gather donations and disseminate information about people who need various organs, an Organ Procurement Program was started in Pittsburgh, Pennsylvania. This program was established to facilitate the matching of donor with recipient and provide a central listing agency for those in need of transplants. Today organ procurement agencies are located in many regions of the country. These groups carry out many activities related to organ procurement including establishing groups for individuals who have received donated organs and their families, publishing newsletters and developing educational materials, increasing public awareness of the need for organs, as well as serving as a clearinghouse for organ procurement and matching. They are connected through the federally funded United Network for Organ Sharing.

Concerns About Individual Property Rights

Concern for an individual's property rights in regard to human tissues has also attracted attention. Biotechnological developments allow profit-oriented companies to use human tissue to generate lucrative products such as drugs, diagnostic tests, and other medically related materials. The modern legal system has consistently held that no property rights are attached to the human body (Swain and Marusyk, 1990). In 1990 a Seattle man sued the University of California, two researchers, and two biotechnology and drug companies. In 1976 he had sought treatment for hairy cell leukemia and subsequently had his spleen removed, which is the standard treatment. It was later discovered that the removed spleen contained unique blood cells that produced a rare blood protein used experimentally in the treatment of certain cancers and possibly the acquired immunodeficiency syndrome. The patient was never told that his cells had great potential value, although he was brought from Seattle to Los Angeles frequently for blood and other tests. His cells were then developed into a self-perpetuating cell line to mass produce the rare blood protein. The patient's suit claimed that the defendants wrongfully converted to their own use his personal property (i.e, the blood cells) and that this was done without his consent. As late as 1991 the courts were still ruling in favor of the University and the drug companies but the issue will undoubtedly continue.

Truth-Telling and Health Care Providers

Although the issue of "to tell" or "not to tell" may not carry the emotional and bioethical impact that one experiences with concerns such as euthanasia, it is one that is frequently encountered in the hospital environment. Despite the fact that informed consent has forced a more straightforward approach between physician and client, the problem of having the patient fully understand the outcome of care still exists. Sometimes the question about telling the patient the expected outcome of care results from a request made by a close relative, but most of the time it results from the persistence of past medical practices.

In such instances the physician operates in a paternalistic role in relation to the patient. Under this model of care, the locus of decision making is moved away from the patient and is now with the physician. "Benefit and do no harm to the patient" is the dictum often cited as the ethical basis for this approach. It rationalizes that complete knowledge of his or her condition would place greater stress on the patient. More recent discussions of medical ethics explore the rights of patients, particularly their right to make their own medical decisions. These discussions emphasize that in our pluralistic society, which has also fostered medical specialization to keep up with advances in knowledge and technology, physicians may be unable to perceive the "best interests" of their patients and act accordingly.

Physicians do not agree on how much patients should know about their condition. We usually experience the major controversy relating to this issue when the patient has a terminal diagnosis such as cancer. Because, ideally at least, physicians are committed to protecting their patients from potential harm, both physical and mental, many have difficulty sharing bad news that will result in unhappiness, anxiety, depression, and fear. These physicians are concerned that if the patients know they are suffering from a terminal illness, they will give up. After all, medical science might be wrong, or research may develop new cures that would change the course of the disease.

Physicians who argue the other side of the issue state that there exists a common moral obligation to tell the truth. They believe that the anxiety of not knowing the accurate diagnosis is at least as great as knowing the truth, especially if the truth is shared in a humane manner. These physicians also argue that one needs to have control over one's life and, if the news is bad, to have time to get personal affairs in order.

Still other physicians choose to deal with the problem in a quasi-truthful manner. Such approaches would include the selection of language that would avoid the word cancer or telling the truth in such a complete and scientific way that the patient would not understand what had been said. For example, if the patient were to be told that he or she has "a neoplasm with the characteristics of leiomyosarcoma with possible secondary metastatic growth," the medical jargon would leave most patients uninformed.

Although to tell or not to tell is a problem that exists between patient and physician, nurses often become involved in it. First of all, the nurse may have definite personal feelings one way or the other. For example, if the physician has decided not to tell the patient, or to delay sharing this information until later, and the nurse believes that the patient has the right to be informed, the nurse may be in a frustrating situation and may even be angry with the physician. Because the nurse is in contact with the patient for a more extended period of time, he or she may be put on the spot by the patient's questions. The nurse may feel that by hedging on a response there is a compromise of the ethics of nursing practice. In such instances a conference, whether formal or impromptu, that would involve the physician, nurses, and other appropriate members of the health team, may help everyone deal with the situation. The nurse who is new to the nursing role in the health care system should realize that anyone can initiate a patient care conference, although appropriate channels of communications should be followed in organizing it.

Thus far we have discussed situations in which information regarding a terminal illness may be shared with the patient and family. At least one other circumstance that involves telling the truth is worth mentioning, although there are many examples that could be included. One that we often see in the obstetrical area of the hospital deals with sharing information with the parents of a newborn who is critical or who has a malformation. Sometimes physicians may want to spare the mother unpleasant news until she is stronger. This occurs frequently enough for obstetrical nurses to have labeled it the *spare-the-mother syndrome*. In other instances the physician may want to delay giving information until suspicions can be validated. If the doctor is waiting for the return of laboratory tests to confirm suspicions of genetic abnormalities, several days may be required. If good communication exists between nurse and physician, so that the nurse is well informed, the nurse can provide emotional support and meet the patient's need for information. Once again, a team approach usually is most effective.

Ethical Concerns and Behavior Control

Before leaving this discussion of bioethical issues, we should say a few words in relation to behavior control. Many people experience extreme discomfort when contemplating research into human behavior. Although it may be one thing to work with atoms, molecules, and genes, it seems quite another to look at the science of human behavior.

Some of the problem seems to center around the fact that people define "acceptable behavior" in different and sometimes conflicting ways. When is behavior deviant? When is the patient mentally ill? An excellent example is that of homosexuality, which at one time was listed by the American Psychiatric Association as a mental illness. Although many people may not approve of homosexuality, they would not classify all homosexuals as being mentally ill. Increasingly, society looks on sexual orientation as a personal matter.

The world has benefited from the work of many people whose behavior might not be looked on as being normal. Van Gogh cut off his ear; Tchaikovsky had terrible periods of depression; Beethoven was known for his uncontrollable rages. Some have suggested that Florence Nightingale's flights into fantasy could better be described as neurosis. Should this behavior have been changed, and by what methods?

We can now change behavior by a variety of methods. Certainly one of the most common methods in which nurses will be involved is the administration of pharmacologic agents. Tranquilizers are now one of the largest classifications of drugs in the United States. Other chemicals, such as alcohol, marijuana, cocaine, and lysergic acid diethylamide (LSD), also change behavior. Some of these are considered socially acceptable, whereas others are not. Some are socially acceptable to some people or to some whole cultures, while unacceptable to others.

Electroconvulsive therapy, known earlier as electric shock therapy, has been used for years to treat severe depression. Although antidepressant drugs are more commonly used today, most nurses who were enrolled in psychiatric nursing courses in the 1950s had some experience assisting with electric shock therapy. Opponents of this form of therapy, who see it as inhumane, are becoming an organized political force. Proponents point out that with the current safeguards, it can be an effective therapy.

Psychosurgery, for example, frontal lobotomy (portrayed in *One Flew Over the Cuckoo's Nest*), has been used since the 1930s. This is undoubtedly one of the most criticized of treatment modalities because of its effect on the person. Its use has greatly decreased.

Psychotherapy can change other behavior. This technique includes verbal and nonverbal communication between the patient and the therapist. Although psychotherapy requires considerable time, it is widely used.

When are any of these methods justified? Who makes the decision? What behavior is beyond the realm of acceptability? Who determines this? How does behavior control mesh with our beliefs about the autonomy of the individual or with concepts of self-respect and dignity? The issues of power and coercion pose a concern at this point. Problems related to involuntary commitment have moved this from the arena of ethics to that of legal determinants.

Halleck (1981, p 268) has defined behavior control as treatment "imposed on or offered to the patient that, to a large extent, is designed to satisfy the wishes of others. Such treatment may lead to the patient's behaving in a manner which satisfies his community or his society." Halleck goes on to point out that the question of behavior control has become more critical because newer drugs and new behavior therapy (such as aversive therapy and desensitization) make it possible to change specific behavior more rapidly and effectively. Traditional psychotherapy, which works slowly, offered the patient time in which to contemplate the change and reject it if it was unacceptable.

Dworkin (1981, p 278) has proposed a set of guidelines that preserve autonomy in behavior control. Briefly stated here, these guidelines include the following:

We should favor those methods of influencing behavior that support the self-respect and dignity of those who are being influenced.

Methods of influence that destroy or decrease a person's ability to think rationally and in his or her own interest should not be used.

Methods of influence that fundamentally affect the personal identity of the person should not be used.

Methods of influence that deceive or keep relevant facts from the person should not be used.

Modes of influence that are not physically intrusive are preferable to those that are (such as drugs, psychosurgery, and electricity).

A person should be able to resist the method of influence if he or she so desires, and changes of behavior that are reversible are preferable to those that are not.

Methods that work through the cognitive and affective structure of a person are preferable to those that "short-circuit" his beliefs and desires and cause him to be passively receptive to the will of others.

Rationing of Health Care

As we move into the 21st century perhaps no issue in health care will receive more attention than that which deals with the rationing of health care. Technology has allowed people to live longer and longer. New treatment modalities have become more and more expensive. Dollars do not exist within our current social system to make all forms of health care available to all who may wish to receive it? What should be treated and what should not? Who should receive the treatment and who should not? Should age be a factor? Mental status? Ability to contribute to society?

A number of states have begun to wrestle with these issues. In 1989 the Oregon legislature passed a package of statues that, among other things, created a process by which health care priorities would be established so that Medicaid and state-encouraged private coverage could provide the most cost-effective and beneficial forms of care for the largest number of persons. Implicit in this legislation was the involvement of the public in the process of building consensus on the values to be used to guide health resource allocation decisions.

In Vermont a statewide public education and discussion project was initiated that was designed to explore public attitudes and values that underlie health care and the public's priorities in the allocation of health resources. The project focused on the need for individuals to make known their preferences with regard to personal treatment.

In New Jersey a Citizens' Committee on Biomedical Ethics has taken the position that citizens have the right and responsibility to insist that their preferences and values influence the development of health care policies and the allocation of medical resources. They have launched into a community health program to clarify the ethical and social issues surrounding the provision of health care in that state.

Other states are following the examples set. Citizens are being asked to make informed decisions regarding health care. As a nurse you have a vital role to play in the sharing of information regarding the delivery of services. It is critical that you have anticipated some of the questions you may be asked and have analyzed your own values.

CONCLUSION

There are no easy answers to many of the issues we have presented, and we have only scratched the surface of concerns that face us. In many instances the courts have been asked to help the public make decisions. In some instances the churches have also been asked to assist with ethical issues. Other times the profession as a whole has developed codes of conduct. Currently we see the general public being asked to assume responsibility for some of the decision making.

Many times the decision is made at the individual level. It is not to be anticipated that the issues will grow smaller in number or that decisions will be easier to make; just the opposite should be expected. Technology, longevity, and personal rights all expand the dimensions of the decisions that must be made.

As you consider all the many issues presented in this chapter, we hope that you will endeavor to keep an open mind toward all points of view. You will, of course, make your personal decision, but do not let that blind you to the factors in someone else's life that may bring her or him to another decision. There is an old saying that we cannot really understand what it is like for another person until we have "walked a mile in his moccasins." This is especially true with ethical issues. Nurses must strive to remain open to other people if they are to function most effectively in their professional role.

REFERENCES

Backmun H: Majority opinion in Roe vs Wade. *In* Mappes TA, Zembaty JS: Biomedical Ethics, 2nd ed, pp 478–482. New York, McGraw-Hill Book Company, 1981

Capron AM: Death, definition and determination of: Legal aspects. In Reich WT: Encyclopedia of Bioethics, vol 1, p 300. New York, Free Press, 1978

Colby WH: Missouri stands alone. Hastings Center Rep 20(5):5–6, 1990

Dworkin G: Autonomy and behavior control. In Mappes TA, Zembaty JS: Biomedical Ethics, 2nd ed, pp 273–280. New York, McGraw-Hill Book Company, 1981

Fromer MJ: Ethical Issues in Health Care. St Louis, CV Mosby, 1981

Fry ST: New ANA guidelines on withdrawing or withholding food and fluid from patients. *In* Lindeman CA, McAthie M: Readings: Nursing Trends and Issues, pp 499–507. Philadelphia, Springhouse, 1990

Gustafson JJ: Mongolism, parental desires, and the right to life. Perspect Biomed, Summer 1973, p 529

Halleck SL: Legal and ethical aspects of behavior control. *In* Mappes TA, Zembaty JS: Biomedical Ethics, 2nd ed, pp 267–273. New York, McGraw Hill Book Company, 1981

Hayt LR: Medicolegal Aspects of Hospital Records, 2nd ed, p 397. Berwyn, IL, Physicians' Record Company, 1977

Hellegers AE: Bioethical debates in gynecology and obstetrics. *In* Romney SL et al: Gynecology and Obstetrics: The Health Care of Women, p 36. New York, McGraw-Hill Book Company, 1975

Hosital sued for "wrongful life." Am J Nurs, May 91(5):111, 1991

Macklin R: Artificial means of reproduction and our understanding of the family. Hastings Center Rep 21(1):5–11, 1991

Mancini M: Nursing, minors, and the law. Am J Nurs 78(1):124–127, 1978

Roe v Wade, 410 U.S. 113 (1973)

Rothman DA, Rothman NL: The Professional Nurse and the Law. Boston, Little, Brown & Co, 1977

Rothstein MA: The challenge of the new genetics. Natl Forum 69(4):39–40, 1990

Thomas CL: Taber's Cyclopedic Medical Dictionary, 16th ed. Philadelphia, FA Davis, 1990

Swain MS, Marusyk RW: An alternative to property rights in human tissue. Hastings Center Rep 20(5):12–15, 1990

Veatch RM: Death, Dying and the Biological Revolution. New Haven, CT, Yale University Press, 1976

FURTHER READINGS

Arras GJ: Crazy making: Embryos and gestational mothers. Hastings Center Rep 21(1):35–38, 1991

Arras JD: Anencephalic newborns as organ donors: A critique. JAMA 259:2284–2286, 1988

Bailey LL: Organ transplantation: A paradigm of medical progress. Hastings Center Rep 20(1):24–28, 1990

Battin MP: The least worst death: Biotechnology and the right to die. Natl Forum 69(4):36–38, 1989

Chervenak FA, McCollough LB: Justified limits on refusing intervention. Hastings Center Rep 21(2):12–18, 1991

Colbert T: Public input into health care policy: Controversy and contribution in California. Hastings Center Rep 20(5):21, 1990

Cranford RE: A hostage to technology. Hastings Center Rep 20(5): 9–10, 1990

Crawshaw R: A vision of the health decisions movement. Hastings Center Rep 20(5):21–22, 1990

Daniels N: Duty to treat or right to refuse? Hastings Center Rep 21(2):36–46, 1991

Ellman IM: Can others exercise an incapacitated patient's right to die? Hastings Center Rep 20(1):47–50, 1990

Fowler MD: The role of the clinical ethicist. Heart Lung 15(5):318–319, 1989

Garland MJ, Hasnain R: Health care in common: Setting priorities in Oregon. Hastings Center Rep 20(5):16–18, 1990

Gaylin W: Fooling with mother nature. Hastings Center Rep 20(1):17–21, 1990

Guido GW: Legal Issues in Nursing: A Source Book for Practice. Norwalk, CT, Appleton & Lange, 1988

HHS stands by "Baby Doe" policy despite court's ruling on regs. Am J Nurs, June 1983, pp 83(6):851, 868–869

Hill TP: Giving voice to the pragmatic majority in New Jersey. Hastings Center Rep 20(5):20, 1990

Jecker NS, Pearlman RA: Ethical constraints on rationing medical care by age. J Am Geriatr Soc 37(11):1067–1075, 1989

Lauritzen P: What price parenthood? Hastings Center Rep 20(2): 38–46, 1990

Lippman H: After Cruzan: The right to die. RN 54(1):65–68, 73, 1991

Lynn J, Glover J: Cruzan and caring for others. Hastings Center Rep 20(5):10–11, 1990

Macklin R: Ethical principles, individual rights, and medical practices. Natl Forum 69(4):25–27, 1989

Moss RJ, La Puma J: The ethics of mechanical restraints. Hastings Center Rep 21(1):22–25, 1991

Nurses seek a voice in right-to-die cases. Am J Nurs, March 91(3):26, 1991

Overall C: Selective termination of pregnancy and women's reproductive autonomy. Hastings Center Rep 20(3):6–11, 1990

Pence T: Ethics in Nursing: An Annotated Bibliography, pt 2. Publication No. 20-1989. New York, National League for Nursing, 1986

Powledge TM: Capital report—springtime for fetal tissue research? Hastings Center Rep 21(2):5–6, 1991

Robertson JA: Cruzan: No rights violated. Hastings Center Rep 20(5):8–9, 1990

Rousseau PC: How fluid deprivation affects the terminally ill. RN 54(1):73–74, 1991

Veatch RM: Bioethics discovers the bill of rights. Natl Forum 69(4):11–13, 1989

Vernale C, Packard SA: Organ donation as gift exchange. Image 22(4):239–242, 1990

Wendling EM: Anencephalics as organ donors. Imprint, April/May 1990, pp 47–48

Wurzbach ME: The dilemma of withholding or withdrawing nutrition. Image 22(4):226–230, 1990

Unit III
Economic and Political Aspects of Health Care Delivery

Health care in the United States is part of the overall economic and political life of the nation. It reflects much of what is best about life in the United States but also serves to point out those areas where serious problems exist.

In this unit we try to help you understand the health care delivery system in a basic way. The complexity of the system as it exists cannot be completely explained in one short chapter, but we have tried to focus on those aspects that will best help you put health care issues into context. From an overview of the system, we move to the issue of collective bargaining and how it affects nursing. The political process and how that relates to health care is the final chapter in this unit. Our hope is that you will find an understanding of the political process relevant to your professional life.

8

The Health Care Delivery System

Objectives

After completing this chapter, you should be able to

1. *Define primary health care provider.*

2. *Outline some of the problems related to the use of the nurse practitioner and the physician's assistant as primary health care providers.*

3. *Differentiate between the terms* technologist *and* technician *and* therapist *and* therapy technician.

4. *Describe the various agencies and institutions that provide health care to the community.*

5. *Identify problems related to the distribution and supply of health care providers.*

6. *Discuss the reasons for people using means other than the conventional health care system to meet health needs.*

7. *Describe the distribution of power in the health care system.*

8. *Discuss the impact of cost containment on health care delivery.*

9. *Define prospective payment and discuss how diagnosis-related groups are used in relationship to prospective payment.*

We refer to the health care system as if it were an organized entity, with each part relating to another in a systematic way. In reality it is often more like a nonsystem of many diverse people and organizations, each going in its own direction. There is no central authority in the U.S. health care system, no setting of overall priorities, and no general planning for the use of resources. There are private components and governmental components, nonprofit sectors and profit-making sectors, and individuals and groups all operating independently.

Although this nonsystem is chaotic, it has produced some of the most significant advances in medicine and health care ever seen. At the same time there is a maldistribution of the benefits of those advances, as attested to by such factors as the high infant mortality rate in the United States, which exceeds that of many other major industrialized nations (Hughes et al., 1989). Some people receive outstanding health

Figure 8–1. Many different factors are affecting the health care that can be provided.

care in the most modern of settings. Others receive no health care. Health insurance grows ever more expensive, and many working people are unable to afford coverage for their families (Hudson Institute, 1987). Society appears to stagger under the increasing costs of governmental programs such as Medicare and Medicaid (Kenkel, 1990).

To help you understand some of the concerns regarding the health care delivery system, we first introduce the various categories of care providers in the system and then will explore the organizations that help to shape the system. Issues and trends related to each of these areas are discussed as they arise.

COLLEAGUES IN HEALTH CARE

Many different groups of individuals deliver health care. All of these providers exist because they meet the needs of our society in some way. Some of these groups are believed to be valuable, but others are the subject of considerable debate.

More than 230 types of health care workers have been identified within the United States. It is not within the scope of this book to discuss each of these occupations individually, but we do attempt to outline the general categories of health care providers with whom you may be working.

Primary Health Care Providers

The primary health care provider furnishes entry into the health care system. This person is consulted by the patient for routine health maintenance, as well as for care of episodic illness. This health care provider has traditionally been a medical doctor, osteopathic physician, or dentist. These professionals are licensed in all states and are authorized to treat illness, including the prescribing of drugs. Some nurses are moving into this area of practice as *nurse practitioners*.

Medical Care Providers

The differences between traditional (allopathic) medicine and osteopathic medicine are becoming less distinct. Historically, the philosophy of care and remedial techniques of osteopathic physicians included more treatments such as back manipulation and nutritional counseling, while fewer drugs were prescribed and less surgery was performed. Osteopathic physicians and allopathic physicians practiced entirely independently of each other and used separate hospitals; a visible antagonism between the two groups was often apparent. Recently the move has been toward greater cooperation, with physicians from both traditions practicing side by side in hospitals. The osteopathic group is considerably smaller, has far fewer specialists, has fewer resources for research, and is less well known. However, the educational patterns for both are the same.

Undergraduate medical education may vary in focus, but a strong science background is required. This is followed by 4 years of medical school. During this time formal education is stressed, with patient contact occurring most often at the latter part of the program. Some medical schools are beginning to provide patient contact earlier in the educational process. After completion of medical school, licensing examinations are taken.

Once individuals are licensed as physicians, they then participate in a residency program. These programs are developed by hospitals and primarily focus on patient care. Their length varies depending on the specialty. The resident is paid a salary by the hospital. In state, county, and city hospitals the resident physician may serve as the primary physician for some patients. For patients who are responsible for their own medical bills (either directly or through insurance), the admitting personal physician usually remains in charge and the resident serves a supporting role in the patient's medical care. At the end of the residency, the physician is able to practice independently.

An issue of current concern in medical education is the demands made on resident physicians. When they are "on call," they sometimes find themselves working 24, 36, and even 48 hours without sleep. Residents have questioned the safety of this practice in the complexity of modern health care. Legislation has been introduced (but not passed) in some states that would limit the number of hours a resident could be required to remain on duty. Nurses working with residents have a responsibility to help maintain safety when pressures are high.

After residency training is completed, the physician is prepared to write examinations to become certified in the specialty by passing an examination. The person who successfully passes the specialty examination is termed *board certified*. It is not legally required that a physician be board certified to practice in a specialty area.

Subspecialty training takes place after completion of specialty training. Given this pattern of education and training a physician may have a total of 10 or more years of postsecondary education and training before beginning to work independently.

Podiatrists (formerly called chiropodists) are educated in the care and surgery of the foot. They care for corns, bunions, and toenails; prescribe and fit corrective shoes and arch supports; and perform surgery on the feet, such as correction of deformities, removal of bunions, and removal of small tumors. A podiatrist does not prescribe systemic medication or care for any generalized disease condition.

As demands on the system have increased, additional people have been added to the group of primary care providers. Nurses working in specialized roles as primary care nurses or nurse practitioners are one example. These nurses have obtained education in addition to that required for basic licensure and have earned certification in a particular specialty. Nurse practitioners may work with a physician in an office or clinic, or they may function independently in a nurse clinic. Some states grant nurse practitioners who meet special guidelines the authority to write prescriptions. This type of authority is the subject of heated debate in other states.

Another primary caregiver is the physician's assistant. This person, also called the *medex,* often has medical and emergency training, such as from the military service or other health occupations, and has completed a university program. Physician's assistant programs vary from 1-year to 4-year baccalaureate programs. Physician's assistants must work under the direction of a physician at all times.

Physician's assistants usually see patients with commonly recurring health problems such as colds, flu, and minor trauma, such as cuts needing suturing. Physician's assistants may also provide some primary health care such as routine physical examinations. If the patient needs referral to a specialist or hospital admission, the physician's assistant first refers the patient to the physician with whom he or she works. In some instances the physician's assistant may work with a specialty physician such as an orthopedic physician and have different responsibilities, such as applying and removing casts.

The use of physician's assistants is sometimes controversial. Some patients believe that they are receiving less than quality care if they are treated by a physician's assistant instead of seeing the physician. Within the health care team, the appropriateness of physician's assistants writing prescriptions and orders on the charts of hospitalized patients has been questioned. Nurses have been concerned because their own licensure laws state that they can administer medications only on the order of a licensed physician, osteopath, or dentist, and in some instances they have been asked to give medications on the order of a physician's assistant. In the state of Washington a court decision stated that nurses should not give medications ordered by a physician's assistant until those orders are countersigned by a physician.

Another area of concern has been whether nurses working in expanded roles should be classified as physician's assistants and be governed by the board of medicine rather than the board of nursing. Some nurses have enrolled in and completed the regular physician's assistant programs and are working in this capacity. Other nurses believe strongly that the role of the nurse is an independent one and that the nurse in primary care should not be considered a physician's assistant but rather an independent nurse. The American Nurses Association (ANA) has supported the view that the nurse in primary care is more than a physician's assistant and should not be included in that classification.

Other Primary Care Providers

Social workers and clinical psychologists also perform a primary care role by providing a person's entry into the mental health care system, serving as the supervisors of care, and furnishing referral as needed. Because they are not able to treat physical problems, they often work in cooperation with physicians or nurse practitioners who are able to manage this aspect of care.

Optometrists provide vision testing and prescribe glasses, contact lenses, and corrective exercises for eye problems. They have a general background in assessment of eye disease so that they can screen and refer patients to an ophthalmologist (a physician who specializes in eye disease) when diagnosis and treatment are needed. Because ophthalmologists offer some of the same services as optometrists there is some disagreement between the two groups over scope of practice.

Dentists provide for primary care of the teeth and mouth. Many dentists are beginning to include general health screening, such as examining the mouth and throat for tumors or disease and taking blood pressure in their basic examination. The patient is referred to a physician if an abnormality is noted. Dentists have an educational background similar in length to that of the physician—4 years of baccalaureate education followed by dental school. There is no residency period, and dentists begin independent practice after passing state licensing examinations. Dentists are empowered to prescribe medications in addition to providing care for the mouth and teeth. There are specialty areas in dentistry, such as orthodontics (the application of devices to change the occlusion of the teeth), just as there are in medicine. Education for specialties takes place in universities that have dental schools. After the student has graduated, his or her diploma indicates competence in the specialty. There is no legal requirement for advanced education to practice a dental specialty, although there are strong professional constraints.

Issues Related to Primary Health Care

One of the problems in U.S. health care is maldistribution of private care providers. Urban areas have proportionately more health workers of every kind than do rural areas. Within large cities, care providers are concentrated in more affluent areas. Many programs that would provide an incentive to establish a practice in an area that is insufficiently served have been attempted. Some of these programs include educational loans that are forgiven or canceled if the person works in an underserved area after completion of the course of study. In other instances schools have tried to recruit students from underserved areas, hoping that after graduation the student would return home to practice. Some schools incorporate into their programs learning experiences in rural or poorly served areas in the hope that graduates may be attracted to the area and return later to work.

Despite these efforts the problem still exists for several reasons. Physicians prefer to practice where there is access to specialized medical centers and where opportunities for consultation are readily available. Another factor that deters physicians from practicing in rural areas is the tremendous physical strain involved in being the only care provider. The rural physician often receives little respite from 24-hours-a-day, 7-days-a-week availability to the community. Incomes of rural physicians also tend to be less than incomes of physicians in urban areas. Nurse practitioners increasingly are providing health care to underserved populations and have been more willing to relocate in rural or poverty areas.

The large number of specialty physicians compared with the number of physicians in family practice is another problem in the system. The current emphasis on family practice in many medical schools and the increase in numbers of family practice residencies are helping to alleviate this situation.

The trend in private medical practice is toward group practices. Several specialties may be represented within the group. Although patients may have a private physician, they may easily receive care from other members of the group. Group practice assures the individual physician of more time for personal and family life.

Care in private practice usually is based on fee for service. Although some physicians may attempt to make adjustments for those with less ability to pay, one of the serious health care problems of our day is the cost of health care for even middle class individuals. Insurance may pay for some outpatient care, and it funds most of the care given during hospitalization, but increasing numbers of people have inadequate or no insurance.

Allied Health Care Workers

Allied health care workers are categorized in many ways. Frequently the term *technologist* is used to refer to those with baccalaureate preparation and *technician* is used to identify those with 2 years of education or less. The term *therapist* usually denotes more advanced functioning than *therapy technician*. Most of the allied health care professions provide diagnostic and treatment services for patients. Some, such as those who work with records, serve roles to support the system.

Laboratory and Diagnostic Services

Included in the category of laboratory and diagnostic occupations are those who work in the clinical laboratory, such as the medical technologist and medical laboratory technician, as well as those who work in all the specialized diagnostics fields, such as nuclear medicine technician, electroencephalograph technician, and radiologic technician. They assist with all of the tests that are now used to diagnose and monitor progress in illness. As new sophisticated diagnostic technology is introduced, new technicians are created to operate and monitor the equipment. Some technicians, such as the medical technologist, require a baccalaureate degree. Others, such as the radiology technician and medical laboratory technician, usually have 2-year associate degrees. Still others, such as the electrocardiographic (ECG) technician, may be trained on the job.

Administrative and Business Personnel

As health care facilities have become more complex, the administrative and business aspects have similarly become more demanding. Many people are needed to maintain and retrieve information from the medical record. These workers include the medical record administrator, the medical record technician, and the medical secretary.

The posts of hospital administrator and assistant administrator are undergoing change. In the past these posts may have been filled by a physician, an attorney, or a businessman. Because the health care system now has such specialized demands, the administrative positions are increasingly being filled by those with a baccalaureate or master's degree in health care administration. A special certification is required of those who administer nursing homes.

Community Health Care Workers

As a growing field, community health has required an increasing number of workers. The major focus of community health care is the promotion of health rather than care of illness. Some workers, such as the health educator and community health visitor, work directly with individual clients. Others, such as the sanitarian, are engaged in assisting the community as a whole toward better health through maintenance of standards related to cleanliness and infectious disease control.

Other community health care workers are those who help individuals with health and personal care after discharge from the hospital. Although some of these positions are held by registered nurses who provide skilled care, many more are held by home health aides who assist with nontechnical aspects of care and may even help with household tasks and shopping. Education for home health aides is almost entirely conducted as on-the-job training.

Makers of Prosthetic and Assistive Devices

With technological advances, the number of different types of prostheses and assistive devices increases. Those who make and fit devices such as eyeglasses, braces, and artificial limbs need specialized education. They do not usually have licenses. Most are employed by health care institutions, although some (e.g., dispensing opticians who make eyeglasses) may be in private business.

Dietary Services

The nutritionist or dietitian spends a large percentage of time planning for the special dietary needs of patients as a group, that is, determining the menu for those on a diabetic diet, a low-salt diet, or any other special diet provided by the facility. In addition, dietitians work with individual patients in planning appropriate diets and teaching nutrition. Registered dietitians have 4 years of college plus an internship. Dietetic technicians have a 2-year associate degree education.

Respiratory Care

Those who provide direct care related to respiratory treatments and the use of respiratory devices are called respiratory therapists, respiratory technicians, and inhalation therapists. Many are educated in associate degree programs. Some have on-the-job training only; others have baccalaureate degrees. They are employed by hospitals and may provide patient teaching, as well as specific treatments in respiratory care.

Pharmacy Services

The pharmacist has a baccalaureate degree in pharmacy. In many universities a pharmacy program includes clinical work in a hospital or other patient care setting. Although pharmacists are principally involved with dispensing medications, they also provide drug therapy consultation to physicians and nurses and directly teach patients how to comply with their drug regimens. Many pharmacies also employ on-the-job trained pharmacy technicians to complete certain routine tasks in the pharmacy.

Physical Therapy

The physical therapist is educated in a 1-year postbaccalaureate program or a 4-year baccalaureate program. The focus of physical therapy is the restoration of normal function of large muscle groups, bones, and joints. Treatment includes exercise, heat and cold therapy, electrical stimulation, and the use of other physical agents. The physical therapist also teaches the patient to use crutches, prostheses, and other assistive devices. There is a strong movement within the profession that advocates the master's degree as the requirement for practice as a physical therapist. Physical therapy technicians are educated in 2-year associate degree programs and work with registered physical therapists in carrying out planned therapeutic regimens.

Occupational Therapist

The occupational therapist focuses on restoring fine motor skills and the ability to accomplish activities of daily living. Treatment includes exercise, the making of splints and assistive devices, and identifying ways to modify the environment to make the performance of daily living activities possible. Meaningful activities such as crafts and games are often used to provide needed exercise. Occupational therapists also provide diversional activities that are appropriate to the patient's strength, ability, and interest or that are designed to achieve physical or psychosocial goals for the patient. The occupational therapist has a baccalaureate degree and a 1-year internship. Occupational therapy technicians have associate degrees and carry out plans for therapy that have been established by the registered occupational therapist.

Other Specific Therapies

Many health occupations involve the provision of specific types of therapy. The speech pathologist and radiation therapy technician are among these. Also included in this group, but more rarely seen, are the music therapist, the bibliotherapist, and the art therapist.

Only a few of the many different health occupations have been mentioned here. Table 8-1 outlines some common health occupations and identifies the educational level and credentialing of each.

(Text continues on page 301)

Table 8–1. Occupations in Health Care With Corresponding Level of Education and Type of Credential

	Educational Requirement					Credentialing		
Occupational Group	*Less Than 1 Year*	*1 Year*	*Associate Degree*	*Bacca-laureate*	*Post-bacca-laureate*	*Professional Certification or Registration*	*Legal License*	*None*
Primary Care Providers								
Clinical psychologist					4 yr plus		X*	
Dentist					4 yr		X	
Doctor of medicine					5 yr plus		X	
Doctor of osteopathy					5 yr plus	X	X	
Doctor of podiatry					3–4 yr	X	X	
Nurse practitioner			X		1 yr		X	
Optometrist			X	plus	4 yr		X	
Physician's assistant	X———————			X		X	X*	
Administrative and Business								
Hospital administrator					1–2 yr			
Medical records administrator				X——	1–2 yr	X		
Medical records technician			X			X		
Medical transcriptionist			X			X		
Medical secretary		X				X		X
Medical assistant	X					X		X
Ward manager	X———		X					X

(continued)

Table 8–1. *Occupations in Health Care With Corresponding Level of Education and Type of Credential (continued)*

	Educational Requirement					Credentialing		
Occupational Group	Less Than 1 Year	1 Year	Associate Degree	Bacca-laureate	Post-bacca-laureate	Professional Certification or Registration	Legal License	None
Laboratory and Diagnostic Services								
EEG technician	X————		————X					
ECG technician	X————		————X					
Cytology technician						X		
Medical technologist				X		X		
Medical laboratory technician			X			X		
Radiologic technologist			X————	————X		X		
Direct Care Services								
Registered nurse			X————	————X		X	X	
Practical nurse		X					X	
Nursing assistant	X							X
Dietitian					1 yr	X		
Dietetic technician			X			X		
Emergency medical technician	X					X		
Paramedic	X————	————X				X		

(continued)

Table 8–1. *Occupations in Health Care With Corresponding Level of Education and Type of Credential* (continued)

Occupational Group	Educational Requirement					Credentialing		
	Less Than 1 Year	1 Year	Associate Degree	Bacca-laureate	Post-bacca-laureate	Professional Certification or Registration	Legal License	None
Specific Therapies								
Child life worker (play therapist)				X				X
Occupational therapist				X		X		
Occupational therapy technician			X			X		
Pharmacist				X			X	
Pharmacy technician	X							
Physical therapist				X —— 1 yr		X		
Physical therapy technician			X			X		
Speech pathologist				X		X		
Radiation therapy technician		X —— X				X		
Recreation therapist				X				X
Respiratory therapist			X			X		

(continued)

299

Table 8-1. **Occupations in Health Care With Corresponding Level of Education and Type of Credential** (continued)

Occupational Group	Educational Requirement					Credentialing		
	Less Than 1 Year	1 Year	Associate Degree	Bacca-laureate	Post-bacca-laureate	Professional Certification or Registration	Legal License	None
Makers of Prosthetic and Assistive Devices								
Prosthetist				X				
Prosthetics technician			X					
Optician	X		X			X	X*	
Community Health								
Health educator				X				X
Community health worker	X							X
Environmental technologist				X				X
Environmental technician			X					X

X——— X indicates that preparation varies between categories marked.
* Licensure in some states, not all.

300

AGENCIES AND ORGANIZATIONS PROVIDING CARE

Many different institutions are involved in providing various types of health care within our communities. It has been estimated that there are over 7000 hospitals, 26,000 long-term care facilities, and 4000 community health agencies in the United States (American Hospital Association, 1987).

Acute Care Hospitals

The traditional hospital is changing in many ways because of the demands of modern health care. More and more the hospital is used only for those in need of short-term acute care, a situation that is largely due to the increasing cost of care in the highly technological environment of the hospital. These costs reflect the vast amount of specialized equipment that is used, the number of laboratories needed, the specialized operating rooms and treatment facilities, and the many people employed in the modern hospital. For each hospitalized person, more than four people are employed (Williams and Torrence, 1988). This includes maintenance, kitchen, and office workers as well as health care personnel. Although at one time hospital workers were poorly paid in comparison with the rest of the community's workers, collective bargaining has changed this. Hospital workers are no longer willing to subsidize the cost of health care by receiving substandard wages.

After World War II health care moved more and more into hospitals and large medical centers. The diagnostic and treatment methods used required a high degree of skill, and everyone was in favor of using the best technology. However, having those in this environment who did not need the technology created enormous cost burdens. A desire to limit these cost burdens resulted in changes in reimbursement that created incentives for early discharge to home or to long-term care facilities and the provision of more services on an outpatient or ambulatory care basis. The acute care hospital of today has become a center for delivering specialized care to a severely ill population.

The demands of accrediting bodies, state governments, third-party payers, and patients have all helped to shape today's hospitals. Also, through financial support for building hospitals and the regulations regarding the use of the federal funds such as Medicare and Medicaid, the federal government has gained a great deal of control over the operation of health care institutions.

Each hospital must be licensed by the state in which it is located. The licensure requirements vary among states. In addition to the required state licensure, almost all hospitals adhere to national standards through seeking voluntary accreditation by the Joint Commission for the Accreditation of Healthcare Organizations (JCAHO). This organization is often referred to as the "Joint Commission." Many third-party payers, such as Medicare and Medicaid, require that a hospital be accredited by the JCAHO to receive reimbursement for care provided. The JCAHO has been effective in influencing hospital construction, operation, and evaluation by means of its criteria for accreditation.

The JCAHO is composed of members of the American College of Surgeons, the American Hospital Association, the American Society of Internal Medicine, and the American Medical Association. A consumer representative also serves on the board. Although nursing is a major focus of hospital care, there is no designated seat for nursing. The ANA has tried many times to become part of the JCAHO but has repeatedly been refused. Nurses have testified about nursing practice standards, served on subcommittees of the JCAHO, and have been employed individually by the JCAHO in a variety of positions related to accrediting. Continuing efforts are being made by both consumer and professional groups to broaden the representation on the JCAHO board.

Public hospitals are those owned by state or local governmental agencies. These hospitals often provide low-cost or free care to those without financial resources and may serve as the primary source of care for those receiving assistance under the Medicaid program. The federal government also operates hospitals for specific groups, such as veterans, the military and their dependents, and certain Indian tribes. These hospitals are administered through different branches of the federal government, which works against any system-wide planning. Private hospitals include both proprietary (profit making) and voluntary (nonprofit) hospitals. Private nonprofit hospitals may actually make a profit on operations, but any profit must be used for hospital maintenance and expansion whereas the profit-making hospital directs profits to stockholders.

Policy and direction for a hospital are usually provided by a governing board. In the public hospital this board may be composed of elected officials or may be appointed by elected officials. Federal hospitals do not have individual governing boards but are directed by the rules and regulations of the federal agency responsible for their function. Proprietary (profit making) hospitals are directed by the board of the corporation owning the hospital. Nonprofit hospitals often have boards composed of influential members of the community. The board, itself, may recommend and elect any new members. In many areas consumers are seeking greater representation on hospital governing boards. This is especially true if the hospital is supported by public donations. The governing board of a hospital has ultimate responsibility for its legal and financial management.

The actual functioning of the hospital is directed by a chief administrator, or executive officer, and a wide range and diversity of divisions and departments and their administrators. Acute care hospitals are complex, big businesses. The budget of one hospital patient care unit may be over $1 million a year.

The medical staff of a hospital, composed of those primary health care providers with authority to admit patients, governs medical practice within the facility. Although the ultimate responsibility for all hospital matters rests with the board, the usual practice is for the medical staff to make recommendations in the area of medical care for board action. This includes establishing rules that govern the medical staff and monitoring and evaluating medical care. The medical staff consults with and advises the administration in regard to other concerns such as the need for new equipment. Any person who wants to admit patients must apply for membership on the medical staff. In some areas nurse practitioners have been seeking authority to admit patients to hospitals. Physicians and their organizations (such as the American Medical Association) have generally opposed opening staff privileges to additional categories of health care providers.

Historically the deliberations and decisions of a medical staff in regard to individual health care practitioners have been confidential. For example, a physician whose privileges to practice were removed for substandard practice would be free to go to another community and seek hospital privileges knowing that the records from the first hospital would not be shared.

The federal government, in 1990, established a National Practitioner Data Bank to address this concern. The goal of this data bank is to prevent the relatively small numbers of physicians who have been unsafe from having a large effect on health care by moving frequently and thus escaping the consequences of their own behavior. Whenever a hospital awards, denies, or removes practice privileges from a physician, the National Data Bank must be notified. Additionally, when a physician applies for hospital privileges or to take the licensing examination in another state, the hospital or state board must check with the National Data Bank to learn whether there have been previous problems and concerns reported. Insurance companies must report all monetary awards paid on the behalf of any physician regardless of whether any finding of malpractice was made. In addition, the medical staff must check on current members every 2 years. Eventually, this data bank is expected to be expanded to cover other licensed health care providers as well as physicians.

Those opposed to the National Practitioner Data Bank have emphasized that although the goal is laudable, the mechanism is cumbersome, is expensive, and may result in more, not fewer problems. Without the cloak of confidentiality, members of a medical staff may be more reluctant to deny privileges for fear of being the object of a suit for defamation of character. In addition, the majority of malpractice actions are currently settled out of court without an admission of malpractice. Insurance companies often have encouraged this practice because it is more expensive and time consuming to defend against a claim in court than to make a modest award. If this will result in a report to the National Data Bank, most physicians would be unwilling to do this. Therefore, courts might be stressed with additional cases. They also see the potential for errors that could ruin an individual before being corrected (Grad, 1991).

Long-term Care Facilities

The majority of long-term care facilities are nursing homes. These institutions traditionally provided care for people—most of whom were elderly—who had stable problems and needed custodial, rather than highly skilled, care. The situation has rapidly changed with the decreased lengths of hospital stays and the increasing emphasis on not using the acute setting for anything that can be accomplished elsewhere. Nursing homes may have as patients people who are still receiving chemotherapy for cancer, intravenous nutrition, or long-term ventilator support, as well as traditional residents. Our understanding of the needs and problems of the elderly has expanded, and we are beginning to recognize that skill in care involves not only technical procedures but also skill in perceiving a person's unique needs and planning care that supports continued independence and prevents deterioration whenever possible.

One development in the area of long-term care has been centers for developmentally disabled young adults. These centers allow young people who are physically or intellectually disabled to live in community-type surroundings with other young people who have similar problems. Efforts are made in these settings to increase independence and foster self-care. Group homes for the disabled may house eight or 10 people in a homelike setting.

Other long-term care centers have been established to offer rehabilitative services to those who have had strokes or spinal cord or head injuries. In these centers it is possible to provide the kinds of comprehensive coordinated services that achieve the best results in terms of restoration of function and optimum life-style.

The area of long-term care continues to grow rapidly for several reasons. More people are surviving acute illnesses, injuries, and congenital problems that would have been fatal a decade ago. Many of these people need care for a long period of time. Advances in nutrition and health care contribute to longer life spans, and many very old people who have disabilities require care and support. Social changes have made it more difficult for families to provide care at home, and an alternative setting for care is sought. Because of its rapid growth, long-term care offers many opportunities for nurses.

Standards for long-term care have been constantly rising. Many of the facilities are now accredited by state or national groups and therefore meet established criteria for sound care. It has been suggested that the nursing home industry is the most regulated industry in the United States. Some nursing homes provide exceptionally fine care, but unfortunately there are some long-term care facilities that still provide minimal or marginal care. This is often related to funding difficulties.

Funding for long-term care is a serious concern within the health care community. Many elderly and dependent people who need permanent total care in nursing homes have minimal financial resources. Few insurance companies cover long-term care. Medicare coverage of such care is limited to specific and narrowly defined situations and conditions and is also limited in the length of time that coverage is available. Many people must rely on the federal Medicaid program that is administered by the states for financial support of long-term care needs.

The federal government also has enacted strong regulations in regard to staffing, record keeping, and standards of care for any nursing home that receives funds through any federal program. These regulations are much more stringent that those that govern acute care hospitals. These include such things as requiring that nursing assistants complete an approved educational program; meeting specific criteria before using restraints (either physical or chemical); and limiting psychotropic drug use to conditions outlined in regulations. These were enacted as part of the Omnibus Budget Reconciliation Act of 1987. By tying requirements for care to reimbursement, the federal government was able to legislate many standards for nursing homes that would ordinarily be considered state responsibilities.

Although Medicaid regulations have demanded more services, better training for nursing assistants, and a greater number of licensed nurses, funds have not been increased proportionately. For example, the funding of nursing homes does not permit them to pay registered nurses the prevailing wage in the community. Therefore, the shortage of nurses has had a serious impact on nursing homes.

With increasing pressure on budgets from taxpayers and from inflation, dependent people in long-term care have often not had a strong enough voice to make an impact on decision makers. Those involved in long-term care delivery constantly strive to inform the public of the need and seek the funding necessary to provide high-quality care.

COMMUNITY HEALTH CARE AGENCIES

Within each community there are many organizations, groups, and individuals who offer health care. Some of these are funded publicly, and others are funded privately. Within the past few years there have been severe cuts in the federal funding of all community social and health services. In addition, many states have diminished funding for such services. This has created a situation in which demand for services has often been greater than the ability of agencies to meet the need. More funding is being sought from private sources, but many groups are seeking support from the same sources. It is often difficult for nurses when they find that there is no source of health care for a particular client's needs.

Community Mental Health Centers

Community mental health centers were established to allow those with psychiatric problems to remain in their own communities. There is strong evidence to support the belief that those psychiatric clients who remain in their communities on an outpatient basis, with family and community ties intact, have more successful treatment outcomes. For those who must be hospitalized, the community mental health center provides a resource so that early discharge from the hospital setting is possible. Another advantage is that people seek help more readily when it is available within the community. These centers usually employ a variety of mental health workers including psychiatrists, clinical psychologists, social workers, marriage and family counselors, psychiatric nurses, and community workers. Services may include individual counseling and therapy, group or family counseling, evaluation, and referral.

In actual practice, community mental health centers have not been adequately funded to meet the many and varied needs of those with mental health problems. The mentally ill are often not eligible for care that can maintain their health but are eligible for care only when they have again become acutely ill. Some people are not eligible for help because of the complex rules and regulations governing funding. Still others do not continue with prescribed treatment, and thus relapse but legal constraints do not allow involuntary treatment. While this recognition of the rights of the mentally ill has been important, there is also concern that society is expecting people to make rational decisions about their own best interests when they are not mentally capable of understanding the consequences of their own actions. The entire area of community mental health has many problems and challenges.

Day Care Centers for the Elderly

Day care centers have been established for elderly people who could not safely be alone throughout the day. There they receive a variety of social and health services while continuing to live in their own or a family member's home. A variety of maintenance and rehabilitative services are usually available, including exercise classes, medication education and supervision, recreational activities, mental health care, and an opportunity to interact with other people. Some of these centers provide "drop in" or intermittent services for those who need one aspect of the program. Others provide care each day for those who need continuing supervision while family members are at work or school.

Public Health Departments

Public health departments usually have the responsibility for maintaining the health of the community as a whole. This involves such diverse duties as inspecting restaurants for sanitation, licensing food handlers, providing for immunization programs, and treating venereal disease and tuberculosis. The exact responsibilities are specific to the laws and funding of each community. Some public health departments also provide nurses who make home visits to offer a variety of supportive services. These services usually are directed at health maintenance through assisting with well-child management, teaching people how to manage their own care, or following up on communicable disease treatment. Some public health departments also provide direct care services. Care through public health departments is usually free or provided at cost. Many of the services are delivered by nurses.

Home Health Care Agencies

Home health care is growing dramatically. Individuals and their families may need assistance with direct care, supervision of health status, and education related to self-care. With early discharge, intensive support may be needed for a period of time. Increasingly, these agencies employ a variety of personnel, ranging from nurses for skilled care to home health aides who can cook, clean, and provide personal care. Personnel assignments are based on the client's needs. These agencies may be either nonprofit or profit making. In the nonprofit agency, fees may be based on the client's ability to pay. In profit-making agencies, payment usually is based on a preset fee schedule.

Traditionally, much of home health care has been nursing centered. However, reimbursement programs for home care of all kinds require that a physician authorize the services. Although physicians are the experts in regard to medical care and its delegated activities, plans for home care are often made by discharge planners and nurses before the patient's discharge from the hospital and the plan is continued and expanded by the home health care nurse. Home health care nurses often believe that they should be recognized as independent planners for needs of patients at home.

Health Maintenance Organizations

Health maintenance organizations (HMOs) have been in existence in the United States for more than 50 years, but their growth in numbers was slow until the federal government provided the impetus to start new HMOs through legislation passed in 1972 and 1974. Although HMOs differ from one another in the extent of care provided, they have many similarities. Fees are a flat rate per month. This fee usually covers routine preventive health care, care for illness, and hospitalization and, in some instances, is designed to cover prescription costs, outpatient care, and other items. Primary health care providers are often employees of the organization and receive a salary that is not related to the number of patients seen or procedures performed. In other instances a group of primary health care providers contracts with the HMO to provide services for a preset fee per individual in the program. HMOs also employ many other health care workers, including nurses. In some HMOs clients have a choice of care providers; in others they do not. Because the HMO receives the same income regardless of whether the client requires extensive care or very little care, there is a built-in incentive to emphasize preventive care and avoid costly hospitalization.

The Kaiser Permanente Health Care organization in California and Oregon is one type of HMO. This organization owns and operates its own hospitals. The physician are members of a group that contracts with the organization to provide medical services. The fee for membership provides for almost all health care costs, including both outpatient and inpatient costs.

Group Health Cooperative of Puget Sound, located in Washington State, is a consumer-owned and operated cooperative that owns and operates its own hospitals and clinics and employs physicians and other health care providers. People who join the cooperative as members pay an entry fee as their share in the capitalization of the program and thereafter pay a monthly fee for comprehensive health care, which includes both outpatient and inpatient services. The governing board is elected by the membership, members serve on policy-making committees, and some issues are determined by a vote of the entire membership. In addition, Group Health Cooperative contracts with employers to provide comprehensive, prepaid coverage for employee groups. Members of the employment groups do not pay a capitalization fee and are not voting members of the cooperative. Their monthly fees may be paid by the employer or the employee.

Preferred Providers

In an attempt to contain costs, some insurance companies have negotiated with individual and organizational providers of health care to provide certain kinds of care at an agreed-on, usually lower, price. The insurance company then provides an incentive for clients to use these "preferred providers." This incentive may involve the waiver of co-payments by the insured or coverage of additional conditions or situations. Preferred provider organizations (PPOs) may include corporations employing care providers or groups of care providers who have joined together to negotiate more successfully with insurance companies for these special contracts. The advantage to the provider is the assurance that all bills will be paid in full and that the size of the practice is ensured. In a time of competition in health care, this may be a significant advantage. Each PPO operates independently and is not regulated by the government; therefore the exact structure and contractual arrangements are individual.

Nontraditional Ambulatory Clinics

After their initial rise as a counterculture phenomenon in the 1960s, many nontraditional ambulatory clinics have become well established parts of their communities. Most of these clinics are characterized by informality and a warm accepting environment. Some of them began as community movements to seek better and more responsive health care for people residing in a certain area. Others were started to provide an alternative to conventional health care systems for those whose life-style or philosophy was incompatible with the current highly organized structure of modern health care. Some provide a wide range of outpatient services; others are specifically for women's health care, well-child care, or care for the elderly.

Funding for many of these clinics has been a continuing difficulty. Clients usually are asked to pay what they can afford. Many of the clinic workers may be volunteers or work for minimal salaries. A large number of the paid staff are usually nurses. Private contributions may be one source of funding. Federal grants have been used by many, but this source of funding has been unstable. Some clinics have been short lived, but the ones providing a needed service and having sound management and planning have survived to become an important part of the health care delivery system.

Commercial Ambulatory Care Centers

The number of profit-making corporations moving into the health care arena has been increasing in all areas. The profit-making ambulatory care center (sometimes called emergency centers) provides walk-in care for minor accidents and commonly occurring illnesses. They advertise the speed and convenience of their services. Locations are often in or near shopping malls or on major thoroughfares. Some people think that their presence has added choices for consumers and that they have introduced much needed competition into health care. Others believe that they are draining off the profitable segment of ambulatory care and leaving hospital emergency departments with only the most expensive critical care. This creates more financial concerns for the acute care hospital. Some physicians have also expressed concern that people who use these clinics will not have a stable primary health care provider and that this may lead to a lower quality of care.

Alternative Health Care Resources

Professionals in health care often ignore the many alternative avenues of health care that people use, such as health foods, vitamins, chiropractors, and faith healers. When professionals consider these alternatives at all, they often dismiss them as quackery, with little recognition of why people turn to these resources.

One of the reasons for the appeal of these alternative health care routes is the caring and personalized response that clients often receive. To the person who has felt intimidated by a very business-like clinic and who was made to feel unimportant by an impersonal professional, the

Figure 8–2. Clients are often uncomfortable receiving care from persons who do not meet their expectations.

warm, concerned, accepting atmosphere of the nonconventional setting may meet many personal needs. If you understand the major role that stress and anxiety play in any health problem, you may understand why many people are helped by therapies that may or may not be based on sound scientific knowledge.

The Health Food Movement

The health food movement in the United States is very popular. There are countless books written and innumerable products produced for this market. One of the appeals of this approach to health care is that it focuses on the normal and natural, as opposed to science and technology. Many people are helped by paying attention to good nutrition. In addition, medicine is beginning to identify that some may benefit from using food and vitamins in therapeutic ways. Often it is possible to work with clients who rely on this approach to health care by accepting what they believe helps them, as long as it is not detrimental to their well-being. When you are willing to acknowledge their philosophy and values, they may be willing to consider what you have to say about health care.

Chiropractic Care

Many people seek medical help from chiropractors, who are licensed in most states. Chiropractic care is a method of treatment that is based on the theory that disease is caused by interference with nerve function. It uses manipulation of the body joints, especially the spinal vertebrae, in seeking to restore normal function. The chiropractor may also use a variety of other treatments commonly associated with physical therapy, such as massage and exercise. There are definite differences among chiropractors. One group recognizes that there are illnesses that they are not competent to treat and do recommend that clients seek medical care. Another group believes that all illnesses may be treated by chiropractic methods and do not refer clients for medical care. Many people with joint and muscle strain and tension find that chiropractic treatments relieve discomfort. The major concern is for those who have more serious illnesses that may be missed altogether or not recognized in time to be given optimal medical attention.

Naturopathy

Naturopathy gets its name from the natural agents used in treating disease, such as air, water, and sunshine. The naturopath treats people by recommending changes in life-style, diet, exercise, and the use of vitamins. For many this is successful. The danger lies in the possibility of delaying treatment of more serious disorders. Naturopathy is licensed in some states.

Herbal Medicine

The herbalist treats illness by prescribing a wide variety of natural herbs. Many of the herbs are imported from around the world. Herein lies one of the difficulties. Rules and regulations regarding labeling and content purity may not be as strict in some countries as in the United States. This means that herbs sold may contain contaminants. We know that plants often may have active ingredients that affect the human body. Digitalis, for example, was originally a dried leaf of the foxglove plant.

It was indeed a potent and effective medication when used as an herb, but dosage was not accurate and there was little scientific information regarding its effects at that time. It is wise to recognize the potential problems inherent in the use of herbal medicines. Patients taking such products should be encouraged to share this information with their physician.

Ethnic Health Care Traditions

Native Americans, Hispanic Americans, Asian Americans, and many other ethnic groups have traditional health care resources that are still used by many. Often termed *folk medicine,* these traditions usually are handed down by word of mouth and relate to treating common health problems. Treatment often involves the use of herbs and foods as well as traditional ceremonies. Little is understood about many of the herbs used, but some have demonstrated therapeutic effects. Within an ethnic group there may be people who are designated as healers or people of special knowledge and ability in regard to illness. The advice of such a person may be sought instead of consulting a physician.

Those who support the conventional, official methods of health care have long ignored or repudiated the value of these nonorthodox health care traditions. It is important that we recognize that the traditions have persisted because people have found them to be valuable. Acknowledging these health care methods and working cooperatively usually is much more productive than trying to oppose them.

POWER IN THE HEALTH CARE SYSTEM

In trying to understand any system you need to examine some of the unique sources of power and authority within it. Some sources of power unique to health care are the authority to decide who may enter and leave the system, the authority to decide who may practice within the system, and the ability to control funding. These sources of power present problems for the client because the client is excluded from them. Clearly the client determines only the most basic entry into the system. The client cannot enter any institution without the express approval of a physician. Additionally, the client has no control over who practices and with the advent of HMOs and PPOs may have little choice of physician. Funding is usually controlled by third-party payers, and the client is often powerless to determine who will be paid, how much, or when.

Regulatory Agencies

The primary regulatory agencies in health care are governmental bodies. These agencies administer licensing laws that govern who is allowed to practice. There are also agencies that approve or accredit institutions that educate personnel for health care and those that provide services. Through regulation these agencies have a profound effect on how institutions operate.

Nongovernmental agencies such as the JCAHO have a great deal of power. For example, although nursing experts had taught for years that individualized nursing care plans were important for patients, they were often not written. When the presence of nursing care plans was required by JCAHO standards, hospitals began putting time, energy, and money into systems for keeping care plans up to date. With the removal of this standard, practice may change.

Third-Party Payers

Because they represent the financial interests of large groups of people and control payments for services, third-party payers have the power to demand changes in the system. When initially established, these agencies did not see their role as anything beyond a financial relationship. As health care costs rose these agencies began to look for ways of controlling costs to maintain their competitive place in the insurance market. They have set increasingly rigid criteria for payment for services. The standard rates set for payment for procedures have tended to place some restraints on charges (although actual fees often are slightly ahead of payment schedules). By determining whom they will pay for services, insurance companies reduce the choices available to those who carry insurance and do not wish to find their care outside of that program where reimbursement would not be available. Third-party payers thus have more power with institutions and with care providers than an individual has.

Physicians

Physicians have historically had almost unlimited power within the health care system. They determined who entered and when, decided if and when all other services and personnel would be used, and determined when someone would leave the system. Where other agencies and individuals have obtained some power or independence, the overall power of the physician has often diminished. As a whole, physicians have opposed changes that would disperse power in health care, arguing that they are the most educated and knowledgeable of all health care providers and that their professional judgment should be accepted. Those favoring increased distribution of power have argued that increased competition, increased choice for consumers, and judgments of others will make the system more balanced and more responsive to the individual consumers. Despite changes, physicians are still very powerful in the health care system as a whole. For example, although the consumer through a third-party payer may pay the costs of health care, the physician is the "customer" whom the facility tries to please by providing those services, supplies, and schedules preferred by the physician.

Consumers

Consumers do have rights in the health care system. These are stated in different ways by different institutions and groups but all revolve around the recognition of the health care consumer as an adult with the ability and right to be self-determining. As a general rule, consumers are not aware of these rights and even when aware may be reluctant to demand them. The consumer is in a particularly vulnerable place in the health care system. Because he or she depends on those within the system for life itself there is often a reluctance to complain or request changes for fear of offending those on whom one depends. When consumers try to exert power within the system, they may be met with resistance and comments such as "Well, you really do not have the background to understand this issue." Consumers are most often effective in exerting power in the system by working in groups and through established committees and agencies.

Nurses

Nurses have historically had limited power in the health care system, a situation that has roots in many aspects of nursing. Most nurses were women, employees of institutions, and economically unable to take risks. In addition, nursing education did not prepare nurses to try to affect the system, but rather to function within it. However, things are changing in nursing. Nursing education programs try increasingly to educate nurses into a role as patient/consumer advocate and agent of change. Nursing organizations are working to provide nurses with a voice at higher decision-making levels in health care. Collective bargaining has provided nurses with a mechanism for demanding recognition of the importance of their role and for being participants in the decision-making processes.

Nevertheless, change does not occur rapidly and nurses are often frustrated because of their inability to influence the system. Many new

Figure 8–3. To have power and exert influence in the health care system, it is essential that nurses develop effective group action.

graduates are especially distressed to learn that, as individuals, they cannot affect the system. Somehow they expected that if they spoke with a voice of reason and acted in the patient's best interests, others would respond positively. By understanding the political realities and the ways in which decisions are made, and by working together to speak with a united voice, nurses are gradually increasing their power within the system. Mechanisms for this are discussed in Chapter 10.

ECONOMIC INFLUENCES IN HEALTH CARE

The cost of health care for the nation as a whole has risen at a faster rate than has the general inflation. A wide variety of factors has been responsible for this phenomenon. Much effort and attention have been given to cost containment.

Causes of Cost Increases

One important factor in cost increase is the cost of new technology. New and more sophisticated diagnostic and treatment devices are being invented each year. This type of cost is found in every area of the health care field from the cardiac care unit to the laboratory.

Another area contributing to rising costs has been the construction of new care facilities. An increasing population needs additional facilities, but in addition the nature of facilities has changed. More space is needed for the various technologies both at the bedside and in the many other hospital departments. More offices and conference rooms are needed. The regulations governing hospital construction have also become more stringent, requiring more fire safety, infection control measures, and protection against environmental hazards. All of these factors combine to make the "per bed" cost of new hospital construction enormously high.

The average hospital stay for standard diagnoses has been steadily decreasing. The typical patient in today's hospital is rapidly discharged to convalesce at home or in a long-term care facility, leaving behind only the very acutely ill. Many patients who would have died quickly in years past are saved but require long and intensive care. All of these factors make the acuity level of a patient today much greater. This in turn requires more intensive observation and care and the use of more specialized equipment.

The population as a whole is growing older and, statistically, the elderly have an increased incidence of all chronic illnesses. Thus a greater percentage of the population requires health care on a regular basis and may be dependent on medications, treatments, and therapies for continued functioning.

As mentioned earlier in the chapter, salaries of health care workers (except physicians) were far below that of the general society. To remedy this, for a time health care salaries rose more rapidly than the general inflation rate. Physicians have also had an increase in income greater than the relative inflation rate.

Companies that manufacture health-related devices and drugs have reportedly some of the highest profits in industry. This has been justified by these manufacturers as being appropriate to the relative risk and cost involved in their research and development activities; however, some critics think that they have taken advantage of the public's dependence on their products.

Lack of competition in the health care field is a factor that has been included in some discussions as contributing to higher costs. Physicians have remained primary gatekeepers in the system. The advent of other primary care providers, such as nurse practitioners, has offered alternate and less costly care for many routine problems or normal life processes, such as pregnancy and childbirth. There has been opposition to allowing these practitioners to operate in collaborative rather than dependent or subsidiary roles.

One attempt to increase the availability of alternative care has been the movement to obtain legislation requiring that government agencies and third-party payers (e.g., insurance companies) pay the nonphysician, such as the nurse practitioner, who provides service. The current pattern requires that payment always be directed to a physician, who then pays the provider. Although some progress has been made in regard to third-party reimbursement for nurses in primary care, in most areas physicians are still the only ones with access to third-party payment for primary care.

Cost Containment

In an attempt to slow the rapidly increasing costs of health care, the various governmental agencies have established rules, regulations, and procedures aimed at decreasing the rate of inflation in health care. There has been no expectation of cost reductions or even of cost maintenance, but rather the aim has been to control the rate of increase. This effort is termed *cost containment*.

To add new high-cost equipment or additional patient care facilities, a health care institution may be required to apply for a certificate of need. This establishes that there will not be unnecessary duplication of services in an area and that a need for them exists. For example, if each hospital were to purchase magnetic resonance imaging equipment and it was used to only one fourth or one third of capacity, the cost per use would have to be higher to cover the investment and maintenance costs than if the device were used to capacity.

Nonprofit hospitals must make application for rate increases. In their applications, they must document all the factors contributing to the increase. Hearings are held, and permission for rate increase is given only when there is evidence that all possible economies are being taken.

Within facilities, personnel are being asked to become cost conscious. This includes such ordinary things as being conservative with telephone line use, canceling meal trays when patients are discharged, and using expensive supplies with care. Physicians are being asked to carefully judge the necessity of diagnostic studies and costly procedures. In some hospitals physicians are asked to consult with pharmacists before prescribing certain very high cost drugs to determine whether a lower cost alternative exists. Many physicians are upset about these cost-containment measures because they may interfere with the physician's independent decision making. Hospitals with a high population of extra-risk patients (e.g., the very elderly or poor) have expressed concern that discharging a patient for convalescence in a home with a caring family, good food, and a clean environment is very different than discharging a person to a poverty environment and that this should be considered in the regulations for length of stay. The proponents point out that these cost-containment measures have contributed to shortening hospital stays and thus to containing costs and that health care should not be used to solve social problems.

The federal government has sought to control costs for Medicare and Medicaid by establishing higher deductibles that the person must pay and by limiting the fees that the government will pay. Because the elderly or the poor are often unable to pay these deductible amounts, they become liabilities that health care providers must meet from higher fees collected from those who do pay their bills. Medicaid costs have also been limited by tightening eligibility requirements. This shuts more people out of the health care system altogether.

Statistically, HMOs have shown lower costs for health care than the conventional fee for service systems; therefore, the federal government has subsidized the creation of new HMOs and has encouraged employers to offer an HMO as an alternative to a traditional health insurance plan. This has speeded the development of new HMOs. Another purpose in subsidizing HMOs is to help contain costs in all health plans as a result of the competition.

All of these efforts at cost containment certainly have had effects on the health care system in many areas beyond costs. They have affected decision-making processes, power structures, the kind of care provided, and the practice of individual health care providers. It is important to recognize the impact that cost containment has had.

Diagnosis Related Groups and Prospective Payment

A major change in the method of payment for health care services began at the end of 1983, when the federal government introduced a prospective payment system for Medicare using diagnosis-related groups (DRGs) to determine the payment level. This change was designed to stop the spiraling costs of Medicare and to correct the inequities in which the costs of care in one facility were very different from the costs in another facility.

A prospective payment is a reimbursement amount for a procedure or illness that has been determined in advance of the provision of the service. This predetermined amount is paid without regard to costs in the individual situation. If the costs were less than the prospective reimbursement, the hospital will make a profit, and if they are more, the hospital will lose money. This is designed to be an incentive for hospitals to control costs. Hospitals had previously been paid by Medicare on a retrospective system, in which they were able to bill for each item of care independently; thus there had been a reverse incentive—the more care items, the more the hospital received.

DRGs, the method chosen to determine the rates to be paid in the prospective system, were a result of a computerized analysis of the costs that had been billed in the past. Categories of medical diagnosis—467 in all—were formed. In addition, a decision was made to increase the payment if other illnesses or conditions, called *co-morbidities,* were present. These were factors such as heart failure in the person with a fracture. Hospitals also receive an additional amount for cases that are determined to be "outliers." An outlier is a case in which the patient stay significantly exceeds the average. The number of days that qualify a case to be considered an outlier is predetermined. For example, if an average stay is 6 days, the stay might have to reach 35 days for the case to be considered an outlier.

Most hospital costs are included in the DRG reimbursement. Some costs are still being reimbursed separately. These include costs for nursing education, medical education, and research. These areas will be reevaluated in the future. The goal is to include all aspects of cost in one reimbursement figure. Physician costs are also being paid separately, and some suggestions have been made that eventually these should be included in the single rate.

Most of the controversy surrounding DRGs has not been an argument with the basic aim of providing an incentive for cost control, or even with the prospective reimbursement system itself, but with how the payment amount is determined and how the system is being administered. There are conflicting studies regarding whether the DRGs adequately reflect the intensity of nursing care required (Halloran et al., 1985; McKibbin et al., 1985). Another concern is that patients are reported to be discharged after much shorter stays and needing more care (the "quicker and sicker" concern). It is expected that some alterations and modifications of the system will continue to be made but that the basic prospective plan will remain in place.

There are a variety of implications for nurses in the current DRG system. The importance of charting that will reflect the acuity level and multiple problems of the patient when records are audited for compliance has been emphasized (Hoke, 1985). The need for discharge planning is always present but is more critical as the length of stay becomes shorter. Added length of stay is a crucial component in increasing the costs to the hospital; therefore, nursing actions that prevent complications, that avoid inappropriate scheduling, and that facilitate early discharge are important. Nurses in home health agencies and long-term care facilities have identified that they are caring for patients with complex nursing needs. A major concern is whether the DRG reimbursement provides adequate funds for quality nursing care to be delivered and whether hospitals, in their attempt to cut costs, will cut quality of care as well.

In addition to the patients currently covered by Medicare, many states are considering systems similar to DRGs, and some private insurance carriers are looking at ways the basic concepts could be used in their cost control efforts. Therefore, this will continue to be an issue of concern to nursing.

Patient Acuity

Patient acuity describes the relative severity of a person's current health problem. A variety of ways of measuring acuity in both general hospitals and psychiatric settings have been devised. Most consist of categories that reflect the kind of care needed. These categories are then assigned numerical values. All applicable category values are then summed and compared with a standard. For example, an acuity measuring system might have one category reflecting the need for assistance in personal hygiene. As the person needs more assistance, more points are assigned. Another category might reflect the amount of time needed for monitoring vital signs. The more time that is required, the more points are assigned. Each category is assigned appropriate points, and the total is computed. The points identified for the individual patient are then compared with a standard and the patient is assigned an acuity level. Those with the least points are level 1 and require the least care. Those with the most points are level 4 and require the most care. Each system in use has its own scale for determining acuity. These measures are also called "intensity measures" because they reflect the intensity of care needed.

In some settings acuity levels or intensity measures are being used as a mechanism for determining the staffing needs of a patient care unit. Acuity levels have also been used as a means of billing for the level of nursing care needed, rather than have nursing be a constant part of the room charge for the patient. It has also been suggested that prospective reimbursement might be based on acuity level rather than on medical diagnosis because acuity level more closely reflects the real impact on resources than the medical diagnosis does (DRG's Reflect Nursing Resources, 1985).

The state of New Jersey pioneered in the use of relative intensity measures (RIMs) as a mechanism for determining the cost of providing care (Joel, 1984). In long-term care settings similar systems have been used for determining costs for billing. In New York a system called resource utilization groups (RUGs) has been developed for this purpose (Mitty, 1987).

FUTURE CONCERNS

In 1984 a study funded by the American College of Hospital Administrators was reported in which a large number of experts in the health care field were polled as to what they expected to be true of health care in the 1990s (Arthur Andersen & Co., 1984). Six groups of experts were consulted: hospital leaders, physicians, other providers, legislators and regulators, suppliers, and payers. Nurses were not separated out but were included in the "other providers" category. The study examined social philosophy relative to health care, governmental regulations in health care, payment systems, competition and marketing, human resources, corporate structure, and finance. Some of the changes they identified are actually occurring. In addition to identifying concerns, they also identified strategies that may emerge to cope with those concerns.

Some changes they saw were the move toward defining a minimum level of health care that is a right. This could lead to a two-tiered system in which those who are able to pay, either through insurance or private means, receive a high level of care and those who are unable to pay receive a minimum level of care. Those polled believe that there will be increasing governmental regulation in health care and that PPOs and HMOs will provide an increasing share of care. They identified increasing competition and marketing of health care services. No health care occupations will have a shortage of personnel; there may actually be a surplus of physicians, leading to changes in the way physicians work.

There will be an increasing number of profit-making health care agencies, and much greater business skills will be demanded of all those associated with health care. The emphasis will be on providing ambulatory services, and the hospital share of the health care will decrease. Although no prediction system can be relied on, this study provides food for thought and is worth thorough study by those who have an interest in how the system is changing.

Figure 8-4. Clients often need assistance in finding their way through the modern health care system.

During 1987 it became apparent that a nursing shortage was present and that nursing supply was going to continue to fall further behind the demand. Many large hospitals began offering recruitment bonuses and bounties to attract nurses and to increase salaries. Several bills designed to assist in alleviating the nursing shortage were introduced into Congress in 1987. Senate bill S.1402 authorized demonstration projects and also designated $5 million to support five regional nurse recruitment centers (Morrissey, 1987).

CONCLUSION

The health care systems of today are complex. When even the professionals cannot keep all the parts of the system organized, is it any wonder that the public is completely baffled when dealing with health care? Part of the role of the nurse is to assist consumers in finding a way through this maze so that they can make informed and careful decisions about personal health care.

REFERENCES

American Hospital Association: Hospital Statistics. Chicago, American Hospital Association, 1987

Arthur Andersen and Company: Health Care in the 1990's: Trends and Strategies. Chicago, American College of Hospital Administrators, 1984

DRG's reflect nursing resources. Hospitals 59(19):56, 1985

Grad JD: The feds take aim at bad doctors and hit everyone in sight. Med Econ 68(4):22–24, 1991

Kenkel PJ: Pointing the finger: Who's to blame for high health care costs? Med Healthcare 20(48):22–25, 1990

Halloran E et al: Exploring the DRG equation. Am J Nurs 85(10):1093–1095, 1985

Hoke JL: Charting for dollars. Am J Nurs 85(6):658–660, 1985

Hudson Institute: Workforce 2000: Work and Workers for the 21st Century. Indianapolis: Hudson Institute, 1987

Hughes D et al: The Health of America's Children: Maternal and Child Health Data Book. Washington, DC, Children's Defense Fund, 1989

Joel LA: Relative intensity measures (RIMs) and the state of the art of reimbursement for nursing service. In Shaffer FA: DRGs: Changes and Challenges. New York, National League for Nursing, 1984

McKibbin RC et al: Nursing costs and DRG payments. Am J Nurs 85(12):1353–1355, 1985

Mitty E: Prospective payment and long-term care: Linking payments to resource use. Nurs Health Care 8(1):14–21, 1987

Morrissey KL: Congress turns attention to nursing agenda. Nurs Health Care 8(7):378–379, 1987

Williams SJ, Torrence PR: Introduction to Health Services, 3rd ed. New York, Wiley Medical, 1988

FURTHER READINGS

ABC's of DRG's: Basic glossary. RN 48(6):55–58, 1985

Adams R, Duchene P: Computerization of patient acuity and nursing care planning. J Nurs Admin 5(5):11–17, 1985

Brazda J: Little-noticed law should bring hospitals good cheer. Modern Healthcare 20(5):37–38, 1990

Breo DL: Severe allied health shortage cause for concern. Am Med News 31(47):10, 1989

Foegelle WE, Couch GC Jr: A study of passage rates: Hospital vs. college programs. Radiol Technol 61(5):393–395, 1990

Fosbinder D: Nursing cost/DRG: A patient classification system and comparative study. J Nurs Admin 16(11):18–23, 1986

Hassanein SA: On the shortage of registered nurses: An economic analysis of the RN market. Nurs Health Care 12(3):152–156, 1991

Martin BG: Lab personnel shortage: The growing crisis. Med Lab Observer 20(7): 28–32, 1988

Mathews JS: Preparation for the twenty-first century: The educational challenge. Phys Ther 69(11):981–986, 1989

Mathews LR: The future? The respiratory therapist in the year 2000. Can J Respir Ther 26(2):18–19, 1990

Mitchell PH, Krueger JC, Moody LE: The crisis of the health care nonsystem. Nurs Outlook 38(5):214–217, 1990

Rogers JC, Brayley CR, Cox RC: The educational preparation and professional activities of occupational therapists. Am J Occup Ther 42(10):642–646, 1988

Some hospitals offer higher salaries to attract RN's. Am Nurse 19(6):12–13, 1987

Spitzer RB et al: Cost containment: Impact on nursing services and nursing education. *In* The Impact of Changing Resources on Health Policy. American Nurses' Association publication No. G-149. Kansas City, MO, American Academy of Nursing, 1981

Taylor MB: The effect of DRG's on home health care. Nurs Outlook 33(6):290–291, 1985

Thompson JD, Diers D: DRG's and nursing intensity. Nurs Health Care 6(8): 434–439, 1985

Timmreck TC, Cole GE: Health services administration skills: An overlooked need of community health education and health promotion. Health Ed 20(1): 36–44, 1989

9
Collective Bargaining

Objectives

After completing this chapter, you should be able to

1. *Define the term negotiate.*
2. *Discuss the effect of federal labor legislation on collective bargaining for nurses.*
3. *Define the terms commonly used in collective bargaining and use these terms appropriately.*
4. *Identify at least two aspects of arbitration.*
5. *Explain the purpose of a contract.*
6. *List three items that should be considered in a contract for professional nurses.*
7. *Discuss the grievance process.*
8. *Identify the problems related to the role of the nursing supervisor in collective bargaining.*
9. *Present concerns of nurses about joining a bargaining group.*
10. *Identify three advantages of having the state nurses' association serve as the bargaining agent for the state's nurses.*
11. *Discuss issues that should be considered by nurses prior to taking a vote to strike.*
12. *Describe changes seen in the 1980s in collective bargaining practices of nurses.*

In 1974 amendments to the National Labor Relations Act (NLRA) made it possible for employees of nonprofit and voluntary health care institutions to bargain collectively. This means that all health care workers have the right to establish and be represented by a union and have a voice in determining certain employment conditions. Before this time nurses, as well as several other professional groups, were excluded by law from organizing and negotiating collectively for salaries, working conditions, and benefits. First as public employees and later as employees of private, nonprofit health care facilities they were legally exempted from federal collective bargaining laws. Health care, which has come to be regarded as a fundamental right, was seen as an essential service—one that could not be disrupted.

With this type of history, the right to bargain collectively was initially a controversial issue among nurses and other members of the health care team. Nursing had evolved as a profession that was characterized as one of dedication, service to humanity, and altruism. For nurses to work toward changes in their economic status would have been viewed as incongruous with these values.

But nursing has come of age. Today nurses are vitally concerned about such issues as nursing's image, autonomy, comparable worth, advancement of the profession, and economic welfare. They are concerned for patient well-being and want to be included on critical committees that establish standards for patient care. Nurses believe that people who choose nursing as a career should have the opportunity to have some voice in patient care assignments, length of the working day and week, fringe benefits, and wages without losing face with the public at large, members of the medical profession, or other colleagues. This thinking was succinctly outlined in a statement by Janet Muff (1988, p 245):

> We are not in this business out of charity, as altruists and nightingalists would have us believe. We are here to make money, to use our minds and our skills, to provide services to patients on our own terms. We need no longer apologize and feel guilty.

As a new graduate you may enter the job market just as the contract negotiations reach a peak between health care institutions and nursing bargaining groups. It is possible that your educational preparation to date has provided little information about the process of collective bargaining, and you may therefore find yourself poorly prepared to make decisions that involve bargaining issues. If you are like many other nurses, you probably know little about the "rules of the game." Terminology may confuse you. If the negotiation process goes poorly, you might be faced with the decision of whether you want to join other nurses who have decided to strike, an ominous predicament for the new graduate who has just landed a first job.

In this section we provide some information that is basic to collective bargaining, in the hope that as a new graduate you will have a better understanding on which to base decisions and actions. Having some knowledge of the history that surrounds the collective bargaining process in this country will be helpful in applying the process to the health care professions.

HISTORY OF COLLECTIVE BARGAINING

As early as the 1850s, Horace Greeley, a reformer, publisher, and politician, was generating interest in and giving impetus to collective bargaining issues in his editorial columns of the *New York Tribune*. During the early part of the 20th century, efforts by workers to organize were met with opposition from employers, governmental officials, and some members of the public. After the Great Depression that immobilized the United States in the late 1920s and early 1930s, several laws were enacted to help improve workers' conditions. Franklin D. Roosevelt was elected president in 1932, and his New Deal administration saw the passage of the National Industrial Recovery Act. Among the activities that resulted from this act was the creation of the National Recovery Administration, whose purpose it was to administer codes of fair practice within given industries. The nation was called on to accept an interim blanket code that established for workers a 35- to 40-hour work week, minimum pay of 30 to 40 cents an hour, and prohibition of child labor.

On July 5, 1935, the NLRA became the national labor policy of the United States. Also known as the Wagner Act, for Senator Robert F. Wagner who introduced the legislation, the NLRA gave workers federal protection in their efforts to form unions and organize for better working conditions. It listed as unfair practices any actions on the part of employers that would interfere with this process. Senator Wagner wanted management and labor to resolve their mutual problems through a system of self-government. This act also created the National Labor Relations Board (NLRB), a quasi-judicial body that was to ensure that the conditions of that legislation were properly enforced.

National Labor Relations Board

The NLRB has the responsibility for administering the NLRA. It consists of a general council and staff and five members, each of whom has a staff. The NLRB has the responsibility to determine into which of the established groupings of hospital workers the various employees fall, that is, into units for office and clerical employees, units for technical employees, units for service and maintenance employees, and other specified units including nursing. In addition, the NLRB has two primary functions: (1) to conduct secret-ballot elections that will determine that the majority of employees of a unit desire the representation of a given union in collective bargaining procedures and (2) to prevent and rectify unfair labor practices committed by employers or unions.

One of the duties of the NLRB is seeing that elections of union representatives are properly conducted. It is also responsible for investigating charges of unfair labor practices on the part of either employer or employee and judicially making decisions about violations of the NLRA and hearing appeals.

Outgrowths of the Wagner Act

The original act used the term *labor organization*, which was defined in language that could be interpreted to exclude nursing and several other professions, such as teaching and medicine, that were organized through professional organizations. In 1947 the original NLRA was amended through the Taft-Hartley Act (also known as the Labor Management Relations Act). Because of heavy lobbying on the part of hospital management, the act was written in such a way as to specifically exclude nonprofit hospitals from the legal obligation of bargaining with their employees. Although the administration of some hospitals chose to negotiate salaries and working conditions with their employees, many did not and there was no legal action that could be taken to force the process to occur.

By 1931 the American Nurses Association (ANA) was publicly recognizing its obligation with regard to the general welfare of its members and developed, within their organization, a legislative policy speaking to this concern. Some suggest that this effort was spurred by the fact that other groups, particularly the Service Employees International Union (SEIU), an affiliate of the American Federation of Labor/Congress of Industrial Organizations (AFL/CIO), was actively working to organize health care workers. Other factors also were important. Prior to 1930 most nurses were employed in public health, visiting nurse, or private duty positions. Much of the care within hospitals was delivered by students, aides, and orderlies under the direction of a head nurse. As more and more care was delivered in the hospital setting, the number of nurses employed by these facilities increased. The existing working conditions affected more people.

In 1945 a committee was appointed by the ANA to study employment conditions. This study culminated in 1946 in the creation of an ANA Economic Security Program. This action was followed by the enactment of a resolution that would encourage state nurses' associations to act as exclusive bargaining agents for their respective memberships in the important areas of economic security and collective bargaining. In this same year, 1946, the SEIU formed its first RN Guild in New York City.

The concept of professional collectivism, which emphasizes that good care is dependent on satisfactory working conditions and satisfaction with nursing itself, began to take shape. However, concern for the image of the nurse and nursing prompted a no-strike policy to be officially adopted by the ANA in 1950, and it remained in effect until it was rescinded in 1968.

By 1947, with the impetus provided by the Economic Security Program of ANA, collective bargaining between nurses and hospital administration had been implemented in several states and negotiated contracts were in effect. Many hospital employers were voluntarily developing contracts with employees and were showing genuine concern about working conditions. Some states were mandating that state hospitals negotiate with all employees. But there was no federal requirement that this process would occur.

Federal legislation passed in 1962 enabled employees of federal health care institutions to participate in collective bargaining. In 1967 investor-owned hospitals and nursing homes were also included, and the ANA was identified as the bargaining agent for the nurses of the Veterans Administration hospitals. Legislation passed in 1970 saw the inclusion of nonprofit nursing homes in the collective bargaining process. Concurrently, SEIU and other labor-related organizations were also bargaining for nurses.

Finally, on August 25, 1974, Public Law 93-360 was put into effect; it amended the Taft-Hartley Act to provide economic security programs for those employed in nonprofit hospitals.

This change brought health care facilities and their employees under the jurisdiction of the NLRB. Finally nonprofit hospitals were legally required to bargain with nurses for better wages, hours, staffing conditions, patient–nurse ratios, and a voice in hospital governance in general.

In the health care industry, a strike or concerted work stoppage could have serious implications for the public. In an effort to ensure the least possible disruption of service, several amendments were attached to the NLRA passed in 1974. In general these conditions required a longer period of notification prior to work stoppage or termination of contract and established the provision that parties would be required to participate in mediation.

UNDERSTANDING THE BASIC LANGUAGE

Intelligent bargaining begins with an awareness of the process itself. The neophyte must understand that, as the word "bargaining" implies, it consists of a set of procedures by which employee representatives and employer representatives negotiate to obtain a signed agreement (contract) that spells out wages, hours, and conditions of employment that are acceptable to both. A key word in this definition is *negotiate*.

Bargaining and Negotiating

To negotiate means to bargain or confer with another party or parties to reach an agreement. *Bargaining* implies a discussion of the terms of the agreement and suggests that there will be give and take, that neither party will obtain all items asked for in the contract. The usual approach in negotiations is for representatives of the employees to ask for more than can be expected and for representatives of management to offer less. Some believe that if either party were to start from a realistic position, it would not allow room for bargaining and might be seen as a sign of weakness. Ideally, negotiations would proceed in a somewhat philosophical vein, moving toward reasonable compromises that could allow each side to win, but this does not always occur.

Union and Collective Action

Collective bargaining allows employees working together as an organized unit to negotiate. A *union* is an organized group of employees that negotiates and enforces labor agreements. Its major concern is the improvement of wages, hours, and working conditions of its members. When a branch or part of a professional association assumes this responsibility, as often occurs in nursing, the negotiating group may be known as a *collective action division*. The activity of the group may be referred to as *professional collectivism*, which supports the premise that the quality of patient care is directly tied to working conditions and that collective action is a professional responsibility (Bloom, 1977). A professional organization must work under the same legal constraints as unions. It provides legal counsel and representatives to assist with negotiations, may lobby on behalf of issues, or may take part in other activities that would further the economic welfare of nurses. It oversees the development of the contract.

The Contract

The conclusion of the bargaining process should result in a signed contract that converts to writing the agreements that have been reached. A *contract* is "a legally binding agreement made between two or more persons to do or to refrain from doing certain actions" (Guido, 1988, p 167). In most instances a contract need not be in writing, but it is much easier to implement if it is written and signed by all involved. The contract remains in effect until breached or terminated. Most negotiated contracts define the period of time to be covered by the established conditions, usually 2 or 3 years.

Before being put into effect a contract must be *ratified*. This means that the terms of the contract must be accepted by the members of the bargaining group. This is usually done by a vote of the membership.

Some Rules Governing Labor Relations

When two parties agree to begin the negotiation process, it is understood that both will *bargain in good faith*. Bargaining in good faith is a poorly understood term, but generally it means that the parties will meet at regular times to discuss, with the intent to resolve, any differences over wages, hours, and other employment conditions. Failure to carry out these activities could fall into the category known as an *unfair labor practice*.

An *unfair labor practice* is any action that interferes with the rights of employees or employers as described in the amended NLRA. It is not possible to discuss all of these in detail; however, some examples follow. An employer must not interfere with the employee's right to form a union or other organized bargaining group, join the group, or take part in the group's activities. The employer may not attempt to control a group, once organized, or to discriminate against its members in regard to hiring or tenure. Most important, the employer must bargain collectively and in good faith with representatives of the employees.

Likewise, labor organizations have constraints placed on their activities. They, too, must bargain in good faith. They must not restrain or coerce employees in selecting a bargaining group to bargain collectively. They may not pressure an employer to discriminate against employees who do not belong to the labor organization.

One of the issues frequently brought up in negotiations that usually results in a dispute is that of *agency shop*. If an agency shop clause is in effect, all employees are required to pay the dues for membership. If, because of religious or philosophical beliefs, they are unwilling to pay dues to the bargaining group, provisions are made to pay the same sum to a nonprofit group such as a church or foundation. The obvious advantage of this requirement, from the workers' point of view, is encouraging membership in the union. Because the union is required to represent all employees, members or not, their desire to have a greater percentage of paying members is also obvious.

SETTLING LABOR DISPUTES

When labor disputes arise, several actions can be taken to help resolve the differences. As we discuss the various options we will continue to provide explanations of the terms that are most frequently used.

When the parties doing the negotiating cannot come to agreement on an issue they are considered to be *at impasse* or the two groups are *deadlocked* on the issue. One method of reaching solution is to employ an *authoritative mandate*, by which a peaceful settlement will be encouraged by a president, secretary of labor, or other high-ranking or influential person.

In other instances, an *injunction* may be requested. This results in a court order that requires the party or parties involved to take a specific action or, more commonly, to refrain from taking a specific action. This measure can forestall a strike.

In still other instances the institution or company may be subjected to *government seizure and operation*. Government employees are then used to run the plant, firm, or industry in question. This is seldom seen in the health care industry for obvious reasons. However, this option was used in Montana in 1991 when state employees decided to strike. The National Guard was called in to replace striking state patrolmen.

Mediation and Arbitration

Perhaps the most commonly used method of seeking agreement between parties is through *mediation* and *arbitration*. A *mediator* is a third person who may join the bargainers in early sessions to assist the parties to reconcile differences and arrive at a peaceful agreement. Mediation involves finding compromises, and the mediator is to assist with this. He or she must gain the respect of both parties and must remain neutral to the issues presented.

An *arbitrator* is technically defined as a person chosen by agreement of both parties to decide a dispute between them. Thus the primary difference between a mediator and an arbitrator is that the mediator assists the parties in reaching their own decision whereas the arbitrator has the authority to actually make the decision for the parties if necessary. However, the terms *mediator* and *arbitrator,* and *mediation* and *arbitration* often are used interchangeably, and, in fact, a mediator may also serve as an arbitrator.

Arbitration may take several forms. It may be mediation-arbitration, in which a third person joins the parties in the negotiation process before there are any serious disputes. This person's role is to act as a mediator who will attempt to keep the parties talking, suggest compromises, and help establish priorities. If an agreement is not reached by a specified date, or if it appears that neither party is willing to compromise on an issue (called a deadlock), the mediator then assumes the role of an arbitrator and gives a decision based on the information gained in the role of mediator.

Figure 9–1. The arbitrator's decision may not really please either side.

Another form of arbitration is called *binding arbitration*. This means that both parties are obligated to abide by the decision of the arbitrator. Some people see this as the least desirable alternative in settling disputes because it may result in a decision that is not satisfactory to either side but one by which both must abide. It has been suggested, in instances in which binding arbitration is to be used, that the parties spell out exactly which of the issues are to be decided by the arbitrator. Binding arbitration has the advantage of resolving deadlocked issues without a strike being called. It also encourages both parties, knowing that the arbitrator's decision may not please either side, to reach a compromise on their own.

The *final offer* approach is a type of binding arbitration. Employer and employee bargaining representatives reach agreement on as many issues as possible. The deadlocked issues and a final position from each side are then presented to the arbitrator, who is obligated to select only the most reasonable package. The arbitrator may not develop a third alternative, which would "split the difference." The final offer approach encourages both sides to come up with a fairly realistic package and serves to close the gap on issues.

One criticism of any type of arbitration is the expense involved. Arbitrators must be paid for their services. It is also criticized because it undermines voluntary collective bargaining and allows parties to avoid unpleasant confrontation with their own difficulties by shifting that responsibility to a public authority. However, this is useful in preventing the disruption of services.

Arbitration may be requested from the American Arbitration Association or from available state public and private mediation and conciliation services. The American Arbitration Association is a nonprofit, nonpartisan organization that, for a nominal fee, will provide a list of qualified arbitrators. Most states also have available groups such as the Public Employees Relations Commission that also can provide a list of mediators and arbitrators.

Strikes and Lockouts

When the negotiation process breaks down, lockouts and strikes are likely to occur. A *lockout* occurs when an employer closes a factory or other place of business to make employees agree to terms. One can readily see how undesirable this would be in the health care system, but it has occurred in some instances.

In technical language, strikes may fall into one of two classifications: those related to strikes that arise from economic concerns and strikes that arise from unfair labor practices. An *economic strike* results from efforts on the part of employees to seek better economic benefits. This is the type of strike most frequently engaged in by nurses and other health care workers. They are striving to improve their own working conditions, salaries, and benefits.

Unfair labor practice strikes may further be divided into two additional classifications: those caused or prolonged by the employer's unfair labor practice and those caused by the employees' unfair labor practice. If employees initiate an economic strike and during the strike the employer commits any of the actions that were described as unfair labor practices, the strike then becomes an unfair labor practice strike on the part of employers. *Sit-down strikes*, in which employees not only refuse to work but also refuse to leave the employer's property, are an example of unfair practices on the part of employees. Sit-down strikes have been uncommon in the health care industry. Employees who engage in unlawful activities during a strike or whose activities cause a strike to become unlawful may not be entitled to reinstatement privileges.

Reinstatement Privilege

A *reinstatement privilege* is a guarantee offered to striking employees that they will be rehired after the strike, provided that they have not engaged in any unfair labor practices during the strike and provided that the strike itself is lawful. The hospital may replace a striking nurse during the strike. If strikers agree unconditionally to return to work, the employer is not required to replace the striking nurse at that time. However, recall lists are developed, and if the nurse cannot find regular and equivalent employment, he or she is privileged to recall and preference on jobs before new employees may be given employment.

As stated earlier, nurses may lose their reinstatement privileges because of misconduct during a lawful strike. For example, strikers may not physically block other nurses and personnel from entering or leaving a struck hospital. Strikers may not threaten nonstriking employees and may not attack management representatives. These types of activities usually do not occur in strikes conducted by nurses but are not outside the realm of possibility.

WHAT TO LOOK FOR IN A CONTRACT

Thus far we have discussed the history of collective bargaining in the United States, the negotiation process, and the language commonly used in the negotiations. We have discussed broadly negotiating wages, hours, and working conditions. As mentioned earlier, this process should ultimately conclude in the development of a written contract that is signed by both the persons representing the bargaining group and representatives from management. In this section we spell out in more detail specific provisions that might be included in a contract.

A contract must meet certain specified criteria to be legally binding. It must result from mutually agreed-on items arrived at through a "meeting of minds," Something of value must be given for a reciprocal promise, that is, professional duties for an agreed-on sum. Contracts can be enforceable whether written or oral, but it is easier to work with those that are written (Rothman and Rothman, 1977).

Although each agreement will differ, most contracts have a fairly general format that will include the following:

- A preamble stating the objectives of each party
- A statement recognizing the official bargaining group
- A section dealing with financial remuneration, including wages and salaries, overtime rates, holiday pay, and shift differentials
- A section dealing with nonfinancial rewards, in other words, fringe benefits such as retirement programs, types of insurance available, free parking, and other services provided by the employer
- A section dealing with seniority in respect to promotion, transfer, work schedules, and layoffs
- A section establishing guidelines for disciplinary problems
- A section describing how grievance procedures will be resolved
- A section that may explicitly state codes of conduct or professional standards.

The contract may also include many other mutually agreed-on items, such as no-strike agreements and an arrangement for using an arbitrator to settle issues that become deadlocked (Werther and Lockhart, 1976).

Several other areas that are negotiable are important and should be incorporated into the contract. These may be included in the section dealing with professional standards or nursing care. Cleland (1981) outlines the following items that should be considered in a contract that involves professional nurses. First of all, the contract should provide for shared governance; that is, that professional policy decisions should be developed by professional staff and administration who work jointly on the policy. This often takes the form of a nursing practice council or a professional performance committee. Second, the contract should provide for individual professional accountability. This would ensure peer

Figure 9–2. As a new graduate, you may find yourself poorly prepared to make decisions that are involved in bargaining issues.

evaluation of a practitioner's competence. Third, the contract should define the collective professional role. This spells out the responsibility of registered nurses as professional practitioners and describes their part in the planning of patient care. The purpose of this is to strengthen nurses' influence on the quality of care.

It is important that, as a new graduate, you know whether there is a contract in effect in the institution from which you seek employment or in the community in which you plan to work. You should also be knowledgeable about the terms of the existing contract so that you might best fulfill your obligations and recognize and benefit from the provisions to which you are entitled. The organization to which you are applying for employment can provide you a copy of the current contract. The state nurses' associations can be contacted for information regarding the organization that represents nurses in a particular hospital or facility. They can also provide a copy of any contracts that have been negotiated for which they represented the nurses.

THE GRIEVANCE PROCESS

Although the grievance process is a somewhat different subject than collective bargaining, it is usually one part of a negotiated contract and therefore deserves some mention here. Effective contracts will include, in addition to wages, hours, working conditions, and other items, a section that spells out the grievance procedure.

A *grievance* is a circumstance or action believed to be unjust and in violation of the contract. The *grievance process* represents an established and orderly method to be used in the adjustment of grievances between parties. In this sense, it represents a problem-solving mechanism. Grievances are usually related to interpretations of the contract. They generally occur as a result of a misunderstanding or difference of opinion about the contract or its language or as direct violations of the contract. Although grievances can be filed by either the management or the employee, most cases are filed by the employee.

The grievance process spells out in writing in the contract a series of steps to be taken to resolve the area of dissension. Initially the employee and the immediate supervisor attempt to resolve the disagreement through informal talk. If no resolution occurs, the discussion moves into the steps of the grievance process. Typical steps are as follows:

1. A written request for the next step is given to the immediate supervisor. Generally a time stipulation (e.g., 10 days) is established for submitting the written request. A written response is required that also carries a time limit. From this point on in the deliberation, a representative from the bargaining unit may be present.

2. Assuming that the written response does not result in settling any problems, the grievance is submitted to a higher authority within the organization for appeal. Again time lines are in effect and failure to comply with those time lines results in the discussion coming to a halt.

3. The employee, his or her representative, the appropriate representative from management (perhaps the Director of Nursing Service), and the grievance chairperson (who may be an officer in the bargaining unit) meet for discussion. The meeting may also

include the personnel director, especially if the grievance relates to personnel policies. Once again, the contract usually specifies the number of days in which this must occur.

4. If no solution evolves following discussion, a neutral third party (arbitrator) is designated and is present at the deliberations. If no agreement is reached the arbitrator will rule on the situation. The decision of the arbitrator is usually binding.

It is important to discriminate between complaints and grievances. Employees may have complaints that are not violations of the contract. For example, Nurse No. 1 may object that she was required to float from the postpartum unit to the nursery. She had been oriented to the nursery but preferred to work in the postpartum unit. Nurse No. 2 was required to float from a medical unit to a surgical unit to which she had

Figure 9–3. It is important to discriminate between complaints and grievances.

not been oriented. If the contract in this hospital stipulated that no one would be floated to a unit to which he or she had not been oriented, Nurse No. 1 had a complaint, whereas Nurse No. 2 had a grievance.

Hoover and colleagues (1990) point out that all organizations have problems. The absence of grievances may not be the best indicator of the health of the organization. It is entirely possible that problems are not being addressed. On the other hand, a high number of grievances is an indication of problems within the organization. These problems often relate to the language of the contract or the education of the employee to the conditions of the contract. Another barometer of the health of the organization is the level at which the grievances are resolved. It is most desirable to settle most grievances at the informal level and without the involvement of an arbitrator.

The grievance procedure may sound like many steps that may take a great deal of time, and indeed this is true. Although most grievances are settled short of arbitration, they are still time and energy consuming. Grievances can be best avoided if everyone has a good understanding of the terms of the contract, and if sound personnel policies are developed and applied consistently and equitably. Open discussions between the employees and management to review mutual concerns and share information help reduce the number of grievances. Mutual respect is a critical element in any organization.

ISSUES RELATED TO COLLECTIVE BARGAINING AND NURSING

The issues of collective bargaining that relate to the nursing profession can be divided into five major points of discussion:

1. The role of the supervisor in collective bargaining
2. The strain that may exist between professionalism and collective action
3. The decision facing nurses about whether they want to join a bargaining group
4. Which bargaining group nurses should choose to represent them
5. Whether the individual nurse will decide to strike if negotiations break down and a strike is called.

These various issues may take on greater or lesser importance depending on the area of country involved, the length of time the nurses in that area have been participated in collective bargaining, and the group that has been chosen to represent the nurses at the bargaining table.

The Supervisor and Collective Bargaining

Historically, nursing has paid little attention to how the term *supervisor* has been used in the health care system. An employee observing another employee carrying out a procedure for the first time might be said to be "supervising" the activity. Likewise, charge nurses, head nurses, and possibly team leaders perform a different type of supervisory activity, that of supervising the care of patients and the actions of personnel. When the Taft-Hartley Act was amended to require nonprofit hospitals to bargain collectively with their employees, problems arose regarding the definition of supervisor as written in the amendment. A supervisor was defined as

> any individual having authority, in the interest of the employer, to hire, transfer, suspend, lay off, recall, promote, discharge, assign, reward, or discipline other employees, or responsibly to direct them, or to adjust their grievances, or effectively to recommend such action, if in connection with the foregoing the exercise of such authority is not of a merely routine or clerical nature, but requires the use of independent judgment (Public Law 93-360, Section 2, 1974).

In this sense, supervisors were not viewed as employees, but as agents of the employer, carrying out actions on behalf of the employer. Therefore, if the person hired as supervisor were to become involved in the collective bargaining group and its workings, it could be ruled an unfair labor practice. The supervisor's participation could be viewed as "dominance" on the part of the employer. Thus any person functioning within the health care system in any manner that met the above definition was excluded from the appropriate bargaining unit.

At least initially this has created some dilemmas for nursing. Those people who, for years, had assumed leadership positions among their peers could not do so when it came to determining working conditions. Membership in the association was not prohibited by law, but it needed to be patently clear that no one in a supervisory capacity represented the staff nurse.

These challenges have posed some problems for the ANA. First of all, the organization had to determine that no person with a supervisory role was involved in directing or advising the activities of the Economic and General Welfare Commission or its committees. In addition, an effort was made to place professional association dues and collective bargaining section dues in separate accounts to ensure that there would be no commingling of funds. This separation of funds tends to further emphasize that supervisors are in no way involved in the bargaining process, although their right to belong to the professional association is valid.

If the association were to represent nurses in the institutions, the directors of nursing service were concerned about their relationship with the organization. In some instances hospital management discouraged directors from belonging to the association. Directors and assistant directors have become increasingly vulnerable, and sometimes they were discharged without notice and with no recourse. In other instances directors resented having part of their professional dues used to fund the Division of Economic and General Welfare of the association when that group could not represent them and, in fact, could make their job more hectic.

Probably the saddest aspect of the issue is the schism that results between supervisor and nursing staff within the hospital. It is the supervisors and directors that usually serve on key committees within an institution, in which they support, define, and encourage greater professional recognition of the registered nurse in the care-giving role. In the negotiation process these leaders are placed on the opposite side of the bargaining table. As supervisors and staff, who, as a total group, have united for quality patient care, align themselves with one side or the other, the terms "we" and "they" begin to carry more meaning than either should. In a heated dispute some bad feelings inevitably result.

Many state nurses' associations are working to keep nurses united, whatever their role in health care delivery, and they are attempting to find methods to represent the welfare of all members. As nurses have become more experienced in the area of labor relations, the process has been handled in a less emotional manner and as just one more aspect of the work environment.

Professionalism and Collective Action

Among the issues related to collective bargaining, the strain that exists between professionalism and collective action has probably received more space in recent nursing literature than has any other.

The argument against unionism has its roots in the history of nursing itself. Nursing was perceived by many, including nurses, as a selfless, all-serving, altruistic calling. The act of caring for others, even if that meant subordination of the individual to the goals of that care, was to be compensation enough for the services rendered. The strong religious influence that pervaded the early development of nursing added to this concept of the profession. Early leaders in nursing espoused this dedication to its arts. In 1893 Lavinia Dock stated

> Absolute and unquestioning obedience must be the foundation of the nurse's work, and to this end complete subordination of the individual to the work as a whole is as necessary for her as for the soldier (cited in Bullough and Bullough, 1966, p 96).

Another factor that has hampered the strong development of unionization in nursing is the fact that nursing is primarily a women's profession. Although more men now enter nursing, only about 3% of the registered nurses in the United States are men.

Early social beliefs that woman's role should be submissive, supportive, and obedient were extremely compatible with pervading concepts of the expectations that our society placed on nurses. The paternalism that has existed in the health care delivery system has also made the process of collective bargaining for nurses a slow one (see Chapter 1). The combination of the role of women and the role of the nurse under earlier paternalistic practices had the nurse caring for the "hospital family," looking out for the needs of all, from patient to physician, and being responsible for keeping everyone happy (Ashley, 1976). The tendency to see the physician as the father figure in the health care system, and the nurse as the corresponding mother figure, and the patients as the children, has done little to promote the autonomy of nursing as a profession. A quote by Campbell (1980, p 1286) demonstrates the use of the family concept in health care: "If we are to keep unions out of the profession we, as nurses, must make every effort to build loyalty and a family feeling among our fellow nurses."

Despite the fact that nursing has a history of ambivalence toward union negotiations, today we see nurses involved in collective bargaining in greater numbers than ever before. Several factors are responsible for this change. Wilson and colleagues (1990) have identified these as the focus on the continued high cost of health care and the need to examine this rise, the scrutiny that has been placed on employee's salaries as part of this process, the fact that nurses comprise the largest number of employees in hospitals (nearly half), and changes in the NLRA allowing nurses to bargain collectively. Various sources differ with regard to whether unionization of hospital employees results in higher hospital costs.

In the early years of collective bargaining by nurses there was some reticence to use the term "unionism." Much of the nursing literature surrounding the issue used appropriate and less emotionally charged synonyms. Today the term "unionism" is used with increasing frequency reflecting a change in sentiment that supports the belief that nurses should be involved in collective bargaining. Unionism to some means gaining coercive powers and thus creating a public image of nurses and nursing that would have a detrimental effect on the profession. Some have feared that their white collars might turn "blue," recalling the traditional association of unionism with blue-collar workers. However, most of the literature of today has stopped quibbling over the word "unionism."

Many have come to believe that the collective action of nurses provides one of the best avenues for achieving professional goals and exercising control over nursing practice. As nurses are called on to assume greater and greater responsibility for complicated decisions, collective bargaining through a professional organization may provide the means to implement the concept of collective professional responsibility.

Certainly the way that collective bargaining will be perceived by the nurse and by the public that is served will be primarily determined by the manner in which the bargaining is conducted. Nurses as a group need to develop the skills that are necessary to communicate to the public the importance of their role in health care delivery. They must be able to handle conflict situations and work toward resolution while maintaining integrity and dignity. Nurses need to become enlightened and informed, and they need more than a superficial understanding of the process of collective bargaining.

Nurses may benefit from broadening their perceptions. This applies to many areas of practice in addition to that of collective bargaining, particularly bioethical issues (see Chapter 7). Many nurses dichotomize issues into categories such as good/bad, right/wrong, best/worst. Nurses need to work toward understanding and accommodating differing points of view and acknowledging that areas of compromise can exist.

To Join or Not to Join

Once the individual nurse has gained an understanding of collective bargaining and has developed a personal philosophy about the professional role, he or she will be ready to make a decision in regard to membership in the bargaining unit.

In working with students who are soon to embark on professional careers, we find that it is easier for them to decide whether to bargain collectively than it is to decide to part with the money that is required for membership. Many nurses want better working conditions and higher salaries but are all too willing to let someone else fund these endeavors and work to achieve them.

It is in response to these concerns that many "agency shop" clauses have been added to contracts. Those who are members and are active in the negotiation process believe it is inappropriate for some to benefit from the labors of the bargaining process without having contributed, at least financially, to the effort. The presence of agency shop clauses may serve as either an asset or a deterrent to recruitment, depending on the applicant's viewpoint.

Representation for Nurses

Of far greater controversy than whether nurses should unionize is the issue of which organization should represent nurses at the bargaining table. As mentioned earlier, this is determined by elections that are supervised by the NLRB. To become the certified collective bargaining representative of a group of employees, the organization in question must receive 50% of the votes cast, plus one.

When nurses first began to organize, the ANA, through the state nurses' associations, was the bargaining representative. This group still represents more nurses than all the other organizations combined. However, there has been a strong movement on the part of other organizations to vie for the representative position. It has been estimated that more than 30 labor organizations represent health care workers (Miller, 1980). The ANA has been representing nurses since 1946. The National Union of Hospital and Health Care Employees (representing nurses since 1977) and the Service Employees International have voted to unite, creating something of a "super union" for health care workers. The Federation of Nurses and Health Professionals began organizing nurses in 1978. Other groups representing nurses in various parts of the country include the United Food and Commercial Workers, the Teamsters Union, and the American Federation of Teachers.

Nurses face a difficult decision when trying to decide which group can represent them best. In recent years, perhaps this decision has occupied more time and effort on the part of nurses than has the actual bargaining. Those who have strong allegiance to the ANA contend that only RNs should bargain for RNs. One of the reasons given for this position is that in collective bargaining, nurses face different issues than do other workers. In addition to concerns about salary, benefits, working conditions, and the like, nurses want also to negotiate questions pertaining to staffing, patient care concerns, and participation on joint hospital committees. Many believe that only nurses can effectively negotiate such items. These people contend that hospital administration, fearing the power of labor unions, will bargain more constructively and positively with nurses themselves. They also believe that the ANA will be a stronger, more united organization if it serves as both the professional association and the bargaining agent.

Others believe that nurses compromise their collective bargaining powers when the recognized union is a group other than the state nurses' association. They think that when nurses do not bargain for themselves, the "organization shrivels and their influence on health care weakens" (Mallison, 1985, p 943).

Some parts of the country are experiencing a trend toward having an organization other than the professional nurses' association represent nurses. Chief among the arguments for bargaining conducted by another group is the issue of supervisor membership in the professional association (discussed earlier in this chapter). Proponents of this position would also contend that it is not realistic for one group (i.e., the ANA) to work with the professionalism aspect of nursing as well as with the issues of wages, benefits, and working conditions.

Some would argue for two organizations, one to represent issues related to professionalism and another to negotiate salaries. If nurses choose to have one group involved in professional concerns (e.g., codes of ethics, standards of care, and updating skills required in the practice of the profession) and a second group representing them at the bargaining table, there are some obvious drawbacks. First and foremost is the matter of cost because both organizations would be collecting dues. Many perceive the cost of belonging to the ANA and the state associations as very high, with dues of approximately $300 per year. Additional membership dues in another organization, which are equally as expensive, might be prohibitive. Second, there are those who believe that the union would become the dominant force between the two groups because money and working environment issues both speak strongly. There are no easy answers to this question, and it will certainly be one of the biggest issues facing nurses in the future.

To Strike or Not to Strike

Nurses, employers, and the public are served best when negotiations are truly in good faith and continue until resolution occurs. Nurses, as a group, do not like to strike. In some parts of the country where a strike has occurred, it took nurses months, and perhaps years, to regain lost salaries. The level of care to the community may have been placed in jeopardy during the time of the strike, and the public image of nursing may have been damaged. These are not desirable outcomes.

The negotiation process does not always move smoothly. The last

Figure 9–4. There are no easy answers to the strike issue.

alternative for the employer in pushing an issue is the lockout or layoff. For the nursing bargaining unit, the last alternative in forcing an issue is the strike. When negotiations reach this point, serious problems can occur. To some nurses the actual withholding of services to a public that needs them is abhorrent and is incompatible with personal definitions of professionalism. These people would favor no-strike clauses in contracts, coupled with binding arbitration. This eliminates the need to consider the strike as an alternative.

Other nurses believe that strikes are a necessary and justified means of achieving desired ends. One of the benefits of striking is to increase the public awareness of matters related to the working conditions salaries, benefits of nurses. The public may have little understanding of the situations facing nurses in the work environment.

In the early 1980s, when organized activities of nurses were embryonic, negotiations that reached the strike stage received fairly wide publicity. Today strikes have occurred frequently enough among nurses' bargaining groups to be no longer treated in a sensational fashion, although they continue to receive some publicity.

It is not always possible to anticipate how the general public will interpret a strike by professionals, especially if professional standards are an issue. Someone needing health care may be aware only that care is not available and may be angered by any disruption that could occur in the usual pattern of health care delivery. On the other hand, if the public perceives hospital management as being unreasonable and causing the change in services, the public sentiment may be supportive of nurses on strike.

One approach that nurses sometimes use to soften the impact of the strike on health care consumers is an agreement to continue to deliver services to critical care areas. Through this mechanism nurses continue to staff those areas of the hospital in which care is of an emergency nature. This often includes coronary and intensive care units, labor and delivery suites, emergency departments, and emergency surgery units.

The decision to strike is one that is voted into effect by the majority of the members of the bargaining organization. When this occurs the individual nurse who is opposed to striking will have to decide whether he or she will abide by the vote of the majority or whether he or she will go against the majority and cross picket lines to continue in the caregiving role. To strike may be contrary to personal beliefs, but to return to work while colleagues are striking may also be in conflict with values. This once again represents one of the issues in nursing to which there are no easy answers.

CHANGING TRENDS WITH REGARD TO COLLECTIVE BARGAINING

At one time economic concerns and working conditions may have been the principal motivators for collective action. However, by the mid 1980s subtle, and at times not so subtle, changes were occurring throughout the United States with regard to collective bargaining, unionism, and labor-management relations. Some working in the area of contract management would report a shift from the adversarial relationship that had historically existed between the employee and the employer, which focused on salaries, work hours, and the like, to one that placed greater emphasis on the quality of work life.

Concession Bargaining

Concession bargaining is a process by which there is an explicit exchange in labor costs for improvements in job security. This has been seen to occur with increasing frequency. An example would be a shift in emphasis from one that asks for increases in salary to one that focuses on eliminating the practice of calling nurses and telling them not to report for work because the census has dropped. On these days the nurses do not receive salary. These changes have been seen in industry more than in nursing, although the strike of 6000 Minnesota nurses was triggered by hospital practices related to the layoff of staff and the involuntary reduction of hours (6000 Minnesota RNs, 1984).

"Union Busting"

A trend seen in health care institutions during the 1980s and persisting in some areas today is an effort toward "union busting." Although technically illegal when referring to methods used to get rid of an existing union, the term *union busting* has been expanded to include a wide range of legal activities that slow down collective bargaining. Pressured by rapidly escalating health care costs and influenced by the changing attitudes toward work, hospital administrators have hired consultants and law firms to assist and advise in discouraging and impeding organizational activities. This is also a counteraction to the courting by unions of the expanding groups of previously unorganized professional groups, such as physicians and nurses. Antiunion organizing campaigns are usually aimed at strategies that will delay and thus drag down the momentum of organizing efforts. This could include challenging unit membership, attempting to decertify elections, and failing to bargain in good faith, thus drawing out the negotiating process (Ballman, 1985).

Issues of Discrimination

As nurses have become more comfortable and knowledgeable about the bargaining process their energies have been directed toward a variety of issues. This would include such concerns as pay equity, discrimination against female employees, comparable worth, and the right of the employee to know the hazards within the work environment (see Chapter 11). In some instances, discriminatory practices against male nurses have also been an issue.

Changes in the Number of Bargaining Units

Within the organization of hospitals there exist many different positions and job titles ranging from the professional staff through office staff to those responsible for hospital maintenance. In nursing alone are groups of registered nurses, licensed practical nurses, and nursing assistants. As these various groups have been granted authority to organize into bargaining units, concern has been expressed about the number of various unions with which any hospital administration must bargain at any given time. Some fairly elaborate estimates have been made regarding the amount of time demanded by the collective bargaining process.

When the NLRA was first passed in 1974, the NLRB specified that seven employee bargaining units would exist within the health care industry (Wilson et al., 1990, p 37). Those seven groups were registered nurses, physicians, other professional employees, technical employees, business office and/or clerical employees, and skilled maintenance employees.

In 1984 the NLRB determined that bargaining units would be decided on a case-by-case basis. This resulted in the number of bargaining units being reduced to three: all professionals, all nonprofessionals, and guards.

In 1989 the NLRB once again proposed new rule changes that resulted in the establishment of eight collective bargaining units. At this time it was also determined that the rule would apply to all hospitals of all sizes. In response the American Hospital Association (AHA) sought and obtained a permanent injunction against the rule. Subsequently, "all-RN" units were legally approved. As might be expected the AHA and the ANA occupied opposite points of view with regard to this issue.

The Workplace Advocacy Initiative

One of the most recent activities has been a move on the part of the ANA to improve their work environment and gain control over nursing practice. Ideally this would result in an assurance that patients would receive the best possible nursing care.

In moving toward this objective, in 1991 the ANA selected 16 states to receive grants to initiate or improve the workplace advocacy programs. Two grants focused on exploring new methods to ensure that nurses are involved in decisions that affect the quality of their work environments in states where the state nurses' association does not represent nurses at the bargaining table. The other grants were used to mount organizing campaigns that would result in strengthening the bargaining programs of the state association.

Other aspects of the ANA Workplace Advocacy Initiative included providing data about salaries and related economic and employment issues; providing information related to health, safety, and other workplace concerns; developing systems of analysis of compensation packages; consultation; and supporting networks for sharing information and providing mutual support.

CONCLUSION

We have attempted to present a comprehensive, although not detailed, explanation of the collective bargaining process and the issues that surround it. Those who want to gain more information will be interested in an NLRB publication entitled *A Guide to Basic Law and Procedures under the National Labor Relations Act*, which explains union shops, strikes, elections and the other issues related to negotiations in greater detail. It may be obtained by writing to the NLRB office at 1717 Pennsylvania Avenue NW, Washington, DC 20570.

Each of you will need to examine these collective bargaining issues and resolve them according to your personal value system and your philosophy. To do so you will need to consider the issues at stake, the ramifications that any action will have on the health care of a given area, and the dictates of your own conscience. We hope that this chapter has provided information to assist you in any decisions related to collective bargaining that you may be required to make.

REFERENCES

Ashley JA: Hospitals, Paternalism and the Role of the Nurse. New York, Teachers' College Press, 1976

Ballman CS: Union busters. Am J Nurs 85(9):963–966, 1985

Bloom B: Collective action by professionals poses problems for administrators. Hospitals 174(March 16):167–168, 1977

Campbell GJ: In Opinions: Is bargaining unprofessional for nurses? AORN J 31(6):1289, 1980.

Cleland V: Taft-Hartley amended: Implications for nursing—the professional model. J Nurs Admin 11(7):18–22, 1981

Dock LL: Nurses should be obedient. *In* Bullough V, Bullough B: Issues in Nursing: Readings Selected From Books and Periodicals to Form a Basis for Discussion of Problems in Nursing Today, p 96. New York: Springer-Verlag, 1966

Guido GW: Legal Issues in Nursing: A Source Book for Practice. Norwalk, CT, Appleton & Lange, 1988

Hoover K, Sanders EM, Colin JM: What's right about grievances? Am J Nurs 90(11):45–46, 1990

Mallison MB: Weathering the economic climate. Am J Nurs 85(9):943, 1985

Miller RU: Collective bargaining: A nursing dilemma. AORN J 31(6):1197, 1980

Muff J: Altruism, socialism and nightingalism: The compassion traps. *In* Muff J: Women's Issues in Nursing: Socialization, Sexism, and Stereotyping, pp 234–247. St. Louis, CV Mosby, 1988

Public Law 93-360, Section 2, 1974

Rothman DA, Rothman NL: The Professional Nurse and the Law. Boston, Little, Brown & Co, 1977

6,000 Minnesota RNs strike back at layoff trend. Am J Nurs 84(7):941, 948, 1984

Werther WB Jr, Lockhart CA: Labor Relations in the Health Professions: The Basis of Power—The Means of Change. Boston: Little, Brown & Co, 1976

Wilson CN, Hamilton CL, Murphy E: Union dynamics in nursing. J Nurs Admin 20(2):35–39, 1990

FURTHER READINGS

Beletz E, Meng MT: The grievance process. Am J Nurs 77(2):256–260, 1977

Browne MN et al: Litigation and collective bargaining: Two pay equity strategies. A D Nurse 3(6):18–20, 1988

Castrey BG, Castrey RT: Mediation: What it is, what it does. J Nurs Admin 10(9): 18–21, 1980

Eldridge I, Levi J: Collective bargaining as a power resource for professional goals. Nurs Admin Q Winter:29–40, 1982

Flanagan L: All-RN rule to have major impact. Am Nurse March:26, 1982

Hudacek SS: Collective bargaining—not a dinosaur of the past. Adv Clin Care 5(1):27–28, 1990

Gross JA: Conflicting statutory purposes: Another look at fifty years of NLRB law making. Indust Labor Rel Rev 39(10):7–18, 1985

McCarty P: ANA launches workplace initiative—SNAs get grants for RN advocacy, new organizing. Am Nurse April:1, 7, 1991

Pettengill MM: Collective bargaining: Impact on nursing. *In* Chaska NL: The

Nursing Profession: Turning Points, pp 454–463. St. Louis, CV Mosby, 1990

Pettengill MM: Multilateral collective bargaining and the health care industry: Implications for Nursing. J Prof Nurs 1(5):275–282, 1985

Smith GR: Unionization for Nurses: An issue for the 1980s. J Prof Nurs 1(4): 192–201, 1985

Stickler KB: Union organizing will be divisive and costly. Hospitals 64(13):68–70, 1990.

10

The Political Process and Health Care

Objectives

After completing this chapter, you should be able to

1. *State reasons why the political process is relevant to nursing.*

2. *Identify seven ways a person might affect the political process.*

3. *Discuss the significance of the Nurse Education Act.*

4. *Explain the major provisions of the Medicare and Medicaid acts that relate to health care.*

5. *Identify four additional federal legislative acts and state their purposes.*

6. *Discuss the various proposals related to a national health care system.*

7. *List common state-level legislative concerns.*

8. *Discuss common local political concerns.*

9. *Identify how politics is relevant to your participation in organizations.*

Politics is the way in which people in a democratic society try to influence decision making and the allocation of resources. Because resources (money, time, or personnel) are always limited, choices must always be made as to their use. There is no perfect process for making optimum choices because in every instance in which one valuable option is chosen, some other option must be left out. Politics is a part of every organization as well as part of government at every level. In this chapter we hope to help you to understand the political process as we discuss some of the current issues in regard to political decisions and describe ways you can play a role in the political arena.

RELEVANCE OF THE POLITICAL PROCESS FOR NURSES

Nurses have always been involved in politics. Florence Nightingale used her contacts with powerful men in the government to obtain supplies and the personnel she needed to care for wounded soldiers in the Crimea (Woodham-Smith, 1967). Hannah Ropes was able to fight incompetence and obtain decent care for wounded Civil War soldiers because she understood where the power in Washington lay and who would be receptive to her efforts on the soldiers' behalf (Donahue, 1985).

Modern times are no different. With all the many different voices competing to be heard in the decision-making circles of any nation, the person who understands power and how the system works is better prepared to achieve desired ends.

Health care is very costly, and public dollars can be and are spent in many ways to provide health care. What part of the federal budget should be allocated to health care? What part of the state budget? The local governmental budget? Of the money allocated, what part should be used for preventive health programs? What part for research? What part for care and treatment? What part for education? These questions are answered by legislation and by administrative decisions made by governmental agencies.

If you have opinions on what is an appropriate government role in health care, then politics is for you. If you think that priorities as they are set currently are incorrect, then politics is for you. If you have ever been blocked in your attempt to provide health care to a client and family because funds or programs were not available, then the political process is relevant to you.

Your practice as a nurse is controlled by a wide variety of governmental decisions. One of the most basic is the nurse practice act of your state. In that document, nursing is defined legally and the scope of nursing practice is outlined. This document affects what you do each day that you practice. All of the philosophical discussions about the role of the nurse must return to the reality of what is the nurse's legal role. Do you care what that role is now, or what changes are made in it? Does it make any difference to you what education is required in that law or if that law requires continuing education? Answering "yes" to any of these questions underlines the relevance of the political process for you.

Many decisions are made within the various nurses' organizations (see Chapter 13). These organizations speak for nurses in a variety of settings. Are you happy with the way they are spending funds paid in dues? Do you agree with all of the public statements they make? Do you support their mechanisms for decision making? Are you happy with the view the public receives of nurses and nursing from these organizations? Do you care what these organizations do with their resources? The political process is an important part of their functioning, too.

AFFECTING THE POLITICAL PROCESS

Once you have decided that the political process affects you and your practice as a nurse in many crucial ways, your next concern is how to influence the process by which those decisions are made. Can you as an individual have an effect on such things as what legislation is submitted, what is passed, and the content of that legislation? The answer is yes you can, but not without effort and concern on your part. Each person must determine his or her own level of personal involvement, but there is, in the broad realm of the political process, a place for everyone to function in a way that is comfortable. Some of the ways are outlined here.

Keeping Informed

To keep informed about legislation and health care, it is necessary to become familiar with the sources of information. Your daily newspaper can be an excellent source regarding significant legislation being proposed. This source is not complete, however, and you often learn of legislation after it has already been passed.

Television and radio news reports are valuable but may give only an overview of a particular piece of legislation being introduced. This overview may be helpful in alerting you to something that you want to study more intensively. Some television programs do discuss issues in depth. These programs usually make an attempt to present both sides of any issue to meet the Federal Communications Commission rules regarding equal time.

Professional journals usually devote some space to current legislative issues. This is done routinely in the *American Journal of Nursing* and in the *American Nurse.* When major issues are being discussed, other nursing periodicals frequently contain articles of interests.

Nursing organizations or other health-related organizations may hold open meetings to present and discuss legislative issues. Often knowledgeable speakers are present who can help you to understand what is being proposed and the various potential effects.

Newsletters or journals of organizations that have a political focus provide information on what they see as current issues. These include consumer groups such as Common Cause, political groups such as Young Democrats and Young Republicans, and nonpartisan groups such as the League of Women Voters.

Copies of legislation are usually available through your congressional representatives (for federal matters) or your state representatives (for state matters). Along with copies of the legislation you may receive other informational material from a legislator. Government agencies affected by proposed legislation may also provide information about its potential effect.

Each source of information is valuable to you but should be weighed in terms of its known biases. Even the most objective-sounding report may be as greatly shaded with meaning by what is not reported as by what is reported. Considering what groups support and what groups oppose a particular viewpoint may help in identifying bias. Speculate whether the group and its members would tend personally to gain or lose by the passage of proposed legislation. Are there special interest groups voicing an opinion? When biases are very evident, be sure to also obtain information from those with divergent points of view. Decision making needs to rest on a firm factual basis.

Once you are informed about the current issues in legislation, you are better prepared to form a personal opinion about them and to try to influence the outcome of the political process. There are many ways you can affect that process.

Voting

Your individual vote on a ballot issue is significant. One of the unfortunate statistics in the United States is the low percentage of those eligible who are registered and voters. Nurses, as a group, have a high percentage who are voters. When legislators hear statistics like "one in

17 women voters is a nurse," they pay attention to the opinions of nurses. Although you cannot vote directly on most legislative issues, you can vote for candidates whose positions you support and who share your values. Absentee ballots are always available for those who cannot be present at their polling place on the day of the election. These must be requested well in advance of the election, however.

It is a common practice to disparage the importance of the individual vote in any election. Recent major elections in this country have demonstrated again how important those votes can be. Recounts were necessary in several elections because the margin between the two candidates was only a few hundred votes out of the thousands cast. Even one-sided votes with overwhelming support for or against one candidate or issue may strongly emphasize the position of the voting public, and thus affect subsequent legislative and governmental decisions.

Figure 10–1. Sharing your opinions is one avenue of political involvement.

Shaping Public Opinion

Public opinion does influence the actions of legislators and regulatory bodies. You may help to shape that public opinion. As a registered nurse, your opinion about matters that affect health care may help others make their own decisions. Share the knowledge you have gained through your personal experience and research. Do not be afraid to state your own opinion, although you must be prepared with evidence to support that opinion to be accepted as a thoughtful health care professional. This does not mean that you must become an orator on every social occasion, but that you should use opportunities that arise to present your concerns to others.

Communicating With Legislators and Officials

Legislators are affected by the views of their constituents. Letters received usually are reviewed by the legislator's staff; views are tabulated, and letters with significant opinions or information are directed to the legislator for individual consideration. Form letters and postcards receive the least attention from a legislator. A carefully written personal letter that reflects thoughtful and informed opinions on an issue that person is competent to evaluate receives the most attention.

As a registered nurse you have expertise in an aspect of health care that can provide a valuable viewpoint. Identify yourself as a registered nurse in your letter, and outline why you are concerned about the issue in question. Legislators often appreciate personal anecdotes from your practice (with identities concealed, of course) that underscore your point.

Concern regarding rules and regulations of a specific department of government can be addressed to officials of that department. It is possible for officials to become insulated from the effects of their decision making. Communication from concerned citizens is important to them as well as to legislators. Letters to officials should reflect the same careful professional view as letters to legislators do to be most effective in influencing regulations.

Telephone calls cannot usually be made directly to a legislator but can be made to the legislator's office. Staff keep a record of all calls and the positions of callers. In some states a toll-free number is maintained for calls to state legislators during the legislative session.

Telegrams are delivered by telephone within 5 hours of being sent. A mailgram is a less expensive type of telegram that is delivered in the regular mail on the next business day after you send it. These are especially useful right before an important vote or committee deliberation.

Visits to congressional or state representatives may also be an effec-

(Text continues on page 366)

HOW TO WRITE YOUR CONGRESSMAN

How to learn
their names . . .

Call your public library, local news-paper, or chapter of the League of Women Voters to learn the names and addresses of your U. S. senators, your representative to congress, your state senator(s), and your state representative(s), (called as-semblyman in California, New Jersey, New York, and Wisconsin; delegate in Virginia and West Virginia).

How to obtain
a copy of a bill

For a Senate bill, write or visit (no telephone requests filled) the Senate Documents Office, Washington, DC 20510; for a House bill, write or visit the Doorkeeper of the House, U. S. Capitol, Washington, DC 20515.

Ask for the bill by number and enclose a self-addressed and gum-med label for fastest service. There is no charge.

Requests are normally filled the day received, unless the bill is out of print, and sent via first class mail. There is a limit of six items per day per person, and of three copies of one bill per person (or of one copy per bill if the bill is 60 pages or longer).

Request a copy of a state bill from the appropriate state legislator.

Copies of hearing record can be requested from the committee con-ducting the hearing, although they usually are not ready for distribu-tion until several weeks after the hearing.

An alternate to the above proce-dures, for federal bills and hearing records, is to request a copy from your appropriate senator or repre-sentative.

(Reprinted by permission of the N.A.A.C.O.G.)

Fundamentals:

1. Address your letter properly: "Hon. _____, House Office Building, Washington, DC 20515", or "Senator _____, Senate Office Building, Washington, DC 20510".
2. Identify the bill or issue. Try to give the bill number or describe it by popular title.
3. Watch your timing. Inform your congressman while there is still time to take effective action.

Write to the right persons:

Concentrate on your own delegation. The repre-sentative of your district and the senators of your state cast your votes in the Congress and want to know your views.

Be brief:

Be reasonably brief. Your views and arguments stand a better chance of being read if they are stat-ed as concisely as the subject matter will permit. It is not necessary that letters be typed — only that they be legible — and the form, phraseology, and grammar are not important.

Do:

1. Write your own views — not someone else's. A personal letter is far better than a form letter or signature on a petition. Form letters often receive form replies.
2. Give your reasons for taking a stand. The ef-fects of a bill on a certain constituency will be far more helpful.
3. Be constructive. If a bill deals with a problem, but you believe the bill is the wrong approach, outline the correct approach. If you have ex-pert knowledge, share it with your congressman.
4. Say 'well done' when it is deserved. Congress-men appreciate this from people who believe they have done the right thing.

Do not:

1. Don't make threats or promises.
2. Don't berate your congressman. If you disagree with him, give reasons for your disagreement.
3. Don't become a 'pen pal'. Quality is more im-portant than quantity.
4. Don't demand a commitment before the facts are in. A bill rarely becomes law in the same form as introduced, it is possible for a writer to change his or her position once a bill reaches a floor.

The above material, excerpted from *Congressional Record, Nov. 2, 1977*, by Morris K. Udall, was prepared by the Washington office of The American College of Obstetri-cians and Gynecologists.

Figure 10–2. How to write your congressman.

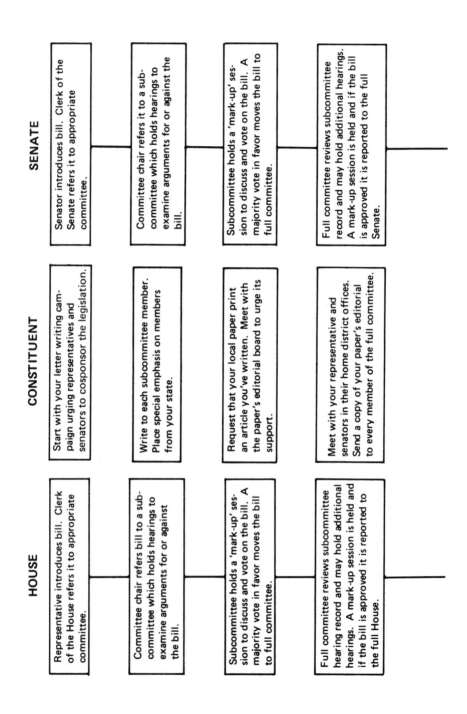

HOUSE

Representative introduces bill. Clerk of the House refers it to appropriate committee.

Committee chair refers bill to a sub-committee which holds hearings to examine arguments for or against the bill.

Subcommittee holds a 'mark-up' session to discuss and vote on the bill. A majority vote in favor moves the bill to full committee.

Full committee reviews subcommittee hearing record and may hold additional hearings. A mark-up session is held and if the bill is approved it is reported to the full House.

CONSTITUENT

Start with your letter writing campaign urging representatives and senators to cosponsor the legislation.

Write to each subcommittee member. Place special emphasis on members from your state.

Request that your local paper print an article you've written. Meet with the paper's editorial board to urge its support.

Meet with your representative and senators in their home district offices. Send a copy of your paper's editorial to every member of the full committee.

SENATE

Senator introduces bill. Clerk of the Senate refers it to appropriate committee.

Committee chair refers it to a sub-committee which holds hearings to examine arguments for or against the bill.

Subcommittee holds a 'mark-up' session to discuss and vote on the bill. A majority vote in favor moves the bill to full committee.

Full committee reviews subcommittee record and may hold additional hearings. A mark-up session is held and if the bill is approved it is reported to the full Senate.

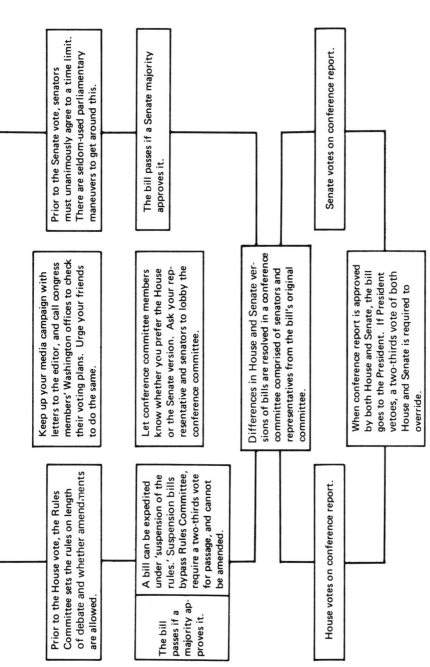

Prior to the House vote, the Rules Committee sets the rules on length of debate and whether amendments are allowed.

The bill passes if a majority approves it.

A bill can be expedited under 'suspension of the rules.' Suspension bills bypass Rules Committee, require a two-thirds vote for passage, and cannot be amended.

Keep up your media campaign with letters to the editor, and call congress members' Washington offices to check their voting plans. Urge your friends to do the same.

Prior to the Senate vote, senators must unanimously agree to a time limit. There are seldom-used parliamentary maneuvers to get around this.

The bill passes if a Senate majority approves it.

Let conference committee members know whether you prefer the House or the Senate version. Ask your representative and senators to lobby the conference committee.

Differences in House and Senate versions of bills are resolved in a conference committee comprised of senators and representatives from the bill's original committee.

House votes on conference report.

When conference report is approved by both House and Senate, the bill goes to the President. If President vetoes, a two-thirds vote of both House and Senate is required to override.

Senate votes on conference report.

Figure 10-3. How a bill becomes a law.

tive means of expressing your concerns. One of the best ways to arrange to speak to congressional representatives and senators is to contact their local offices. Through these offices you may receive assistance in arranging your visit. They may also help you to arrange other interesting and valuable experiences such as attending committee hearings, taking tours, and visiting congress in session. Appointments should always be made well in advance, or the person may not have time to speak with you. If your time is circumscribed (such as a limited visit to Washington, DC), you may have to modify your expectations and meet with a staff member who will relay your concerns. Plan carefully for your visit. It is often helpful to write out concerns and questions. Be sure to leave time for answers to the questions that you pose. Even when you disagree with the position taken by your legislator, be polite and present your concerns calmly. Rudeness will result in an unwillingness to listen to what you have to say.

Group Action

The political process within the nursing profession takes many forms. On one level it is the involvement of nurses in legislative and ballot issues. Nurses can be involved as individuals, but they are far more effective when they work in groups. As the largest single health care occupation, nurses have many votes. This makes legislators pay attention to positions that are held by a group of nurses. In addition, although nurses do not have high incomes, when gathered together their financial contributions can be significant to a candidate or issue.

Nonlobbying Nursing Organizational Effort

Most traditional nursing organizations are nonprofit groups and therefore are limited in their political activity. The major role of these groups in politics is testifying as to facts and concerns within the health care area. The American Nurses Association (ANA) has an office in Washington, DC, and tries to keep the nursing profession informed about legislative matters of importance to health care. The ANA also provides experts in the field of nursing to testify about proposed legislation. Other nursing organizations such as NAACOG: The Organization for Obstetric, Gynecologic, and Neonatal Nurses and the American Association of Colleges of Nursing also testify on pertinent issues before the federal government. Most state and district nurses' associations have legislative committees that serve this function in their area.

The Tri-Council is a coalition of the ANA, the National League for Nursing (NLN), the American Association of Colleges of Nursing, and the National Organization of Nurse Executives that functions at the federal level. This organization provides expert testimony for committees and commissions that are considering health-related legislation. By coordinating efforts, the member organizations are able to present a more united front and a stronger voice for nursing.

Political Action Committees

To take a more active role in seeking passage of desired legislation, defeat of undesired measures, and election of candidates, groups form organizations called political action committees, often referred to as PACs. These organizations are registered as political action groups and are free to try to affect the political process. However, they are not considered nonprofit organizations and donations to them are not tax deductible because they are used for political purposes.

The ANA Political Action Committee (ANA-PAC) is a political action organization formed by the ANA. ANA-PAC actually lobbies for the passage or defeat of bills and supports candidates for public office. Beginning with the 1976 general elections, ANA-PAC has raised funds to support candidates for the Senate and the House of Representatives based on their expressed and demonstrated stands on key health issues, such as national health insurance, funding for biomedical research, extension and funding of the Nurse Training Act, and third-party reimbursement for nurses. Not all endorsed candidates were supported financially owing to the limitations of the funds available. Candidates' successes are attributable to many factors, but the effect of nursing support has been demonstrated. Many state nursing associations also have political action organizations. These groups serve the same function on the state level as the ANA-PAC does on the national level. Many candidates actively seek the endorsement of nursing organizations because they perceive them as influential with voters.

The Nurses' Coalition for Legislative Action is an organization of 28 specialty nursing organizations that works on behalf of those organizations at the federal level. Nurses in specialty organizations have supported this organization as a way to bring a larger voice in support of issues that affect nursing specialty practice.

Although growth in size of these nursing political action groups has not been rapid, it has been steady. In addition, nurses are gaining more sophistication in the political process. Both of these factors result in nurses gaining increased power. There is still a long way to go before nurses have the same kind of power as that wielded by such groups as labor, education, and medicine, but change is occurring.

Figure 10–4. Nurses may lobby to get desired legislation passed by visiting legislators, by presenting information and arguments about the bill, and by writing letters.

Other Politically Important Groups

In addition to these specific nursing related groups, there are other organizations that are concerned about health and social issues. Some are official lobbying groups and others provide information resources. These groups such as Common Cause (a consumer lobbying group), the League of Women Voters, and even church organizations often act to affect the political process. You may support these groups by simply donating money for their needs or by active involvement in the activities and the work of the group.

Testifying for Decision-Making Bodies

Many decisions relative to health care in general and to nursing are made by committees and commissions of the various levels of government.

They frequently have hearings to gather information before decisions are made. As a nurse your testimony may have particular value when certain areas of health care are being considered. A nurse may testify as either an official representative of an organization or an independent individual.

You may learn of opportunities to testify through announcements in the newspaper or through professional publications. In general, you must register in advance to testify. In some instances, this may occur at the door before the meeting begins, but for more formal situations, you may have to notify the committee in advance that you wish to testify.

If you have an opportunity to testify, be sure to make your position clear so the decision makers know whether you speak for yourself or for a larger group. Prepare your testimony ahead of time, but try not to just read a statement. A less formal presentation is usually more interesting for the listener. Be prepared with sources for any facts and figures you present, and explain any technical terms you use. There may be a time limit for each testimony. Check on this ahead of time and make sure that you present your most important arguments and facts first. Most committees will accept written testimony if you cannot be there in person, but the personal presentation is usually more effective.

Individual Support for Legislation and Candidates

As an individual you may choose to support a specific piece of legislation by contributing money for publicity and campaigning or by personally working on a committee that is striving for passage of the proposal. Funds are needed for printing and distributing literature, newspaper ads, and television and radio announcements. Workers may be needed for secretarial tasks, to contact people in a door-to-door campaign, and to speak on behalf of the issue.

Supporting a candidate for public office is done in the same way. In our political system the reality is that those who have actively supported a candidate during an election campaign are listened to more closely when decisions are made. Working for a candidate is one way to make your view known.

Holding Office

Whether you are involved with your local nursing organization or the U.S. Congress, those who have been elected or appointed to office, have considerable power to affect outcomes. Leaders in nursing organizations help to shape the direction and efforts of those organizations. As members of the state legislature nurses have been effective in shaping health policy in their respective states. Although to this date no nurse has been elected to federal office, this may change. Nurses have been appointed to major administrative positions in both state and federal health agencies, have been elected to state office, and in the near future hope to hold office in Congress. Nurses have a promising future in the health policy arena.

Limitations on Your Political Activity

If you are an employee of any governmental agency, such as a public health department or the Veterans Administration, there are restrictions on your political activity that do not apply to the general public. For the federal government, these restrictions are defined in the Hatch Act. The main focus of prohibited activities are those that have to do with supporting a particular political party by being an officer or party spokesperson. The Hatch Act also prohibits any activities on behalf of a party or in support of legislation that could be construed as providing support from the agency that employs you.

This act does not interfere with your rights as a private citizen to support parties and candidates financially, to join political parties, to work for or against measures that will appear on a ballot, or to participate in nonpartisan (i.e., not connected with a political party) elections as a candidate. Each state has its own version of the Hatch Act. If you are employed by a governmental agency of any kind, you should investigate the limitations that it may place on your political activity.

THE FEDERAL GOVERNMENT'S ROLE IN HEALTH CARE

The federal government operates in the health care field in complex ways, as mentioned in Chapter 8. There are literally dozens of federal agencies, some with similar titles. Sometimes identifying which agency is responsible in which area is difficult. The following overview may help you to place some agencies in context.

Department of Health and Human Services

The Department of Health and Human Services (DHHS) is a cabinet-level administrative unit of the federal government. It was originally created in 1953 as the Department of Health, Education, and Welfare. The date of its origin points out how recent has been the view that the federal government should have a major responsibility toward health care or that health should have status equal to defense at the federal executive level. In 1980 a separate department was created for education and the remaining functions were retitled the Department of Health and Human Services. There are four major service divisions of DHHS (Table 10-1).

Office of Human Development Services

The Office of Human Development Services is responsible for four sections. The activities of these sections are primarily in the health prevention and welfare field.

Public Health Service

The PHS encompasses all the activities relating to illness, disease states, and treatment. The sections of this division are much more obviously related to nursing concerns. The Centers for Disease Control (CDC) maintain all statistics relevant to the epidemiology of various disease processes. Research is supported and recommendations are made for the control of communicable diseases both in the institution and in the community.

Table 10-1. Major Service Divisions of the Department of Health and Human Services

Office of Human Development Services	Social Security Administration
Administration on Aging	Systems
Administration for Children, Youth, and Families	Governmental Affairs
	Family Assistance
Administration for Native Americans	Hearings and Appeals
Adminstration for Public Service	Operational Policy and Procedure
	Assessment

Public Health Service	Health Care Financing
Centers for Disease Control	Health Standards and Quality Bureau
Food and Drug Administration	Bureau of Quality Control
Health Resources Administration	Bureau of Program Operations
Health Services Administration	Bureau of Program Policy
National Institutes of Health	Bureau of Support Services
Alcohol, Drug Abuse, and Mental Health Administration	Office of Child Support Enforcement

The Food and Drug Administration

The Food and Drug Administration (FDA) regulates the use of medications and devices for both prevention and treatment of disease. It also sets guidelines for food labeling and for what may be added to foods. The FDA also sets standards for allowable radiation and establishes rules regarding milk and shellfish sanitation, restaurant operation, and interstate travel facilities.

Health Resources Administration

The Health Resources Administration (HRA) is concerned with planning for the agencies and personnel to provide health care in the community. One area of responsibility is planning for nursing, which is done through the Division of Nursing. Because the responsibility for all nursing research endeavors was transferred to the Center for Nursing Research within the National Institutes of Health in 1986, the Division of Nursing has a much more restricted budget than previously experienced. Recent legislation has eliminated many of the other programs that the division used to administer, such as construction grants for schools of nursing and individual assistance for students at all levels of nursing education. There is concern in some circles of nursing that the Division of Nursing will lose much of the influence it has commanded.

Health Services Administration

The Health Services Administration (HSA) provides leadership by supporting the development of health services in communities and providing direct health care to specific groups (e.g., Native Americans, migrants, mothers and children). The Health Services Administration is an area that has received drastic cuts in funding as the federal government strives to transfer responsibility to local and state governments.

National Institutes of Health

The National Institutes of Health (NIH) are agencies established for research and treatment of specific health problems. There are institutes for heart, lung, and blood problems, arthritis, metabolism, and digestive disorders, allergy and infectious disease, neurological and communicative disorders and stroke, and many other areas of concern. It is within this agency that the National Library of Medicine operates as an agency to provide support for research activities.

Alcohol, Drug Abuse, and Mental Health Administration

The role of the Alcohol, Drug Abuse, and Mental Health Administration is to provide research and treatment for these problems. Public education is an important part of its function.

Health Care Financing Administration

The Health Care Financing Administration (HCFA) administers the Medicare and Medicaid programs. As part of this responsibility it establishes policies and procedures for care providers and recipients. This division is charged with the responsibility of researching health care costs and methods of containing those costs. HCFA also provides assistance to the states in their programs to provide health care to the needy. The rules and regulations developed by HCFA in regard to reimbursement through Medicare and Medicaid are a very important factor in whether certain services are available to individual clients and whether an agency or individual is able to be reimbursed for providing health services.

Social Security Administration

The Social Security Administration oversees all of the funds that are dispensed under the Social Security Act. It provides a mechanism for establishing eligibility and dispensing funds and furnishes an appeal system. Medicare is part of the Social Security system.

Center for Nursing Research

In the fall of 1985, against great administrative opposition, including a presidential veto by former President Reagan, legislative supporters of nursing succeeded in establishing a Center for Nursing Research within the National Institutes for Health. All research support was transferred from the Division of Nursing to this new center, and additional funds were authorized for start-up, organization, and research grants. Although the budget for nursing research is still just a fraction of the budgets of the other institutes within the NIH, a great many nurses think that this was a significant move toward putting nursing in the mainstream of research. Nursing needs increased support of its research activities as it strives to establish a broader knowledge base for nursing practice.

FEDERAL LEGISLATION OF IMPORTANCE TO NURSING

In recent years many pieces of legislation have been passed that have critically affected nursing. These legislative acts are not static, however. They are constantly being changed and revised in light of current concerns. A few significant ones are presented here.

The Federal Budget Process

For each federal program the money actually available from the government depends on two separate legislative actions. The first action is the authorization act. This is a bill, passed by both the House of Representatives and the Senate, that describes the program and outlines the rules under which funds can be expended and sets a ceiling on the amount of money that can be provided. It is under these acts (often referred to by the "title" of the section of the authorizing act) that funds are dispensed for all the health-related activities described in this chapter.

The second necessary legislative action is the appropriations act. In the appropriations process the federal budget is established and specific amounts of money are appropriated for actual spending for each program previously authorized. Both the House and the Senate pass a budget appropriations act. Then a joint House and Senate committee meet to achieve a compromise that both will accept. The final result is entitled the "Omnibus Budget Reconciliation Act" (OBRA), which includes the compromises the budget committee has worked out between the House and Senate versions of the budget. The amount appropriated for any program cannot be more than the amount originally authorized, but it can be, and frequently is, less. Sometimes this is confusing because two monetary amounts may be reported in regard to the same act, the authorized amount and the budgeted (or appropriated) amount.

The budget act may also contain requirements or constraints on those people and organizations who receive federal support. It is under this authority that the federal government sets standards for nursing homes that receive reimbursement through Medicaid and Medicare. The rules and regulations for nursing homes included in OBRA '87, the budget reconciliation act for 1987, were very extensive. These rules and regulations were scheduled to take effect in October 1990. This allowed the affected organizations to begin the process of change to meet the new requirements.

Historically, a third factor has affected the amount of money available for a specific federal program. The executive branch makes decisions about how and when funds that are available will be spent. If money that has been authorized and appropriated has not been spent by the end of the budget period it is lost. The funds must then be reauthorized and reappropriated. The executive branch has used this mechanism to withdraw support for programs it opposed.

Nurse Education Act

The Nurse Training Act of 1964 (Title VII of the Public Health Service Act) was a significant factor in the growth of nursing education.

It provided for financial assistance to schools of nursing and to students in those schools for 2 years and was renewed in 1966 for 2 additional years. In 1968 financial assistance to schools and students was continued under Title II of the Health Manpower Act. In 1971 federal aid to nursing education was again expanded. Monies for constructing schools of nursing and for aiding the educational program were provided. Many of you have been educated in buildings or practice laboratories whose construction was funded under this act. Individual financial aid to students was also provided. A large number of your instructors may have had their graduate education made possible by this funding.

Although nurses think that the monies were well used in a responsible manner, continued funding was not automatic. In 1973 and 1974 the Nixon administration made a concerted effort to curtail money spent on nursing education as well as on other health-related endeavors. Later both the Ford and the Carter administrations proposed drastic cuts in nurse training money. Nursing organizations fought long and hard through testimony and through providing public information to achieve passage of the new Nurse Training Act legislation. This was finally accomplished, although there were many compromises over what nurses had originally wanted to see passed.

A new version of the Nurse Training Act was passed in 1979 as Public Law 96-97. At this time it was referred to as the Nurse Education Act. In addition to support for nursing students, nursing schools, and nursing research, this bill provided for an independent study of nursing personnel needs. The total amount of money appropriated was less than previous acts had provided.

Funds currently appropriated through the Nurse Education Act are limited. They support some advanced nursing education and a few specific programs such as nurse midwifery. Each year nurses have supported legislation to reinstitute the Nurse Education Act. Although there has been consistent support from some legislators, it has not been enough to alter the situation. Table 10-2 shows an overview of the Nurse Education (Training) Act and its provisions.

Medicare and Medicaid

In 1965, after years of effort and testimony by many health-related groups, (including the ANA) and with widespread public support, an amendment of the Social Security Act was passed. Title XVIII of the act, which was termed *Medicare,* provided payment for hospitalization and insurance that could be purchased for meeting physicians' fees for people over age 65. Title IX of the act, which was termed *Medicaid,* provided funds for health care for the dependent population. Medicaid

Table 10–2. **Federal Funding for Nursing Education Through The Nurse Education Act (in millions of dollars)**

Year	Authorization	Appropriation
1965	17.1	16.4
1966	42.9	37.5
1967	68.8	61.5
1968	80.3	61.9
1969	88.9	40.1
1970	95.0	49.0
1971	115.0	64.0
1972	201.5	122.8
1973	227.0	122.7
1974	254.5	150.3
1975	254.5	116.7
1976	161.0	127.5
1977	186.0	118.0
1978	206.0	119.5
1979	105.5	100.3
1980	103.0	100.3
1981	103.0	74.3
1982	103.0	46.4
1983	103.0	42.8
1984	70.8	42.3
1985	70.8	50.3
1986	54.1	50.0
1987	55.35	53.2
1988	56.6	54.0
1989	57.4	55.5
1990	56.4	53.6

Authorization figures: 1965–1981 from Kalisch and Kalisch.
1982–1985 from Solomon, 1985.
1986–1988 from Nurses' Coalition for Legislative Action, Correspondence, 1985.
1989–1990 Division of Nursing
Appropriation figures: 1965–1983 from Crosby, Facteau, and Donley, 1983.
1984 from Fy, 1985, December 1983.
1985 from Solomon, 1984.
1986–1990 Division of Nursing

is administered by the states, which determine eligibility and level of coverage.

Medicare and Medicaid have supplied an important health care resource but have not been without problems. Costs have been much larger and have risen faster than anticipated. There has been a great deal of publicity over instances of abuse and even fraud that have occurred in connection with these two programs. The goals of providing adequate health care for elders and the indigent through these programs has yet to be achieved.

The Medicare bill contained many provisions that have made a significant impact on nursing. A definition of skilled nursing care in the original bill was narrow and excluded many important aspects of care needed to maintain health. Through later efforts and testimony, nursing organizations were instrumental in getting legislators to recognize that the definition of skilled nursing was a critical matter, and through a Senate subcommittee the ANA was asked to study skilled nursing care to provide background data for the Senate. Amendments to the Medicare-Medicaid Act of 1972 encouraged increased study of alternative ways of providing health care to contain costs. These alternatives included in-

Figure 10–5. Federal legislation is encouraging hospitals to stop the rapid rise of health care costs.

novation in the use of nurses in expanded roles as well as the use of health maintenance organizations.

Amendments to this act were also responsible for mandating review and evaluation of health care. This was done in the interests of cost containment. Within institutions, records of Medicare/Medicaid patients must be reviewed and compared with specific criteria for care.

In 1982 Medicare was revised by the 97th Congress to prevent the predicted bankruptcy of the system owing to rapidly escalating costs. The premium for Part B of Medicare (the optional portion that provides for out-of-hospital and physician care) and the deductible that the individual must pay for covered service were increased. The system of payment was changed to prospective payment based on diagnosis-related groups. Many items that were previously funded separately were now included in the one prospective rate. A mechanism for reimbursing hospice care was included.

There was still separate support for medical education and nursing education programs that were under the control of the hospital in which they occurred. This was meant to compensate for additional costs related to the teaching responsibilities of and the services rendered by those in such programs. Although the largest share of this fund was for residency programs for physicians, significant support was available for nursing diploma programs. This funding source for nursing education programs in hospitals is now in jeopardy, as increased efforts are being made to cut Medicare costs even further.

Evaluation of Health Services: Peer Review and Quality Assurance

The first provision for the systematic evaluation of health care services provided to the consumer was established through the Professional Standards Review Organization and utilization review set up by Medicare and Medicaid. As part of the 1982 revisions of Medicare the evaluation process was altered. Hospitals are now required to contract with an external medical review organization, called a Utilization and Quality Control Peer Review Organization (abbreviated PRO). These organizations are established through contracts awarded by the secretary of Health and Human Services through competitive bidding. Most of the PROs are statewide in scope and are required to have a substantial number of physicians represented in the organization to effectively set standards and review care.

Evaluation may consist of preadmission, preprocedure, concurrent, or retrospective reviews. The purpose of the reviews is to determine whether the care given was necessary and whether it was given in the appropriate manner. For example, the reviews have resulted in an increase in the number of surgeries performed as day procedures on outpatients rather than as inpatient surgeries. This results in a significant economic saving. The PRO is also required to evaluate outcomes of care to ensure that the changes that are made do not jeopardize clients.

Occupational Safety and Health Act

There has been a great deal of controversy over the provisions of Occupational Safety and Health Act (OSHA), which is designed to improve the safety of the working environment. The act specifies safety devices that must be present, such as goggles, showers, and eye washes, in areas where caustic chemicals are used. Other examples of safety regulations that have been developed under OSHA are safety switches required on machinery to prevent accidental engagement of gears during repair and standards set for air purity and availability of masks and respirators in the working area. OSHA regulations have been used to mandate that hospitals place "sharps" containers in all areas where needles are used to safeguard employees from inadvertent needle sticks.

Many people think that the rules and regulations created by this act are too extensive and cumbersome. For example, the rules regarding ladder safety are extremely detailed and cover several pages. When one considers the enormous number of different pieces of equipment and envisions the quantity of regulations that exist to cover all these items, it is apparent that it would be almost impossible for any one person to know all the applicable regulations.

Nevertheless, the concern for the safety of the working person is of real importance to nurses. Occupational injuries are a major health problem in the adult population. They are costly not only in terms of health and personal loss but also in terms of lost productivity. Nurses are affected by the provisions of this act in their work environments. They, too, are subject to injury and accident on the job.

A major concern in nursing is the high incidence of back injuries suffered by direct care personnel. Another, more recent concern is the potential hazard of the many toxic drugs and chemicals, such as chemotherapeutic agents, that health care personnel may handle. Hospitals are being required to set up procedures for handling and disposing of such agents in a way that will protect staff at all levels. In addition, all employers must identify the toxic chemicals that are present in their work environments, maintain information on those chemicals, and have established procedures for managing their use.

Nurses in occupational health nursing are involved in another way. They may be part of the program for educating workers about job safety. In some situations safety precautions are time consuming and uncomfortable, and workers may be tempted to ignore them. Nurses may be able to help workers understand the importance of following health and safety regulations. Occupational health nurses also work with management in planning to make the environment safe and in establishing appropriate procedures of caring for injuries.

Other Significant Legislation

You may want to investigate other federal legislation and evaluate its impact on health care in general and nursing in particular. A few that have particular relevance to nursing are presented here.

OBRA '87 was briefly mentioned in the discussion of the federal budget process. This legislation contained regulations that for the first time mandated a national standard for quality of care in long-term care facilities. Included in this legislation was the mandate for an admission assessment for every individual admitted to long-term care. As part of this admission assessment, the collection of a "minimum data set" (MDS) to facilitate research in long-term care was required. There were also regulations to limit the use of both chemical and physical restraints and to require programs to maintain individuals at their highest level of functioning. Training for nursing assistants was mandated, and the requirements for supervision by licensed nurses were increased. Although the provisions of this act were set to take effect in October 1990, there has been delay because the state of California has gone to court to block implementation of these regulations. California has taken the position that their state regulations already provide this level of quality and that adding another layer of federal regulations is counterproductive. Other states have asserted that reimbursement is not adequate to support all of the requirements included in the new regulations.

The Maternal-Child Health Act, Title V, was planned to improve health in the nation through benefits such as nutritional support, health supervision, and well-child care to mothers and children. Part of the money appropriated was earmarked for nursing research projects and nursing research training. Nurses who provide care are directly affected in their practice because the provisions of the act outline what care is funded and to whom that care can be provided. Since its inception, the Maternal-Child Health Act has never been fully funded. This means that even those who are eligible for services under the provisions of the act may not receive them because of budget limitations.

In 1983 an "orphan drug" bill was passed and signed into law. The purpose of this bill was to support and encourage the production of drugs that would be of benefit to only a limited number of people and therefore might not be financially feasible without some kind of outside support. As you care for individuals with uncommon illnesses, you may become aware of drugs that are available because of the support provided through this legislation.

The Americans with Disabilities Act of 1990 brought to fruition an effort that had begun 20 years earlier to ensure that those with disabilities were assured of equal access and opportunity. A disability is defined in the act as "a physical or mental impairment that substantially limits activities of daily living" (Watson, 1990, p 325). In 1973 the Rehabilitation Act began the effort by providing the disabled with physical and vocational access to organizations and institutions that received federal funds. The Americans with Disabilities Act moves beyond that basic support and provides the same rights to those with physical disabilities as had been provided to women and minorities under the 1964 Civil Rights legislation. The law requires accessible workplaces, nondiscriminatory practices, and access to public services, such as transportation and telephone, and provides legal avenues for redress when these provisions are not carried out. Nurses are key individuals in educating the disabled about their rights under the law and acting as advocates in the community (Watson, 1990).

The Women's Health Equity Act of 1990 addressed the unmet health needs of the women of the United States. Although women make up 52% of the population, only 13% of the research dollars of the NIH are directed toward women's health issues (Sharp, 1990). For example, although heart disease is the major cause of death in women, no women were included in any of the major heart disease studies. This bill brought together concerns for adequate research into breast cancer, women's infertility and contraceptive needs, and the inclusion of women as subjects in other research studies (Sharp, 1990). When it was not passed, it was re-introduced in 1991.

PROSPECTIVE LEGISLATION THAT WILL AFFECT NURSING

Each year many issues that affect nursing come before the House and the Senate. There are more issues that have never been resolved, and others are attempts to continue (or discontinue) previous provisions related to health care.

National Health Insurance

The United States is the only major industrialized country that does not have some type of government-sponsored health care for all citizens. Public opinion appears to be moving toward support of some type of nationwide health care plan. Costs of hospital and medical care have risen much more rapidly than the general rate of inflation. Part of this rise is caused by advances in treatment that require expensive equipment, laboratory work, and intensive care. People are also beginning to look at health care as a right rather than as a privilege available only to those who can afford it.

Through Medicare, Medicaid, and the widespread effects of the military, public health, and Indian health systems, the federal government is already deeply involved in the provision of health care. How much greater that involvement should be is the subject of serious debate.

One factor that is creating more support for some type of statewide or national health plan is the increasing amount of uncompensated care being provided by some of the nation's health care facilities. When people are unemployed or underemployed they often do not have health insurance. These same people are often not eligible for public assistance for health care. They then do not receive preventive health care or prompt attention to health problems when they arise. When they have major health care needs, bills simply remain unpaid. Hospitals historically have absorbed these costs through spreading them out to those who do pay their bills. As insurance companies and the government become more stringent about reimbursement, this is becoming increasingly difficult and some hospitals will be in serious financial trouble if some method of assisting with this problem is not found soon.

Because the federal government has not acted, many states are beginning to look at the problem from a state perspective. Some questions that are being raised are: Is there a right to health care? If there is a right, what level of health care does this cover, that is, routine preventive services, surgery and hospitalization for all conditions, or only for serious life-threatening conditions? Should catastrophic illnesses, transplantation, and experimental treatments be included? These are difficult philosophical and ethical questions, and there are no simple answers.

The ANA and the NLN are cooperating in presenting a Nursing National Health Proposal to the public. The decision was made to sponsor a plan when research revealed that nurses hold a unique position of trust in the minds of the public. In the Hart survey conducted for the NLN, 77% of those polled believed that nurses took a constructive role in health care and were not solely concerned with their own self interest.

This contrasted to 42% who believed that doctors had a constructive role, 19% who believed the federal government had a constructive role, and 11% who thought insurance companies took a constructive role (National League for Nursing, 1991).

One component of the Nursing National Health Proposal includes a federally defined standard package of essential health care benefits. This would include primary care and prevention and would be financed by a mix of public and private sources. Additional components are improving access to health care by delivering it in schools, workplaces, and the home; controlling costs through managed care; and implementation of the plan in steps. Forty-two nursing groups have endorsed the plan, and more are expected to add their weight to the push for action.

Reimbursement of Nursing Services

One key concern of nurses is whether nursing care will be directly reimbursed. This has been of special concern to primary health care nurses. The availability of funding for the care to be provided by nurses will, to a great extent, determine whether the public is able to use such services. Physicians (through the American Medical Association) have consistently supported provisions that would result in direct payment only to physicians or for care ordered by physicians. Other organizations of direct-care providers, social workers, nurses, psychologists, and so forth are seeking greater breadth in reimbursement possibilities. Third-party payment funds a large percentage of the health care in the United States; if this avenue of funding is closed to nurses and other direct-care providers, then their ability to provide services is severely curtailed. Physicians believe that controlling access to third-party payment will control costs of health care. This limitation also preserves for the physician a unique position of power in the health care setting.

Equal Rights Amendment

The proposed Equal Rights Amendment (ERA) to the United States Constitution has provoked some of the most heated debates of any issue over the years. The proposed amendment simply states that "rights provided under the Constitution shall not be abridged on account of sex." A further statement enables the legislature to enact laws as necessary to support this. Because the vast majority of nurses are women, this amendment would seem to have special significance in the field of nursing. The ANA and the NLN have strongly supported its passage.

Individual nurses do have varying viewpoints. Some see the ERA as crucial to professional recognition and advancement. They cite the historically low salaries of nurses and other women in the health care field and the lack of power that the nursing profession has had in health care as reflections of the status of women in our society. They believe that legal recognition of the rights of women will support efforts within nursing to achieve acknowledgement as a profession and will assist nurses in righting such historical wrongs as the relative salary gap. Concern also is expressed for the mental health of women. Strong arguments have pointed out that the position of women in society creates problems in mental health and in the way women are treated as clients in the health care system.

Other nurses oppose the passage of the ERA for a variety of reasons that seem to center on what they believe will be negative consequences for society if it is passed. Some think that passage of the ERA will further disrupt family life, which will be detrimental to the health and well-being of children as well as of women.

Most polls indicate that an actual majority of people in the United States favored the ERA. The system of ratification gives equal status to states with lesser populations and provides for ratification through state legislatures rather than by popular vote. This is designed to make the passage of a constitutional amendment a difficult process and made the ERA fail despite popular support. Although ratification of the ERA failed, the idea of having a constitutional amendment to guarantee equal rights has not been abandoned. Supporters have changed their strategy and attempts have been made to legislate equality in ways other than through a constitutional amendment.

STATE-LEVEL LEGISLATIVE CONCERNS

Many issues that vitally affect the health care area are decided at the state level. Because issues in each state differ, only some general areas of concern are outlined here.

State Institutions' Budget and Planning

Types of state institutions range from those for the care of the mentally retarded and the mentally ill to penal systems and institutions of higher education. Health care is often a consideration in all of these settings. When budgets are planned, such diverse concerns as immunization and contraception may be included or omitted from the planning. Nurses often can be a voice for those who are unable to speak for themselves in regard to their own health care needs. Sometimes nurses who work in these settings are unable to deliver quality care because of severe budgetary deficiencies. All nurses can support efforts to provide quality health care in such settings.

Nurse Practice Acts

Nurse practice acts are being discussed and revised in many states. The process is long and difficult and requires intense effort on the part of nurses. Once a bill that has been carefully developed has been submitted to the legislative body, nurses must remain alert to changes and amendments that may substantially alter the intent of the original proposal. The bill must be followed through the legislative process until its passage.

LOCAL POLITICAL CONCERNS

The budgetary process always seems to be at the base of any political or legislative concern. Because there is a limited amount of money available, budgets are always developed with a series of compromises. To gain one objective it is sometimes necessary to recognize that there will be no funds for another. In most communities budgets for public health departments, school nurses, and so forth are developed over a period of several months. Hearings are often held, at which members of the public may ask questions and address the issues. Nurses have often found that involvement at this planning stage is most rewarding. Determining priorities for health is essential, and nurses often can speak with authority on these matters. Nurses actually employed in the department under consideration may be much more limited in making their views known because of regulations governing their action in the political sphere. For this reason it is significant that other nurses recognize the importance of community health. It is not only the practice of the public health nurse that is affected by the priorities of the agency. For example, the nurse who is employed in the hospital may wish to refer a discharged patient to a public health nurse for follow-up, only to find that, owing to changes in the ordering or priorities, home visits for the identified purpose are no longer being made.

In many communities decisions about the allocation of federal money are made at the local level. Support for alternative health care centers, blood pressure screening, and senior citizen centers may depend on whether those who are knowledgeable about the benefits of these services are willing to voice their advocacy.

THE POLITICAL PROCESS WITHIN THE NURSING PROFESSION

Any large group of people that is organized into a body has a political process. All of the earlier discussion about the traditional political process is equally applicable to the politics of the profession.

On an individual level one is seldom able to influence such an organization meaningfully unless one is a member. This may create some conflict within the individual. If you do not agree with all that an organization is doing, the usual course of action is to withhold or withdraw your membership. When you are member of a profession, you may find that this course of action presents more difficulties. The organization may continue to speak for the profession. If you are outside of the organization, you may find yourself without a voice on significant issues affecting your professional life. By joining a professional organization and actively involving yourself in it, you may be able to make your concerns and viewpoints heard.

If you decide to join a professional organization, you have an obligation to be an informed and concerned member. Your vote on candidates for local, state, and national office is important. Your activity on a committee or as an officer is necessary for the organization to function effectively. You have an obligation to be informed on issues that are before the organization and make your viewpoint known. The concerned involvement of many individual members will make an organization an effective voice for a profession. Chapter 12 describes many organizations related to nursing.

CONCLUSION

Political and legislative issues are an important aspect of planning for health care in our society. The informed and concerned nurse can make a significant contribution to society's health by actions in this arena of life.

REFERENCES

Crosby L, Facteau L, Donley R: Priorities for nurse training act legislation: A national survey of nursing deans. Image 15(Fall): 107–110, 1983
Donahue MP: Nursing: The Finest Art. St. Louis, CV Mosby, 1985
Division of Nursing, Funding and Application Data for Grant Programs Administered by the Division of Nursing. 1964–1990.

FY '85 health appropriations. Testimony of the American Nurses' Association to the Labor, Health, and Human Services subcommittee of the House Appropriations Committee. Publication No. 34-323. Washington, DC, U.S. Government Printing Office, 1985

Kalisch BJ, Kalisch PA: The Politics of Nursing. Philadelphia, JB Lippincott, 1982

National League for Nursing: Nursing introduces its national health strategy to the public. Public Policy Bulletin, March 1991. New York, National League for Nursing, 1991

Nurses' Coalition for Legislative Action. Correspondence. 1985.

Sharp N: Women's Health Equity Act of 1990. Nurs Manage 21(12):21–22, 1990

Solomon S: Update: Nursing education funds, NIN, DRGs and education. Nurs Health Care 5(6):302–303, 1984

Solomon S: Nursing's legislative agenda, round one. Nurs Health Care 6(6):296–298, 1985

Watson PG: The Americans with Disabilities Act: More rights for people with disabilities. Rehabil Nurs 15(6):325–328, 1990

Woodham-Smith C: Florence Nightingale, New York, Atheneum, 1983

FURTHER READINGS

The American Nurse. Kansas City, MO, American Nurses' Association, monthly newspaper

ANA, AORN testify at OSHA hearing on employee regs. OR Manager 5(11):1, 4, 1990

Archer S, Goehner P: Nurses: A Political Force. Belmont, CA, Wadsworth Health Sciences Division, 1982

Fedor MA: AIDS: Advocacy and activism. Nurs Health Care 12(3):119, 1991

Headline News. Monthly column. American Journal of Nursing

Maraldo P: Politics: A very human matter. Am J Nurs 82(7):1106–1111, 1982

McCormick P: National Center for Nursing Research. Cardiovasc Nurs 24(6):55, 1988

Nornhold P: 90 predictions for the 90s. Nursing 20(1):34–41, 1990

Sharp N, Biggs S, Wakefield M: Public policy: New opportunities for nurses. Nurs Health Care 12(1):16–23, 1991

Simpson M, Hanley B: Nurse policy analyst: Advanced practice role. Nurs Health Care 12(1):10–15, 1991

Stark PL: Health care under siege: Challenge for change. Nurs Health Care 12(1):26–31, 1991

Watts RJ: Democratization of health care: Challenge for nursing. Adv Nurs Sci 12(2):37–46, 1990

See also the official publication of your state nurses' association.

Unit IV

Career Opportunities and Professional Growth

In this unit we present basic information about the employment world you will find in nursing. This will help you as you move from the student role to the role of the registered nurse employed within the health care delivery system. Chapter 11 looks personally at your relationship to this new role, while Chapter 12 is designed to help you understand the organization itself. In Chapter 13, we present the variety of nursing organizations that may help you in your personal growth in nursing. These organizations will also provide you with opportunities to affect the nursing profession and make a personal contribution to nursing.

11

Beginning Your Career as a Nurse

Objectives

After completing this chapter, you should be able to

1. *Discuss societal and educational factors that have caused changes in the expectations of the new graduate.*

2. *Define competency as it applies to nursing.*

3. *List major areas of competence that are of concern to employers.*

4. *List six consistent expectations of employers for new graduates.*

5. *Identify two areas in which expectations for new graduates differ widely.*

6. *Discuss a variety of ways of coping with expectations as a new graduate.*

7. *Set at least one short-term and one long-term personal career goal.*

8. *Write a letter of application and a resume.*

9. *Prepare for an employment interview.*

10. *Write an interview follow-up letter.*

11. *Write a letter of resignation.*

12. *Discuss the concept of burnout and its relationship to stress.*

13. *Discuss two areas of concern relative to sex discrimination in nursing.*

14. *Identify three ways in which occupational health is a special concern for nurses.*

After completing an educational program, you, as a new graduate, will want to get out into the real world and practice your nursing skills. In the past such a goal was rather simple and straightforward, but a nursing career is now much more complex.

HISTORICAL EMPLOYMENT OPPORTUNITIES IN NURSING

Early in the 20th century almost all graduate nurses performed private-duty nursing. The nurse was hired by a patient or family to provide care during a particular episode of illness or disability. Some nurses specialized in maternity cases, in which they cared for new mothers and infants; others specialized in caring for persons with long-term illnesses, such as strokes. The nurse was expected to live at the patient's residence and assume 24-hour responsibility for the patient's care. This might even include preparing special foods for the convalescing patient. Nurses hired as graduate nurses in hospitals usually were head nurses, supervisors, or directors.

By the 1930s the employment situation began to change. More graduate nurses were hired to provide patient care. Employment practices became modernized, and nurses were no longer expected to be on duty for 24 hours a day when engaged in private-duty nursing. Regular work schedules were established in hospitals. Nurses still worked split shifts—morning and evening of the same day with several hours "off duty" in the afternoon. There were few employee benefits (paid holidays, vacations, insurance, and retirement plans), but the beginnings of change were there. Most nurses were employed in a hospital or an institution.

World War II had a major impact on nursing. Because women were essential to the war effort, it became acceptable for married women to continue working. Women nurses were valued members of the armed forces and attained elevated status by becoming officers in the military. Nurses in the Armed Forces had to learn to be assertive in managing their responsibilities, and many brought this quality back to the hospital. Wanting to be of service to a country at war, women who might never have considered nursing because of its previous status now entered the profession.

The expansion of the hospital or institutional job market for nurses was also influenced by population growth; advances in medicine, with more surgeries being performed and special care required that was available only in a hospital; and the dramatic increase in the number of hospitals.

The noninstitutional job market also grew. Since the early 1900s, when Lillian Wald established a visiting nurse service, community health nursing has continued to develop. Nurses were pioneers in bringing health care to people's homes and in focusing on prevention of illness through consumer education.

Other areas of nursing in the community began to widen as well. More nurses were working in industry. Conditions for workers improved, and action regarding their health became part of law, custom, or contract. Nurses also worked in school districts, and the school nursing specialty started to expand.

Nurses began to provide primary health care. Primary care is that segment of health care that furnishes both the initial contact with the health care system and the longitudinal supervision of health care needs. Perhaps the first primary health care was provided by the nurse midwives of the Frontier Nursing Service in Kentucky in the 1920s. These midwives assumed overall responsibility for the care of childbearing women during pregnancy, delivery, and the postpartum period. Nurses who give primary care have been considered to function in an expanded role that requires additional specialized education.

Another early group that expanded practice were the nurse anesthetists who organized the Association of Registered Nurse Anesthetists in 1931 and assumed responsibility for accrediting programs to prepare nurses in this specialty field. Nurses outside of institutions were still a minority.

After World War II, nursing grew geometrically, extending to many areas at once, and the nation experienced a shortage of nurses. Because of this shortage, many other categories of health care workers were created, but roles and relationships were not carefully planned.

EMPLOYMENT OPPORTUNITIES TODAY

The hospital environment today is affected by all that has gone before. In some settings, there are remnants of the paternalistic attitudes that were prevalent in the years when women were expected to accept the hospital as the family surrogate during training and employment. This attitude may coexist with one that expects today's nurse to be an independent decision-maker. Emphasis is placed on the nurse's need for breadth and depth of theory to cope with the complexities of caring for the acutely ill. At the same time pangs of nostalgia may be expressed for the days when nurses "really knew how to work" and did not worry about so much "book learning."

Unlike graduates of the hospital programs of the past, you may be unfamiliar with the hospital as an employer. Your contact with the institution may have been brief as you focused your time on learning. You may have questions regarding employer expectations and your own role as an employee in an institution.

As more and more care is delivered outside of acute care hospitals, the percentage of nurses working outside the hospital has increased. Home health, hospice care, community mental health centers, women's health care delivery systems, maternal-infant care programs, outpatient and primary care, and long-term care facilities are hiring increasing numbers of registered nurses as they care for clients with more complex needs.

The growth of autonomy for the registered nurse has been even more marked outside the hospital setting than in it. Community health nurses have always operated much more independently than hospital nurses. The focus on health care is shifting from illness to health. Because many of these positions require a baccalaureate degree and experience or specialized educational programs, the new graduate is still most often employed in the hospital or long-term care institution.

The number of positions for registered nurses in many settings other than those that provide patient care has also risen. Health care oriented businesses such as insurance companies and medical equipment supply companies have found that it is easier to teach nurses about business than to teach business people about health care. As a result nurses are being employed in what some individuals see as non-nursing positions. Others argue that these, too, should be considered nursing positions because the expertise that makes the individual successful is nursing expertise.

The number of men in nursing, which remained relatively small for many years, is beginning to increase as society reassesses its attitude toward labeling jobs as woman's or man's work. Men have been attracted by the opportunities and improving economic picture of nursing and in turn have not been reluctant to advance it still further.

The economic position of the nurse has improved for a variety of reasons. One reason is the extension of laws governing fair labor practices to nonprofit institutions and the advent of collective bargaining (see Chapter 9). Another major factor affecting the economic position of nurses is the nursing shortage. Since the demand for nurses has risen faster than the supply, employers have begun increasing salaries and benefits to attract nurses. This has been especially notable in urban communities.

All of these factors bring you, as a new graduate, into a world of uncertainty but one also filled with opportunity and promise. Now you must determine how you fit into this world.

COMPETENCIES OF THE NEW GRADUATE

Considerable controversy exists within the nursing profession concerning which skills the new graduate should possess and to what level of proficiency. In diploma programs, which graduated most nurses of the past, students spent enough hours in direct care that, on graduation, they were prepared to accept almost any nursing position in the hospital where they received training and perform with skill all the procedures commonly used in that institution.

Both nursing education and the nature of the hospital have changed. The hospital population is composed of a much higher percentage of acutely ill patients with complex problems. Extended-care facilities now look after many of the more convalescent patients. Complexity of care has increased as many new procedures and techniques have been introduced. Nurses are expected to make knowledgeable decisions about the moment-by-moment care of the patient, day-to-day concerns, and discharge planning. In order to do this competently, nurses need a greater base in theory.

Changes in nursing education that were caused by a variety of social and economic factors have resulted in students spending less time directly caring for patients (see Chapter 2). The clinical time is carefully planned and structured for optimal use, making the students' learning experiences as meaningful as possible. However, there is little chance that every student will practice every skill. Nursing educators have tried to bridge this gap by using practice laboratories and teaching general principles that can be applied in a variety of situations.

Another factor affecting beginning competency is the mobility of the nursing population. Students no longer can expect to work as graduate nurses in the same hospital where they learned their skills. As a result, many nurses begin their careers far from where they were educated. They may find that equipment, policies, and procedures may differ. Nursing administrators believe that because of these factors, new graduates need considerable supervision and direction before they are ready to assume full responsibility. This lengthy time of teaching and orientation places a heavy cost burden on the first employer, and thus on the patient.

The variance between the needs of the employment settings and the ability of the new graduate to perform has created tension between nursing administration and nursing education. Fortunately, in many areas this tension has provoked mutual dialogue and constructive attempts to solve the problems.

Competency Statements

In April 1978 the Council of Associate Degree Programs of the National League for Nursing (NLN) developed and approved a statement of the competencies of the associate degree graduate. Members of the Council were also asked to plan for implementation of the statement. Competency was defined as a combination of demonstrated cognitive, affective, or psychomotor capabilities derived from the activities of the associate degree nurse in the various roles in the practice setting. Stated in broad terms, a competency is the integration of more specific behaviors (National League for Nursing, 1978). The statement identified competencies in assessing, planning, implementing, and evaluating care. The descriptions of behaviors were somewhat general because they were intended for all graduates of associate degree programs from around the country.

The Council of Baccalaureate and Higher Degree Programs of the NLN published a statement of the *Characteristics of Baccalaureate Education in Nursing* (National League for Nursing, 1979b). Part of this statement listed the competencies expected of the baccalaureate graduate. Most of the descriptions are related to cognitive abilities, such as using nursing theory and synthesizing theoretical and empirical knowledge. Attributes such as accepting responsibility and accountability and collaborating with others are included. The descriptions are broad and do not speak to any specific competencies as they have been defined by other groups (Council of Baccalaureate Degree Programs, 1979).

In 1979 the NLN published *Competencies of Graduates of Nursing Programs,* which was accepted by the Board of Directors of the NLN in April 1979 (National League for Nursing, 1979a). A task force examined all four levels of nursing education (practical nursing, diploma, associate degree, and baccalaureate) and were assigned to

- Identify the common core that runs through all levels of preparation
- Identify differences in programs in terms of competencies

- Identify areas of omission or emerging areas for which competencies need to be specified and to which attention must be given at the appropriate program level
- Present a working paper to the board of directors by April 1979

In the task force report, the knowledge base, the practice role, and the competencies of each level of nursing graduate were outlined. The task force concluded that there was still some ambiguity and lack of discrimination in the statements with regard to minimal expectations of new graduates of the various programs. The task force recommended continued study of the topic and discussion among all the groups representing the numerous programs involved so that the differences in breadth and depth could be more clearly identified. In 1982 the NLN published the results of the task force's study (National League for Nursing, 1982).

Many other groups have also worked on statements to describe competencies of new graduates. The deans and directors of associate degree programs in Florida formulated a statement of competencies that was published by the Florida State Board of Education (Florida State Board of Education, 1977). Because the statement was used to describe a more limited group (one state's associate degree graduates), it was more specific than that developed by the NLN.

The New Mexico System for a Nursing Articulation Program developed a statement of the *Minimum Behavioral Expectation of New Graduates from New Mexico Schools of Nursing* in 1977. This statement outlined competencies for graduates of practical, associate degree, and baccalaureate degree nursing programs. Broad categories such as nursing process, communication, change, and management were described in relationship to each level of practice. A detailed list of tasks appropriate to each degree was also included. (S.N.A.P. Project, 1977)

In 1990 the Council of Associate Degree Programs (CADP) of the NLN published a new statement of the roles and competencies of the associate degree graduate. The Council identified three roles: provider of care, manager of care, and member within the nursing profession (National League for Nursing, 1990).

Concerns of Employers Regarding Competencies

Similarities and patterns have emerged from all of these statements. The outline of theoretical knowledge and functioning in regard to the nursing process seems to be the most consistent. The most divergent opinions seem to be in the area of skill or task competency. Employers are often asking for further clarification of skills. Have these graduates only the necessary theoretical knowledge to perform the skill? Have they actually performed the skill? If so, was it in a practice laboratory only, or was it in a patient care situation? Does competence mean that the new graduate can function independently, or will some supervision still be needed?

In addition to theoretical knowledge, use of nursing process, and skill competency, speed of performance is a concern of new employers. As a student, your patient care load may be limited to two or three patients and might not encompass a full shift. This schedule allows you to focus your time on maximum learning, but it may not give you the opportunity to work within the realistic time and workload constraints of the employment situation.

Further complicating the picture is the confusion surrounding competencies of the graduates of the three types of nursing education programs. Although statements have distinguished between levels of functioning, many employers do not differentiate expectations. Some employers state that new graduates have not clearly demonstrated differences in competencies. This has created confusion in the minds of nurses, employers, and the public over the role of the registered nurse prepared in each type of educational program.

THE EMPLOYER'S GENERAL EXPECTATIONS OF THE NEW GRADUATE

What is expected of the new graduate varies in different facilities and in different geographical areas. Expectations are affected by various factors in the community such as whether there are nursing programs in that community and whether new graduates come from one or from many different schools. The acuity of the patient care load and the types of services offered by the facility may also affect expectations.

Most facilities that employ newly graduated registered nurses expect them to demonstrate the following competencies:

1. *Possess the necessary theoretical background for basic patient care and for decision making.* Many employers believe that new graduates of today are very competent in this area. For instance, the new graduate should understand the signs and symptoms of an insulin reaction, recognize it when it occurs, and know what nursing actions should be taken.

2. *Be able to use the nursing process in a systematic way.* This includes assessment, nursing diagnosis, planning, intervention, and evaluation. New graduates should be able to write and use nursing

care plans. Depth and comprehensiveness may be expected to be related to educational preparation (associate degree, baccalaureate degree, or diploma). Some employers ask that a nursing care plan be written as part of employment screening.

3. *Recognize their own abilities and limitations.* Employers may be able to assist if nurses ask for help and direction but cannot accept the risk to patients created by nurses who do not know their own limitations.

4. *Understand the importance of accurate and complete record keeping.* Employers generally recognize that the new graduate must be given time to learn the record keeping system used in the facility. However, the new graduate is expected to recognize the need for recording data. It is anticipated that the nurse would keep accurate, grammatical, and legible records.

5. *Understand and have a commitment to a work ethic.* This means that the employee takes the responsibility of the job seriously and will be on time, takes only the allowed coffee and lunch breaks, and

Figure 11–1. New graduates are expected to know both their own abilities and when to seek appropriate help.

will not take "sick days" unless truly ill. It also means that the new graduate recognizes that nurses are needed 24 hours a day, 365 days a year, and that this may require sacrifices of personal convenience, such as working evening shifts or on holidays.

6. *Possess skill proficiency in the basic nursing care procedures that often are carried out by nursing assistants.* This includes such things as giving baths and performing general hygienic measures. In some settings nurses will be carrying out these tasks, whereas in different settings they will be directing others who do them. In either case, proficiency is essential.

The tasks that are generally reserved for the registered nurse represent the area of widest diversity. These include passing medications to an entire unit of patients, caring for intravenous infusions, performing sterile procedures such as catheterization,

Figure 11-2. Employers are often concerned about an applicant's specific technical skills.

and assisting a physician with such complex procedures as a spinal tap or thoracentesis.

Some facilities provide extensive orientation programs in which every skill is checked before the new graduate is allowed to proceed independently. Other employers expect the new graduate to perform the skill if able or to ask for help if unable to be independent. Often employers are flexible in their expectations, so that it may be acceptable if a given person seems to have proficiency in a reasonable percentage of skills. Other employers have a list of skills in which proficiency is mandatory, although speed may not be expected. Also, there may be a difference between what the employer would wish and what the employer will accept.

7. *Functioning with acceptable speed.* This is another area in which expectations vary greatly. Most employers state that they expect that the new graduate will be slower; however, they may vary in how much slowness is acceptable and how soon they feel that slowness should be overcome. Generally, an orientation period is planned. An acceptable speed of function is reflected by ability to carry out a usual registered nurse assignment within the shift. Thus, if the usual patient assignment for a registered nurse is the care of six moderately ill patients, the new graduate is expected to accomplish this by the end of the orientation period.

PROBLEMS OF TRANSITION FROM STUDENT TO PROFESSIONAL

With all of this controversy, the new graduate often feels caught in the middle. As a student, you may think that you are expected to learn a tremendous amount in an alarmingly short time. The expectations may seem high and in some ways unrealistic. Then, as a new graduate suddenly thrust into the real world, you may feel insecure and think that your educational program did not adequately prepare you for what is expected of you. On one hand you are expected to function like a nurse who has had ten years of experience, but on the other hand your new ideas may not be considered because you have so little experience. You may become frustrated because you do not have time to provide the same type of care you gave as a student. For example, you may not have adequate time to deal with a patient's psychosocial problems or teaching needs.

As a student, you are taught that the "good nurse" never gives a medication without understanding its actions and side effects and that evaluating the effectiveness of the drug is essential. As a staff nurse, you may find that the priority is getting the medications passed correctly and on time and that there is little or no time to look up 15 new drugs. As for evaluation, that becomes a dream. How can one evaluate the subtle effects of a medication in the 2 minutes spent to pass the medication to a patient one does not know? The individually and meticulously planned care that was so important to you as a student may become a luxury when you are a graduate. Often the focus is on accomplishing the required tasks in the time allotted, and it is efficiency in tasks that may earn praise from a supervisor.

It may seem impossible to deliver quality care within the constraints of the system as it exists. New graduates may feel powerless to effect any changes and may be depressed over their lack of effectiveness in the situation. Marlene Kramer has called the feelings that result from such a situation *reality shock* (Kramer, 1979). She states that the new graduate may experience considerable psychological stress, and that this may contribute to the problem. The person undergoing such stress is less able to perceive the entire situation and to solve problems effectively.

When this occurs some nurses become disillusioned and leave nursing altogether. Others begin to "job hop" or return to school, searching for the perfect place to practice perfect nursing as it was learned. Some

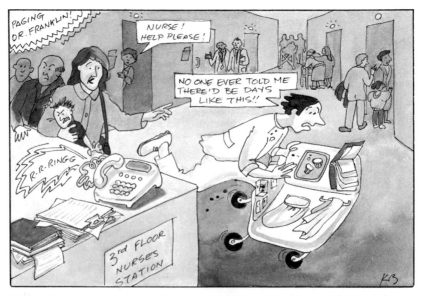

Figure 11–3. Some new graduates are disillusioned by the working conditions that they find on their first job.

push themselves to the limit, trying to provide ideal care and criticizing the system. This may result in their being labeled nonconformists and troublemakers. Still others give up their values and standards for care and reject ideals as impossibly unrealistic expectations that cannot be fulfilled in the real world. These persons simply mesh with the current framework and become part of the system.

There is an alternative to these nonproductive coping methods. It is possible to create a role for yourself that blends the ideal with the possible, one in which you do not give up ideals but see them as goals toward which you will move, however slowly. To do this you need to be realistically prepared for the demands of the real world.

Coping with Expectations

One way of meeting the challenge is to assess yourself as you approach the end of you educational program. Consider what your competencies are. Think about the seven areas of expectation:

1. Theoretical knowledge
2. Use of the nursing process
3. Self-awareness
4. Record keeping
5. Work ethic
6. Skill proficiency
7. Speed of functioning

Second, gain information about what the employers in your community expect from new graduates. This can be done by talking with experienced nurses, requesting interviews with nursing administrators, meeting with the faculty, and contacting recent graduates who are currently employed. Try to get specific information.

After you have gathered this information, try to correlate it with a realistic appraisal of your own ability to function in accordance with the employer's expectations. If you identify any shortcomings, the time to try to remedy them is before graduation. If you identify a lack in certain skills, you might register for extra time in the nursing practice laboratory to increase your proficiency. You could even time yourself and work to increase speed as well as skill. You might consult with your clinical instructor to arrange for experiences that would help you gain increased competence. If you recognize that you consistently have difficulty functioning within a time frame, you might obtain employment in a hospital or other health care facility while still in school; this will give you more experience in organizing work within the time limits that the employer sees as reasonable.

As you plan for your first job, you can examine the psychological challenges to be met. Understanding that you are not alone in your feelings of frustration is often helpful. It may be useful to form a support group of other new graduates who meet regularly to discuss problems and concerns and seek solutions jointly. You can also gain valuable re-inforcement from other nurses in your work setting. Many have successfully dealt with the problems you face and are able to provide support and help. This "mentor" relationship is an important one and needs to be cultivated

When confronted with areas of practice that you would like to see changed, weigh the importance of the issue. Use your energies wisely. The "politics of the possible" is important to you. Learn how the system in which you are employed functions and how to use that system for effective change. You, as a person, are important to nursing, so it is important that you neither burn yourself out nor abandon the quest for higher-quality nursing care; you should be able to continue to work toward improving nursing and bringing it closer to its ideals.

Many hospitals are attempting to help new graduates deal with reality shock. Some are doing it by making orientation programs more comprehensive and by providing an experienced nurse to work as a preceptor to the new graduate. Nurse internships or residencies have been created to provide a planned and organized transition time during which the new graduate participates in a formal program, including classes, seminars, and rotations to various units of the hospital. Some hospitals provide an opportunity for student nurses to work during the summer before the last year of their basic program to become familiar with the hospital and the nursing role. In this type of program the student nurse is employed as a nursing assistant but participates in a planned program that introduces the role of the registered nurse. You may wish to inquire whether hospitals in your area have developed any of these or other programs to assist you when you are a new graduate.

PERSONAL CAREER GOALS

In caring for patients, you are involved in the process of goal setting. Many nurses recognize the value of this in patient care but never transfer the concept to their personal lives. Nursing as a profession offers many career options. Without carefully setting goals, you might drift for years.

Focusing Your Goals

You may want to focus on a broad area of clinical competency, such as pediatric nursing, or on a more restricted area, such as neonatal care. Clinical areas available for concentrated effort become more varied as health care becomes more complex. Emergency care, coronary care, neurological and neurosurgical nursing, and specialties in the care of persons with ear, nose, and throat disorders are just a few of the clinical possibilities. Nurses specialize in aerospace nursing, enterostomal therapy, and respiratory care as well as operating room nursing and post-anesthesia care. Opportunities for additional education and for practice in most clinical specialties are now available for any registered nurse, regardless of his or her initial educational background.

Some specialty areas are in the primary care field, such as the woman's health care specialist, the family nurse practitioner, and the pediatric nurse practitioner. Increasing numbers of these programs require a baccalaureate degree for entry, but some admit registered nurses with experience in that specialty area.

Another approach may be to focus your goals on the setting in which care is delivered, such as acute care, long-term care, or community care. As health care needs expand, these separate realms of care delivery are all demanding more specialized knowledge. Even within the individual area of focus there are differences. For example, within the community there are ambulatory-care settings, public health nursing agencies, occupational health nursing departments, and day-care facilities.

Yet another way of focusing your goals is according to functional categories. Although nurses are initially thought of as direct-care providers, they are needed in many other positions. For example, there is need for those who would move into supervisory and administrative capacities, those who teach, and those who conduct nursing research. Nursing also lends itself to writing, to community service, and even to political involvement.

You may decide to set your goals in relation to all three types of foci. That is, you might identify a clinical area, a care setting, and a functional category.

Setting Your Goals

The first step in setting personal career goals is a thorough self-assessment. Determine how your abilities and competencies correspond to your own expectations as well as to those of the employers. Other factors to explore are your likes and dislikes and the situations or types of work you particularly enjoyed as a student. Also, it is important to recognize the area in which you were most comfortable. Were there areas in which you or your instructor felt that you were an above-average student? Consider your health and personal characteristics in relationship to types of work. Do you have physical restrictions? Do you prefer working independently or with others? How do you respond to close supervision or to relative freedom in the job setting? Do you work well with long-term goals and a few immediate reinforcements, or do you need to see results quickly? Another factor to consider is your own geographic mobility; would you be willing to move or travel as part of a job? Both your personal responsibilities and preferences operate in this arena.

As you plan ahead you need to examine many of the options offered by nursing. What types of jobs and opportunities are open to you? What education and personal abilities are needed in these areas? Are you interested? Does the education you have meet the educational requirement? Are avenues for additional education available to you? All of these considerations are important as you plan for the future.

Career goals need to be both short and long term. They will help you to plan your future constructively. This does not mean that goals are static. Just as patient goals must be realistic, personal, and flexible, so must your own goals.

Short-term goals will encompass what you want to accomplish this month and this year. What do you want to do and what do you want to be in the immediate future? One recent graduate stated that her short-term goal was to have 2 years of solid experience in a busy metropolitan hospital.

Long-term goals represent where you want to be in your profession 5 to 10 years from now. The long-term goal of the graduate referred to above was to work in a small, remote community in which she would have the opportunity to function autonomously.

Although both long-and short-term goals will be revised as your life evolves, they will guide you in making day-to-day decisions more effectively.

MAKING GOALS REALITY

Philosophical questions regarding goals must be resolved by practical approaches. As a new graduate, your first goal simply may be to get a job in nursing (especially if you live in one of the areas of the country that has more limited opportunities for registered nurses).

Whatever the situation, you are more likely to realize your goals if you are prepared to present yourself in the best possible way to a prospective employer. Many of you have held different jobs in the community as students and as adults. You may be familiar with and competent in the "job-search" process. Others of you have never applied for the kind of job that truly could be considered the beginning of a career. Different expectations are held by both employers and prospective employees in such a situation.

Letter of Inquiry or Application

Writing a letter requesting an interview is an excellent way to approach many prospective employers. You can present yourself positively through a well-written letter. In addition, a letter may be dealt with at the recipient's convenience, whereas a telephone call may interrupt a busy schedule. There are fewer chances for misunderstanding if your request is in written form and if you receive a written reply.

Before you write your letter, you should make sure you have information about the prospective employer. What kind of facility is this? What types of clients do they serve, and what special services do they offer? It makes a very poor impression to write to a prospective employer stating your goal is to work in pediatrics if that facility does not provide any pediatric services.

Another part of your advance planning is identifying how you will focus your letter on your special qualifications and what you want to highlight. You will want to focus on the skills or accomplishments that are related to the position you want.

Your letter should be no more than one page in length but be planned to present all essential information. Introduce yourself and your purpose for writing in the first paragraph so that the reader immediately has an understanding of the subject. You may then want to briefly state your reasons for applying for a position with this particular employer. The more specific the reasons, the better the impression you are likely to make.

Briefly highlight your qualifications for the position. This should not be a simple recitation of what is in your resume but should either present the information in a slightly different light or add pertinent detail that is not in the resume. You might include personal qualities that would make you an effective employee in the position.

In the final paragraph, make a summary statement indicating why you want to work for this employer and ask for an appointment for an interview. Be sure to indicate the times you can be available and how and where you can be contacted. Thank the person for considering your application, and close.

Another point to remember is that the letter's appearance as well as its content represents you. You will be judged on spelling, grammar, clarity, and neatness as well as on the letter's content. Your letter of application should be written in standard business form. Make it brief and clear. Ask a friend or family member to double-check your first draft if you have any questions about its correctness (see Sample Letter of Application).

The Resume

A resume is a brief overview of your qualifications for a position. Its purpose is to provide the employer with a way to quickly identify whether you have the basic qualifications for a position and to present yourself in the most positive light to be considered for the position in which you are interested. In some instances you may want to include your resume with your initial letter. You may also choose to take your resume with you and leave it with the employer at the end of your interview.

The appearance of your resume is important, because it presents your initial image to the prospective employer. You will want your resume appearance to reflect a competent, professional image. It is not necessary to have a professionally produced resume. Nursing employers, when asked, have indicated that it neither adds to nor detracts from their impression to read a resume that has been produced by some professional printing method. The important point is that it be a somewhat formal, standard, informative document that is neatly typed without error. This is not usually the place for creative writing.

Your resume should be on standard-sized, white, good quality paper so that it is easy to handle, file, and read. A resume that is individually typed or printed (or reproduced well enough so that is appears to be) usually will be more positively received than a carbon copy or a poor-quality photocopy. If you have access to a computer and word processing, you will find it valuable to create a resume and save it to a disk. In this way, you will be able to easily revise your resume and you may even be able to tailor a resume to an individual job situation.

To achieve legibility, use wide margins, spacing, indentation, and numbering to separate different sections and topics. You might want to underline or bold print important items or highlight them with an asterisk to draw swift attention. When an employer is reviewing many resumes, anything that facilitates review and makes you stand out is an advantage.

The content of your resume is critical. Always include personal information, licensure, work experience, educational background, volunteer or community work, and awards and honors. You might also want to add your career objective and a section for special skills such as computer familiarity or experience with special types of equipment.

In each group of information list the most recent items first. The most common approach is to group information in the categories just mentioned. The sample resume in this chapter is organized in this way.

Sample Letter of Application

16100 Greenwood Avenue North
Seattle, WA 98133
April 15, 1993

Ms. Jane Jancoby, RN, MN
Director of Nursing Services
Pacific Hospital
Seattle, WA 98200

Dear Ms. Jancoby:

After reading the brochure about your hospital that was distributed at Shoreline Community College, I became interested in employment in your new day surgery unit. Your plan for preadmission patient teaching is an excellent opportunity for nurses to make a significant difference for patients. I would like to be a part of that nursing team. Alternatively, I would like to work on a general surgical unit with the potential for transferring to the day surgery unit when that opportunity is available.

I will graduate June 10 and have already applied for my temporary nursing permit, which should be sent to me within two weeks of graduation. I will be taking the licensing examination July 7 and 8 in Tacoma.

In addition to my clinical experience in the nursing program at Shoreline, I have worked as a nursing technician on a surgical unit at Northwest Hospital throughout my last year in school. My responsibilities included preoperative preparation of patients and postoperative care. The experience I gained in that position would be especially helpful to me on any surgery unit. My resume outlines my educational background and general qualifications.

I would like to discuss employment possibilities and will call your office next week to ask for a specific appointment. If you wish to contact me, I can be reached at the above address or at 546-4779. My telephone has an answering machine and I would return any call promptly.

Sincerely,

Elizabeth A. Zartman

Some individuals choose to group information into skill or functional categories. This is more common when you have had several nursing positions and you want to emphasize the responsibilities you have had within those positions.

Under personal information give your name, address, and telephone number (including area code). If you will be moving, indicate the date the move will be effective and provide an alternate method of contacting you after that date. A permanently settled relative or friend who would be willing to forward your mail would be appropriate. Employers are not permitted to ask about age, marital status, and dependents and you do not need to include this information.

You may wish to begin with a brief statement of your career objective. This may include both a short-term goal such as "employment as a registered nurse on a general medical unit" and a longer-term goal such as "with eventual move to employment in coronary care." Be sure that your goal is realistic and does not imply that you are not really interested in a beginning level position. If you state that your goal is to be a nurse recruiter and you have do not have the experience for this kind of position, your application may be discarded. If you state that you want to work in maternity nursing and the only position available is in medical-surgical nursing, you may not be considered for the medical-surgical position that you would have accepted although it was not your first choice.

Indicate the date your license will be effective and whether you have a temporary permit to work as a nurse (if that is required in your state). Your nursing license or permit number and state should be listed. Indicate when you expect to take your licensing examination and have a license.

Work experience should give a complete employment history with no unexplained gaps in time. For example, if you spent 15 years as a homemaker since your last employment, include those dates and state "homemaker" after them. For each job you held include address, dates employed, position, and duties. The prospective employer would be especially interested in a previous nursing assistant position or any other position that demonstrates your knowledge of or experience in some area of health care or the assumption of responsibility.

If you have had only one or two part-time jobs during your educational program, it would be appropriate to include them in detail. However, if during your educational program you held 15 part-time jobs, it is appropriate to list significant ones that offered valuable experience. In one line write, "Various part-time jobs to finance schooling: clerk and waitress. Individual names provided on request." Include the overall dates for this period.

Educational background should cover your nursing education and any specialized courses or postgraduate work you have done. It is appropriate to note any college-level work. Do not include high school information unless you entered your nursing program directly from high school. Then you might indicate your high school and graduation date on one line of your educational information.

If you had experiences in an educational area that especially relate to the position for which you are applying, you might individualize your resume by briefly identifying these special experiences. For example, you might have had a senior leadership practicum on an orthopedic unit and this would be particularly relevant to an application for a nursing position in orthopedics. If you had a practicum in the facility or agency to which you are applying, indicate this in some way. Your familiarity with their policies and procedures would be a valuable asset. If you attended any special workshops, include those as a separate section.

Choose the items you list under volunteer and community work carefully. If you are 40 years old, the fact that you were student-body president in high school would probably be considered irrelevant. However, if you went from high school directly into a nursing program, this information could be important in demonstrating your leadership ability. Your participation in any community organizations such as the Parent-Teacher Association and service in any leadership roles would be significant to an employer.

In some instances you may want to list briefly the skills or abilities gained from a particular activity. For example, if you worked as a volunteer for a Planned Parenthood clinic, you might specify that your duties included individual client counseling in relation to family planning methods. Simply stating that you were a volunteer might not communicate the level of responsibility you assumed. This is an area that you might want to individualize to target the particular skills you think are important to the position for which you are applying. Werning (1991) suggests that you use active verbs to describe skills. Words such as supervised, designed, managed, developed, analyzed, coordinated, documented, planned, delegated, created, completed, and operated give life to your resume and create interest in the reader.

List awards and honors that would demonstrate your competence or leadership ability. You may omit this section if you feel that you have nothing pertinent to enter.

References are typed on a separate page and given to the prospective employer if they are requested. Be selective in choosing the people you will list as references. Consider the people who know you and would be able to speak positively of you to a future employer and who would have credibility with the employer. Seek the person's permission before giving him or her as a reference.

Most commonly you should provide as one reference someone who has known you personally for a relatively long time and who could attest to your ability to relate with others and to such attributes as personal integrity. A second reference should be an instructor or supervisor from your basic educational program. This person would be able to affirm your ability in the nursing field. A third reference should be someone who has employed you and who can describe your work habits and effectiveness as an employee. Include full names with title (if any), addresses, and telephone numbers so that the employer will be able to contact the references easily. When seeking permission to use someone as a personal reference, you might outline what you would like the person to emphasize if contacted; for example, "If you are contacted, I would particularly like you to provide information about my work habits and effectiveness as an employee" (see Sample Resume of a Recent Graduate).

The Interview

The interview should be a two-way conversation in which you will be gaining as well as giving information. Think through the situation before going to the interview and outline information that you want to obtain and questions that you want answered. Writing out your quesions so that they are clearly stated and so that you do not forget items in the tense atmosphere that often exists in an interview situation is advantageous.

Time spent reflecting on your personal views in advance will be valuable during the interview. Remember that an interview is a chance to sell yourself to an employer, a chance to present yourself as a valuable addition to their nursing staff, and an opportunity to determine how you will fit into that work setting.

When planning for an employment interview, consider your appearance, your attitude and approach, and what the content of the interview will be. Your personal appearance is likely to evoke some type of response from the interviewer. Consider what you would like that response to be and dress appropriately. This would mean that what you wear when applying for one type of job might be inappropriate when applying for another type of job. For example, if you were applying for a position at a hospital, you would wear business-like clothing, such as

Sample Resume of a Recent Graduate

Elizabeth A. Zartman
16100 Greenwood Avenue North
Seattle, WA 98133
(206) 546-4779

EDUCATION
Shoreline Community College, Seattle, WA, Associate Degree in Nursing, 1993
University of Washington, Seattle, WA, General Studies, 1988–1990

WORKSHOPS
Ethical Dilemmas in End-of-Life Issues, Sponsored by the Community College-Nursing Home Project, May 2, 1991

WORK EXPERIENCE
June 1992 to present:
Northwest Hospital, Seattle, WA, Surgical Unit

• Title: Nursing technician

• Duties: Assumed responsibility for direct patient care within the skills previously learned in my nursing program. This included preparing patients for surgery, providing postoperative monitoring, and routine patient care.

September 1989 to June 1992:
Crista Nursing Center, Seattle, WA

• Title: Nursing assistant

• Duties: Provided hygiene, feeding, and other personal care to dependent elders in long-term care setting.

VOLUNTEER EXPERIENCE
January 1987 to present:

• Planned Parenthood of King County. Staffed the office, answering telephone questions and making appropriate referrals within the organization. Managed records while maintaining appropriate confidentiality for clients.

COMMUNITY ACTIVITIES
Member Seattle Mountaineers, Chair of Planning Committee

REFERENCES: Available on request

dress pants and shirt or a suit or dress. Being neat and well groomed contributes to a business-like atmosphere. If you were applying for a position in a walk-in health care clinic that offered services to persons who are uncomfortable in a traditional environment, it might be appropriate to wear the casual clothing worn by the workers at the clinic. You need to make a conscious decision about the impression you want to create. Although some may wish that appearances had no effect on the opinions of others, remember that, in reality, appearance often does make a significant difference.

Take a copy of your resume with you to the interview. In addition, be prepared with the names, addresses, and telephone numbers of all references, and your Social Security number. Take along a black pen to fill out any forms and a note pad to make personal notes of important information. This can increase your self-confidence if you have forms to fill out, or if questions about statements on your resume arise during the interview.

Plan to arrive at an interview early. This gives you time to check your appearance and focus your thoughts. When you arrive at an interview be sensitive to the problems and concerns of the interviewer. If it is apparent that unplanned events are demanding his or her attention, state that you are aware of the difficulty and ask whether it would be more convenient if you made another appointment. Your sensitivity to the interviewer's cues are evidence of your sensitivity to patients' cues.

Your manner in the interview is also important. Although the employer expects an applicant to be nervous, he or she will be interested in whether your nervousness makes you unable to respond appropriately. Follow common rules of courtesy. Wait to be asked to sit down before you take a chair. Avoid any distracting mannerisms, such as chewing gum or fussing with your hair, face, or clothes. Be serious when appropriate, but do not forget to smile and be pleasant. The interviewer is also thinking of your impact on patients, visitors, and other staff members.

When you prepare your responses, try to anticipate possible questions from the interviewer. Role-playing an interview situation with a friend or relative may help you to feel more confident in your responses. Another technique is to visualize the interview situation in your mind and mentally rehearse responses to questions.

In most instances be sure to answer questions that are asked rather than skirting them. However, if the interviewer asks a question that is illegal, such as age or marital status, you might want to redirect the question to address what appears to be the concern of the interviewer. For example, in response to a question about your age you might say "Perhaps you believe that I appear to be young and inexperienced. I want to assure you that I have demonstrated my maturity and responsibility both in my nursing education and in my position with (name of employer)." In response to a question about marital status or children, you could reply "Perhaps you are concerned about how long I plan to stay in my first position? I want to assure you that whatever my personal situation, professionally, I am looking for a position in an organization where I can be a long-term employee and plan for advancement within the organization."

An interview usually covers a wide variety of subjects. The interviewer may direct the flow of topics or may encourage you to bring up the ones that concern you. Applicants who focus initial attention on the issues of wages and benefits may be viewed as more concerned about themselves than about nursing. Therefore, if you are asked to present questions, ask nursing-related questions first. Demonstrate that you are concerned about how nursing care is given and by whom, where responsibility and authority lie, the philosophy underlying care, the availability of continuing education, and where you would be expected to fit into their overall picture. However, before you leave be sure to cover such topics as hours, schedules, pay scales, and benefits.

Post-Interview Letter

After your interview, you should write a brief thank-you letter to the person who interviewed you. In that letter, thank the individual for the time and attention to your questions and concerns. Restate any agreement you feel was reached. For example, "I understand that I am to call your office next week to learn whether I have been scheduled for an interview with the maternity unit manager." Close your letter with a positive comment about the organization. Even if you are not offered a job or do not choose to work at that facility, you are leaving a positive impression. You can never tell when that will be important to you in the future (see Sample Interview Follow-up Letter).

RESIGNATION

When you decide to leave a nursing position, it is important that you provide the employer with an appropriate amount of time to seek a replacement. The more responsible your position, the more time the employer will need. For a staff nursing position you should strive to provide 1 month's notice unless an urgent matter requires that less notice be given. Notice of resignation should be in a letter. The letter is directed to the head of your department, often to the director of nursing. Copies

Sample Interview Follow-up Letter

16100 Greenwood Avenue North
Seattle, WA 98133
May 9, 1993

Ms. Betty Hanson RN, MN
Nurse Recruiter
Pacific Hospital
Seattle, WA 98200

Dear Ms. Hanson:

My interview with you on May 8 was very helpful to me in learning about Pacific Hospital and the opportunities for employment as a new nursing graduate. I was especially delighted to learn that you will definitely have an opening on the day surgery unit as well as several openings on general surgery units.

I appreciate your positive response to me. I look forward to the interview with the Unit Manager for Day Surgery, Maxine Reynolds, RN, MN, that your secretary scheduled for me on May 16. I understand that she will make the final determination on hiring for the day surgery position.

If I am not selected for the day surgery position, I will contact your office, as you directed, for an appointment for an interview with a Unit Manager for a general surgery unit.

Sincerely,

Elizabeth A. Zartman

should be sent to other supervisory people, such as the head nurse and the supervisor.

The letter of resignation is important in concluding your relationship with the employer on a cordial and positive basis. The feelings that are left behind when you resign will influence letters of recommendation and future opportunities for employment with that agency. Give a reason for your resignation as well as the exact date when it will be effective. If you have accrued vacation or holiday time and want to take the time off or be paid for it, clearly state that. Comment about positive factors in the employment setting and acknowledge those who have provided special support or assistance in your growth.

If your are resigning because of problems in the work setting and want to note them, do so in a clear, factual, unemotional way. Avoid attacking anyone in a personal way and do not make broad, sweeping negative comments. Try to make the letter a clear and reasonable statement of your position as a professional (see Sample Letter of Resignation).

MAINTAINING COMPETENCE

Every nurse has an obligation to society to maintain competence and continue practicing high-quality, safe care. Continuing education

Sample Letter of Resignation

16100 Greenwood Avenue North
Seattle, WA 98133
June 8, 1994

Mr. Gerald Scott
Director of Nursing
Northwest Hospital
Seattle, WA 98115

Dear Mr. Scott:

I have just received notice of my acceptance into the Air Force Nurse Corps. Therefore, I wish to resign effective August 15, 1994. My time spent with Northwest Hospital has been a growing and professionally rewarding experience. I especially want to thank the staff of the surgical unit for all they have done to help me become an independent professional. The skills that I developed here will be invaluable to me as I move forward in nursing. Although I look forward to my career in the Air Force, I do leave with some regrets.

Sincerely,

Jean R. Johnson, RN

cc: Myrtle Moore, RN
Unit Manager, Surgical

may occur through learning on the job, through reading of professional publications, or through attending classes. There are television courses, programmed instruction programs, and examinations related to journal articles. Any of these avenues may be appropriate, depending on the circumstances. Some nurses may want to advance through specialty or higher education.

BURNOUT

Burnout is a form of chronic stress related to one's job. It can be identified by feelings of hopelessness and powerlessness, accompanied by decreased ability to function both on the job and in personal life. Burnout primarily occurs in nurses who work in particularly stressful areas of nursing, such as critical care, oncology, or burn units. It also occurs in other areas when staffing is inadequate or interpersonal relationships are strained.

Symptoms

Symptoms of burnout include both physical changes and psychological distress. Exhaustion and fatigue, frequent colds, headaches, backaches, and insomnia all may occur. There may be changes in disposition, such as being quick to anger or exhibiting all feelings excessively. As burnout progresses, ability to solve problems and make decisions decreases. This frequently results in an unwillingness to face change and a tendency to block new ideas. There may be feelings of guilt, anger, and depression because one cannot meet the expectations for doing a "perfect job."

In response to these feelings, some nurses quit their jobs and move on to other settings. These other settings may not even be in nursing. Others remain in their jobs but develop a personal shell that tends to separate them from real contact with clients and coworkers. The person may become cynical about the possibility of anyone doing a good job and may function at a minimal level.

Causes

Many causes of burnout have been discussed in the literature. Prominent among them is the conflict between ideals and reality. Just as this is a problem for the new graduate, it is also a problem for the experienced nurse. In trying to achieve the ideal, the nurse drives harder and harder and becomes critical of environment and of self. Nurses see themselves as being responsible for all things to all people and often take on more and more responsibility, thus increasing their own stress level.

Another cause of burnout is the high level of stress that results from practicing nursing in areas that have high mortality rates. Continually investing oneself in patients who die can take a tremendous toll on personal resources. In addition, the demand is constant for optimal functioning.

Institutions that are inadequately staffed may also place great stress on nurses. The patients are in need of care, the nurse has the skills to provide the care, and yet the patients do not receive good care. The nurse typically tries to accomplish more, staying overtime, skipping breaks and lunch, and running throughout the shift. Despite this effort, there is little job satisfaction because the things that are left undone or that are not done well seem to be more apparent than all the good that was accomplished.

Preventive Actions

Burnout can best be prevented by mounting a stress-reduction effort involving the nursing staff, supervisory personnel, the hospital administration, and other health care workers. The most important aspect seems to be bringing burnout into the open and acknowledging the existence of the problems. This alone helps the individual nurse move away from the feelings of separation and alienation that often accompany burnout. Whatever the problems, they seem less frightening if they are defined as "normal" and if the individual nurse does not see himself or herself as the only person not performing as the "perfect nurse." A second step is to provide for group discussions during which nurses can share feelings and specific concerns in an accepting atmosphere. This sharing may lead to concrete plans to reduce the stress created by the setting. For example, if one source of stress is conflicting orders between two sets of physicians involved in care, a plan might be developed whereby the nurses no longer take responsibility for the conflict but refer the problem to some authority within the medical hierarchy. This type of resolution is possible only when the problem of burnout is being addressed by the whole health care team.

Giving nurses more control over their own practice often decreases stress. This action is limited by the constraints of the setting, but it may involve flexible scheduling, volunteering for specific assignments, and participation in committees that determine policies and procedures.

Rotating nurses out of high-stress areas before they become "burned out" may allow them to rebuild resources and return to the job with enthusiasm. This can be done only if there is no stigma or blame attached to the need to rotate and if other nurses are available for replacement. In patient care areas that are known to be stressful, it is helpful to have a counselor available for nurses. Consulting with this counselor should be viewed by the staff as a positive step and not as an admission of some lack or fault. The counselor needs to be someone who understands the setting and who has the skills to assist people in coping with stress.

As an individual nurse, you also can take actions to prevent burnout. These are the same general actions that are designed to control stress in any aspect of life. Paying attention to your own physical health is an important preventive measure. This includes maintaining a balanced program of rest, nutrition, and exercise. Another important point is not to subject yourself to excessive changes over short periods, because changes increase stress. You may decide, for example, not to move at the same time you change to a different shift. A period of "wind down" or "decompression" after work helps you to avoid carrying the stress of the workplace into your private life. This period may be physical exercise, reading, meditation, or any different activity. The activity you choose should not create more demands and increase stress. An important resource is someone who is willing to listen while you ventilate your feelings and talk about your problems. Sometimes this is a family member or personal friend, but it may be more appropriate for this to be a coworker.

Burnout is a serious concern in the nursing profession, but there are strategies for managing it. If you are in a high-stress situation, you need to plan for prevention before you become burned out.

SEX DISCRIMINATION IN NURSING

There are two major areas in which there is concern about sex discrimination in nursing: the issue of comparable worth and discrimination against men in nursing.

Comparable Worth

Nursing has been, and still is, a profession composed predominantly of women (see Chapter 1). Laws exist in many states that prohibit explicit sex discrimination in salary for a given job. For example, if both men and women are hired by an airline as flight attendants, they must be compensated on the same basis. This principle has been expanded to encompass jobs that are essentially the same work, although the titles may differ. The janitor and the maid may have different titles, but if they have essentially the same tasks, then they must be paid on the same basis.

The next step that many women would like to see accepted is the principle of compensation based on comparable worth. Jobs may be studied and assigned points or rank based on educational requirements, skills required, level of responsibility, and authority. Those with the same points or rank are considered to be of comparable worth, although the actual substance of the work may differ. Alaska has a law barring discrimination in pay for work of comparable character.

Many women believe that differing jobs of comparable worth are not compensated equally because of sex discrimination. Most jobs that are found to score high in education, skill, and responsibility and that have low salaries are those jobs that have historically been held by women. Nursing is one example of such a job. Secretaries and teachers are other occupational groups that have traditionally had low wages relative to the level of responsibility required.

Groups of women have brought suit against employers charging sex discrimination based on failure to provide equal pay for jobs of comparable worth. One such suit was filed by a group of public health nurses in Alaska (PHN's win. . ., 1982). They complained that their salaries were significantly lower than those of physicians' assistants, whose educational qualifications were not as high. Because the physicians' assistants were primarily men and the nurses were primarily women, the nurses claimed that they were being discriminated against because of their sex. Even though they were not successful in their suit, they have not given up their stand.

A federal judge in Washington state ruled that the state must pay jobs of comparable worth comparable wages, and that the state is moving ahead with plans to alter its compensation schedules. There is strong opposition to the concept of comparable worth throughout many segments of society. Therefore, any gains in this area will not be made without a great deal of effort. Continued action, both nationally and statewide, to obtain legal recognition of comparable worth as a basis for compensation can be expected (House tackles. . ., 1983).

Discrimination Against Men

Men in nursing have also expressed concern about sex discrimination. Their concern is not monetary but is related to being allowed to practice in all areas of nursing and being accepted within the profession. Anti-male sexism in the United States was discussed by Kus (1985), who pointed out that society stereotypes men just as feminists have criticized that it stereotypes women. He makes a strong case for the importance of nurses examining the stereotypes they hold about men. Stereotypes narrow our thinking and interfere with people being able to develop to their fullest potential. It is appropriate for women in nursing to examine their own behavior and identify whether they have been guilty of perpetuating outmoded stereotypes of the nurse and supporting a type of discrimination toward men that they would fight to eliminate for women.

In some facilities or areas men are not allowed to care for women patients, or if they are allowed to care for women, restrictions are placed on them in terms of obtaining consent for care from each patient. Those who support the limitations on the practice of men in nursing state that it is a matter of providing for the modesty and privacy of the woman patient. This position was upheld by a court decision in favor of a hospital that refused to assign a man to a nursing position in labor and delivery (Arkansas. . ., 1981). The argument was made that the patient did not have free choice of a nurse but rather was assigned a nurse for care, and therefore the restrictions were appropriate.

Those who oppose limitations on the practice of men in nursing state that as a professional, whether man or woman, the nurse should always consider the privacy and modesty of a patient of either gender. This can be done without excluding anyone from providing care in any area. By careful assessment the nurse can determine the true needs of the patient and plan for appropriate avenues to deliver that care. Furthermore, the point has been made that men as physicians have not been excluded from any branch of medicine and this has not created problems. Physicians are not always chosen by the patient either. House staff are assigned, referrals are made to specialty physicians, and many group plans designate a physician to provide care. Women nurses care for men patients in all situations. This has been accepted because women are seen in a nurturing, mothering role that the public associates with nursing.

The American Assembly for Men in Nursing (see Appendix B) provides a forum for the concerns of men in nursing and opposes any limitations on opportunities available to men.

OCCUPATIONAL SAFETY AND HEALTH FOR NURSES

Nurses have expressed concern regarding safety in the working environment for many years. Employees have a right to expect their employers to provide the safest working environment possible. Some hospitals employ an occupational health nurse to examine the working environment and employment practices in order to promote health and safety on the job. Nurses themselves, however, have often been lax in recognizing on-the-job hazards and acting for self-protection. This can be likened to the response of those who continue to smoke, regardless of their knowledge of the health hazards of smoking, or those who fail to wear seatbelts, although they know that the statistics show decreased fatalities in auto accidents when seatbelts are worn. Some people continue to do those things that they know are detrimental to their health and well-being. Unfortunately, nurses are no exception.

Infection as an Occupational Hazard

Transmission of infection is a major concern when caring for infected patients. The presence of resistant organisms causes extra concern and makes treatment difficult. All hospitals have an infection-control officer, usually a registered nurse, who has the expertise to guide the staff in planning appropriate infection control procedures.

Figure 11–4. Personal safety and health in the work environment are important concerns for nurses.

The hidden danger for nurses lies in those patients who have not been diagnosed as having an infection and for whom specific infection-control measures have therefore not been prescribed. The acquired immunodeficiency syndrome (AIDS) has created a reevaluation of all approaches to infection control and of health care workers' obligations to provide care for those with communicable diseases.

AIDS remains a serious concern for all health care workers. Using "Universal Precautions" as described by the Centers for Disease Control has become the standard for all health care situations. The individual nurse must assume responsibility for his or her own protection through conscientiously carrying out appropriate measures at all times. Employers must be held accountable for providing the supplies and environment to make this possible.

Although the details of infection control are beyond the scope of this text, we would remind you that you hold the key to protecting yourself in many ways. Often health care workers become lax in their attention to the use of gloves or eye protection because these measures are inconvenient. It is your responsibility to maintain the very best of technique for self-protection. Your employer also has obligations for protecting you from infection. One of the first employer actions toward preventing AIDS and other blood-borne diseases was the provision of "sharps" containers wherever needles were used. Another important employer responsibility is the provision of a supply of gloves and protective eyewear for employee use. Increasing attention is now being given to designing needles and other sharp devices in new ways that provide greater protection. For example, a needle with a protective plastic housing is available for use with secondary lines. These needles are unlikely to injure an individual even if they are not handled properly. Syringes are being designed that have a protective cover that the needle retracts into immediately after use. Nurses can request that hospitals provide safer equipment.

Nurses who have frequent contact with blood and blood products and those engaged in intravenous therapy have a special risk for exposure to hepatitis B. Although a vaccine exists to protect against this disease, the vaccine itself is not without side effects; therefore, a discussion with a physician regarding risks versus benefits for you as an individual is appropriate before undertaking immunization. The Occupational Safety and Health Administration (OSHA) has developed standards that require employers to pay for hepatitis B immunization for those employees with significant exposure to blood and body substances that can transmit blood-borne organisms.

Hazardous Chemical Agents

Anesthetic gases can increase the risk of fetal malformation and spontaneous abortion in pregnant women who are exposed to them on a regular basis. Standards exist for waste-gas retrieval systems and the allowable level of these gases in the air. Nurses working in operating rooms should seek information on the subject and expect that hospitals will provide a safe environment.

Chemotherapeutic agents used in the treatment of cancer are extremely toxic, and nurses who work in settings where such agents are prepared and administered should seek additional education regarding their administration, not only in relationship to the patient's safety but also in relationship to personal safety. The employer is responsible for providing the equipment needed to maintain safety when handling these agents.

Contact with many medications, especially antibiotics, during preparation and administration may cause the nurse to develop sensitivity. This may not only create transitory problems, such as a hand rash, but may also be a threat if treatment for a serious infection is compromised at some later date. Other medications are absorbed through the skin and may produce an undesirable effect. Nurses who understand this hazard will handle all drugs with discretion and be careful to not expose themselves to these agents.

Cleaning agents and disinfectants used in the hospital may also be hazardous if used improperly. Employers are now required by OSHA to maintain a list of all chemicals used in the work environment, along with information on their possible effects, and the appropriate treatment if individuals are accidentally exposed to them.

CONCLUSION

Many new graduates suffer from reality shock when they are confronted with their first position as a registered nurse. This is caused by the wide discrepancy they find between the ideal world of nursing as they learned it and the real world of nursing in which they attempt to practice. New graduates can ease their transition through this time by gaining an understanding of the world of employment, the forces that have helped to shape it, and some of the factors that exert pressure on that setting. The world of nursing practice is not without its problems for the practicing nurse. Knowing about some of those problems before you begin may help you to be more effective as you seek to make nursing a satisfying career.

REFERENCES

Arkansas judge rules male nurse out of labor/delivery. Am J Nurs 81(7):1253, 1981

Florida State Board of Education: Competencies of the Associate Degree Graduate. Tampa, FL, State Board of Education, 1977

House tackles pay equity issue. Am J Nurs 83(1):7, 1983.

Kramer M: Reality Shock. St. Louis, CV Mosby, 1979

Kus RJ: Stages of coming out: An ethnographic approach. West J Nurs Res 7(2): 177–194, 1985

National League for Nursing: Competencies of Graduates of Nursing Programs. Publication No. 14-1905. New York, National League for Nursing, 1982

National League for Nursing: Working Paper of the N.L.N. Task Force on Competencies of Graduates of Nursing Programs. Publication No. 14-1787. New York, National League for Nursing, 1979a

National League for Nursing, Competencies of the Associate Degree Graduate on Entry Into Practice. Publication No. 23-1731. New York, National League for Nursing, 1978

National League for Nursing, Educational Outcomes of Associate Degree Nursing Programs: Roles and Competencies. Publication No. 23-2348. New York, National League for Nursing, 1991

National League for Nursing, Council of Baccalaureate Degree Programs. Characteristics of Baccalaureate Education in Nursing. New York, National League for Nursing, 1979b

PHN's win first round in equal pay case. Am J Nurs 82(7):1028, 1982

S.N.A.P. Project: Minimum Behavioral Expectations of New Graduates from New Mexico Schools of Nursing. Albuquerque, University of Albuquerque, Division of Nursing and Allied Health, 1977

FURTHER READINGS

Bellocq JA: Comparable worth: Implications for nursing. Prof Nurs 1(3):131–137, 1985

Buechler DK: Help for the burned-out nurse? Support groups. Nurs Outlook 33(4):181–182, 1985

"Career Guide." Nursing '90, Nursing '91 (monthly feature)

Career Planning Guide. New York, National Student Nurses Association (annual publication)

Dailey AL: The burnout test. Am J Nurs 85(3):270–272, 1985

Heine CA: Burnout among nursing home personnel. J Gerontol Nurs 12(3): 270–272, 1986

Hicky JV: How to reduce stress and avoid burnout. Nurs '85 15(4):7–9, 1985

Lender KL: When you're stretched to the limit. RN 53(7):53–55, 1990

Lindquist KD: Finding the perfect match. Healthcare Trends Transition 1(1):6–8, 1989

Lovejoy RL: When are you entitled to worker's compensation? RN 53(3):81–83, 1990

RN Nursing Opportunities. RN Magazine (annual publication)

Styles MM: The uphill battle for comparable worth: How it can be won; why it won't be easy. Nurs Outlook 33(3):128–132, 1985

Tammelo AD: Don't be afraid to blow the whistle on incompetence. RN 53(6):61–66, 1990

Vance C et al: An uneasy alliance: Nursing and the women's movement. Nurs Outlook 33(6):281–285, 1985

12

Understanding the Traditional Health Care Settings

Objectives

After completing this chapter you should be able to

1. *Discuss the early development of hospitals and nursing homes.*

2. *Explain the factors that affected the development of hospitals in the United States.*

3. *Describe the three general classifications of hospitals.*

4. *Identify the role of the hospital board of governors and the hospital administrator.*

5. *Describe the relationship of the hospital medical staff to the hospital and its governance structure.*

6. *Discuss the position nursing occupies in the hospital organizational structure.*

7. *Discuss the purposes of a mission statement, philosophy, and goals and objectives.*

8. *Define terms used in describing organizational structure including channel of communication, chain of command, centralized structure, decentralized structure, and organizational chart.*

9. *Describe the process of quality improvement.*

10. *Describe three patterns of patient care delivery.*

11. *Discuss the role of the case manager in health care.*

12. *Discuss the clinical ladder for staff nurses.*

The majority of all nurses are employees of health care institutions and organizations. Some are employed by physicians or small businesses, but relatively few are engaged in private practice. This means that as a new graduate you will need to function within an organization. Some understanding of health care institutions and their history as well as a brief introduction to organizational function will help you to assume that role with more comfort and effectiveness.

ACUTE CARE HOSPITALS

Most of you, on graduation, will seek your first job as a registered nurse in an acute care facility. Your instructors have probably suggested that this would provide the best orientation to the health care system and would allow you to become efficient in the skills you have learned as a student. Many other employment situations stipulate at least one year general hospital experience as a prerequisite for the position.

The modern hospital may be viewed as the hub or center of the health care delivery system. The "workplace" of the physician, these facilities are central to the health care of the community. They also provide education to a wide variety of health care workers and, in many cases, are centers for research and its dissemination. Hospitals are "big business," employing three fourths of all health care personnel and consuming 39% of the nation's health expenditures (Haglund and Dowling, 1984).

It is therefore important that you have some understanding of the environment in which you will be seeking employment. This chapter provides an overview of the structure and function of the general hospital setting. Let us look first at the historical development of hospitals.

Early Hospitals in Europe and the Middle East

The word "hospital" is derived from the Latin word *hospitalis,* which means to be concerned with *hospites* or guests. In early times these "guests" were persons who needed shelter. As a result, our early hospitals were built to accommodate pilgrims and other travelers. As they grew in number they began to provide assistance to those who were sick and needed care.

From about the fourth century many hospitals were founded as part of the Christian movement. These facilities were associated with a religious group and were staffed by deaconesses, sisters, bishops, brothers, monks, and other groups who had devoted their lives to charitable work. The facilities housed the poor, the orphaned, the aged, the lepers, and the insane as well as those who were ill from other causes such as contagious diseases.

Much of the progress made toward delivery of health care was stopped during the Dark Ages, which lasted from around AD 500 to 1000 following the collapse of the Roman Empire in AD 476. This period of time, which might also be referred to as the early Middle Ages, witnessed the development of three different movements during its early years: feudalism, Islam, and monasticism.

During the period of feudalism the ill were cared for in the home by the "woman of the house," whose life was very difficult. Marrying young and often against her will, she bore and cared for the children; managed the entire household, often serving as hunter and soldier in her husband's absence; and cared for the ill and infirm, often being both nurse and physician. There were very few doctors (Donahue, 1985).

Islam was practiced by the Arab people who followed the prophet Mohammed (AD 570–632) in the worship of Allah. Arab influence extended as far away as India and China as well as into Spain, through northern Africa and western Asia. The Arabs encouraged the study of medicine and built large well-constructed hospitals to house the ill. Many had a host of modern conveniences when viewed according to the time, including such things as streams of running water, treatment with drugs, and separation of patients into wards. Patients were cared for by both male and female nurses (Donahue, 1985).

The period of monasticism witnessed the development of monastic orders exemplified by the Orders of St. Basil, Augustine, Benedict, and Francis. These orders, which provided retreat from the chaos occurring in society at the time, soon became centers of learning and culture. They also eventually began nursing the sick and developed a *hospitalarius* just inside the gates of the monastery to provide care to the sick and the needy of the community. Initially they provided food and shelter more than health care, but as time passed the need for care of the ill grew and became the responsibility of the monastic order. Nursing was done by a monastic sisterhood (Donahue, 1985).

Later hospitals were built outside monastic walls. Three of these hospitals are still in existence; the Hotel Dieu of Lyons (founded in AD 542), the Hotel Dieu of Paris (founded in AD 650–651), and the Santo Sirito Hospital of Rome (founded in AD 717).

The Crusades were also a part of the Middle Ages. Crusaders traveled routes from European countries to Jerusalem raising armies, making pilgrimages to shrines, and attempting to regain control of the Holy Land. Military nursing orders were an outcome of the Crusades that appeared as military brotherhoods. Four of these groups were the Knights Hospitallers of St. John of Jerusalem, the Knights Templars, the Teutonic Knights (Deutsche Orden), and the Knights of St. Lazarus. These groups set up hospitals and carried out various services. The Knights of St. John are recognized for their early ambulance services. The Knights of St. Lazarus were outstanding in the treatment of leprosy. These groups became quite powerful during the Crusades and had their own rivalries.

During the later Middle Ages (AD 1000–1500) religious orders continued. An increase in hospital founding is said to be attributed to monastic and papal reform movements taking place at the time. Over 700 hospitals were founded in England during the middle of the 16th century (Kalisch and Kalisch, 1986). Like other early hospitals they offered accommodations to travelers, the poor, the aged, the orphaned, as well as to the sick.

The Middle Ages were followed by the Renaissance years (1438–1660) with the rebirth of learning and an advance of medicine. Physicians became concerned about hospitals and hospital conditions. Hospitals could not meet the increasing demand for services. As they grew in number they declined in the quality of service provided. Mortality rates increased. Descriptions of the late 18th century hospital characterized situations in which four, five, or six patients might lay, side by side on a single bed in a head-to-toe positioning. The time was right for reform.

The Development of Hospitals in the United States

The history of hospitals in the United States can be traced back to the mid 1700s when most cities had built *almshouses*, also called "poorhouses," to provide food and shelter for the homeless poor. These structures became the home to the aged, disabled, mentally ill, and the orphaned. Also operating at this time were *pesthouses*, which were built to isolate people with contagious diseases, especially those who contacted the disease while aboard ship. In these facilities were persons suffering from cholera, smallpox, typhus, and yellow fever, to name a few. Pesthouses might open and close as the need dictated.

Neither the almshouses nor the pesthouses represented an institution from which most individuals would want to seek or receive care. They were crowded, unsanitary, and poorly heated and ventilated. Cross-infection was common and mortality was high. Those with the financial means were cared for in their homes.

The first hospital in the United States was the Pennsylvania Hospital in Philadelphia built in 1751. The impetus for its founding is attributed to Benjamin Franklin, who maintained that it was the public's responsibility to provide the same quality of care to native citizens who were sick, poor, mentally ill, and homeless as was being afforded to immigrants. The New York Hospital in New York City was to follow in 1773, Massachusetts General Hospital in Boston in 1816, and New Haven Hospital in New Haven, Connecticut, in 1826.

These early hospitals cared for people with acute illnesses and injuries but did not admit the mentally ill. Therefore, during the same period, a number of governmental hospitals were established to house the mentally ill. The first such facility was established as a department of the Pennsylvania Hospital in 1752. The second was founded in Williamsburg, Virginia, in 1773. By 1840 eight hospitals to treat the mentally ill had been established. The forms of treatment of patients in these early mental hospitals is legend, often being cruel and inhumane. Some of you may have studied about Dorothea Dix, a soft-spoken schoolteacher, who campaigned vigorously for and brought about much reform in the area of mental health treatment.

The early hospitals left much to be desired. They were dirty, rank with infection, and poorly ventilated. Linen was used for several patients before it was laundered. Draining, suppurating wounds were commonplace. The stench was overwhelming, and it is said that nurses used snuff to make working conditions more tolerable (Kalisch and Kalisch, 1986). Nursing was not an attractive career, and most of the nursing care was delivered by women who could find no other source of employment; alcoholics, prostitutes, and those convicted of criminal offenses. There was no formal training for their roles nor were there any standards for care.

Factors Affecting the Development of Hospitals

Six major developments can be cited that represented major forces in the continued development of hospitals and patient care. Each one played a unique role in the changes.

The Advance in Medical Science

The first of these major developments related to advances in medical science. By the end of the colonial period two medical schools had been established in the United States. Prior to that time physicians learned their skills through an apprenticeship with a practicing physician. As medicine became more of a science, advances occurred. One of the most significant was the discovery of anesthesia and the rapid advances in surgery that were to follow. The germ theory also did much to advance the practice of medicine because it was soon followed by the development of agents or techniques that would sterilize or serve as antiseptics. The growth of hospitals in the United States was a direct result of these advances that made hospitals safer and more desirable. The discovery of sulfa and antibiotics in the mid 1930s and mid 1940s, respectively, heralded even greater changes.

The Development of Medical Technology

The development of specialized medical technology was a natural successor to the advances in medical science. The first hospital laboratory was opened in 1889, and x-rays were used in diagnosis in 1896. The electrocardiogram (ECG) was discovered in 1903 and the electroencephalogram (EEG) was discovered in 1929 (Haglund and Dowling, 1988).

Changes in Medical Education

Advances in medical education also had a significant impact on the development of health care in this country. The Flexner Report was completed in 1910, and it led to changes in the structure and content of curricula in medical schools. It also expanded the role of hospitals to include education and research and resulted in internships and residencies for medical students.

Development of the Health Insurance Industry

The growth of the health insurance industry is another factor responsible for the development of hospitals. Although there were some antecedents, most sources indicate that the first hospital insurance plan was initiated at Baylor University Hospital in 1929 to serve the need of schoolteachers of Dallas, Texas (Raffel and Raffel, 1989). The approach used there was to form the model for Blue Cross plans around the country.

Today figures vary as to what percentage of the population is protected against costs of medical care by some type of insurance. They range from 85% to 90%. Concern continues to be voiced for the 35 million or so individuals who have no protection (Raffel and Raffel, 1989). Prior to the advent of hospital insurance the financial solvency of many facilities was threatened. The security of funds from insurance policies made hospital expansion of facilities and resources a reality.

Greater Involvement of the Government

The government's role in health care delivery has also impacted the development of hospitals. In early times the government was involved primarily at a local level building almshouses and facilities for the insane. By 1935, the government was providing grants-in-aid to assist in the establishment of public health and other programs to furnish health assistance to citizens. In 1946 the Hill-Burton Act resulted in the construction of many hospitals and other health facilities. The initiation of Medicare and Medicaid in 1965 made another significant impact on the health care industry.

The Emergence of Professional Nursing

The last, but certainly not the least, force significantly influencing the growth of hospitals was the development of professional nursing. Following in the wake of work done by Florence Nightingale in England (see Chapter 1), the first school of nursing opened in the United States in 1873. By 1898 there were 400 schools with 10,000 graduates. Haglund and Dowling (1989, p 165) cite two ways in which the advances in nursing contributed to the growth of hospitals. First it "increased the efficacy of treatment, cleanliness, nutritious diets, and formal treatment routines" that resulted in patient recovery. Second, it resulted in considerate, skilled patient care that made hospitals acceptable to all people, not just the poor. The role of the nurse and nursing impacts the health care delivery system more today than ever before.

Many of the factors that affected the development of hospitals in the early 1900s are still affecting the structure and function of hospitals today. Advances in medical technology continue to create major changes in the ways hospital operate. For example, the development of cardiac monitors led to the critical care unit as we know it today. Surgical techniques in cataract surgery have almost completely eliminated the need for a hospital stay for those patients. Instead they are cared for as outpatients. The addition of techniques such as laminar air flow to create environments almost free of pathogens has created the demand for expensive patient care units that can be used to house severely immuno-compromised patients.

Government involvement in the hospital industry has probably never been greater. In recent years nothing has affected the financing of hospitals as severely as the changes in Medicare. Medical payments, originally designed to provide funds to support both capital improvements and debt retirement, became a greater and greater part of the hospital income on which the hospital became dependent. When the Medicare payment system was changed to diagnosis related groups (DRGs), there was no additional support for capital improvement and debt retirement for the specific hospital, creating more problems for hospitals with a greater amount of debt.

Medical and nursing education continue to undergo significant change. The role of each of these professionals is changing, and their interactions as members of the health care delivery systems is moving toward one of collaboration.

CLASSIFICATION OF HOSPITALS AND HEALTH CARE FACILITIES

Because the hospital industry is so large, so diverse, and so complex, it is difficult to describe. Generally hospitals are classified in one of three ways. It should be remembered that any one of these classifications is somewhat arbitrary and a facility may be placed in more than one classification.

Classification According to Length of Stay

One way of classifying hospitals is according to length of stay. This would include short-stay or short-term hospitals and long-term hospitals. Short-stay facilities provide services to patients who are suffering from acute conditions that usually require less than 30 days of hospitalization. The average length of stay has been declining steadily over the past few years and has become significantly less since the implementation of DRGs in 1983.

Long-term hospitals would include those that offer services to patients with major rehabilitation needs, chronic disease, or mental illness. The average length of stay extends of over several months. State institutions for the mentally ill are usually considered long-term hospitals as are the facilities the federal government operates for veterans' in need of rehabilitation. However, in many cases, long-term rehabilitation is located on one unit of an acute care hospital.

Classification by Type of Service

Hospitals may also be classified according to type of service provided. The most common type is the general hospital that offers medical, surgical, obstetrical, emergency, and other services. Specialty hospitals offer only a particular service such as that provided by psychiatric hospitals, women's hospitals, or children's hospitals. Specialty hospitals tend to be less common than general hospitals.

Classification of Hospitals According to Ownership

The final method of classifying hospitals is according to ownership. Hospitals may be classified as government or public, proprietary (also known as private for profit), and voluntary (private nonprofit or religious).

Public Hospitals

Public, or government, hospitals are owned and operated by federal, state, or local governments. The federal facilities usually serve the needs of a special group of individuals such as veterans, military personnel, American Indians, or inmates in our federal prisons. State hospitals often are represented by state mental facilities or hospitals that are operated by the state as part of the state university medical school that controls the operation of the facility. Local hospitals may be city, county, or hospital district institutions. They may be large or small but most tend to be small.

Proprietary Hospitals

These for-profit hospitals are investor-owned and are operated for the financial gain of the individual or group that owns the facility. Historically, these hospitals were owned and operated by a small group of physicians but over the years have often been sold to community groups. In the past few years there has been a significant trend toward the acquisition of hospitals by investor-owned corporations and the formation of multiunit, for-profit hospital systems. Examples would be The Hospital Corporation of America, which is based in Nashville, and Humana, Incorporated of Louisville. Both of these groups own more than 80 hospitals and operate a number of others. Not all investor-owned hospitals are general hospitals.

Voluntary Hospitals

Nonprofit or voluntary institutions are owned and operated by community associations or religious organizations. More than 50% of the nation's short-term hospitals fall into this classification. The term *nonprofit* may be something of a misnomer in the sense that all facilities must make a sufficient profit to continue to exist and to maintain facilities and services.

A term frequently used when referring to hospitals is *community hospital*. A community hospital is usually an acute short-term hospital, either voluntary or proprietary, that may or may not be owned and operated by the public. They are called community hospitals because they serve the needs of the entire community and meet the needs of most citizens of the area for hospital services. Raffel and Raffel (1989) state that community hospitals constitute 83% of the total number of hospitals in the United States and account for 90% of all hospital admissions each year.

THE LONG-TERM CARE FACILITY

Long-term care is the assistance with care and health care needs identified for people of any age who have conditions that require that they have help with the activities of daily living. These conditions may be physical or mental and may extend over a period of time or may last a lifetime. Some examples would be the person who is mentally retarded, the person suffering from cerebral palsy, or the individual who has had a severe head injury that has resulted in compromised mental and physical functioning. Care usually involves coordination between health and social care systems to make a variety of services available to these individuals and their families, such as special counseling, transportation, nursing care, rehabilitation, and perhaps special education programs. Long-term care facilities include nursing homes, chronic disease hospitals, psychiatric hospitals, tuberculosis hospitals, and psychiatric and mental retardation facilities. The majority of long-term care facilities are nursing homes that care primarily for the elderly.

The Nursing Home

According to Collopy, Boyle, and Jennings (1991), there are at the present time more than 19,000 nursing homes in the United States, of which approximately 75% are proprietary, 20% are nonprofit, and 5% are government operated. The average cost per resident ranges from $28,000 in the Northeast to $20,000 in the South. An estimated 51% of this cost is paid directly by the elderly and their families, about 44% by Medicaid, 2% by Medicare, and 1% by private insurance, and other government resources pick up the remainder.

The fastest growing age group in the United States are those 85 years of age and older. It has been estimated that one in four citizens will spend some of their lifetime in a nursing home, very often the last years. Women outnumber men in these facilities, with the population composed of 75% women and 25% men. The age of elderly nursing home residents ranges from 65 to older than 100, with the average age about 84.

History of the Nursing Home

Like our acute care facilities, the nursing home has a rather harsh beginning. In the 19th century almshouses and poorhouses were constructed by the government to shelter the destitute elderly. These facilities attracted a strange mixture of residents, including those that needed asylum and detention, as well as the poor, the chronically disabled, and the mentally ill. The morality that prevailed at the time tended to see poverty and disability as indications of an undisciplined, improvident, and even profligate life. A person who was housed in a "county poorhouse" often had no family to provide care and assistance and no funds and endured a certain social stigma. In time these almshouses became the community dumps for all of society's cast-offs. These early facilities for the country's dependent elderly offered the same grim surroundings of the early hospitals. They were unsanitary, overcrowded, and poorly ventilated. Residents were expected to work to assist with their keep if they were able. Care was provided by individuals who sought employment there as a last resort. Appropriations to manage these facilities were meager because the majority of the citizens had no identification with these institutions that housed the poor and the transient, who probably had no previous history of contributing to the community.

As the United States grew as a society, various groups became concerned about the conditions that existed in the poorhouse. Gradually, patients tended to be separated according to condition and the mentally and chronically ill were reassigned in different hospitals. Nursing homes began to evolve under different sponsorship as churches and fraternal organizations started homes to care for their elderly members. As a result of the Social Security Act of 1935, private (for-profit or proprietary) nursing homes emerged during the 1930s. Raffel and Raffel (1989, p 205) state, "The original exclusion of benefits for patients in public institutions (since repealed) apparently stemmed from congressional concern about conditions in county poorhouses and a desire to get them closed."

In the postwar period, the Hill-Burton Act of 1948 that supported hospital construction was expanded to include voluntary (nonprofit) nursing homes and some states also developed grant programs. Since 1950, government funding for nursing homes has increased steadily and culminated in the 1965 Medicaid program, which now covers 40% of all nursing home costs (Collopy et al., 1991). Governmental regulation of nursing homes has become increasingly involved and complex.

As changes in funding occurred and as short-term acute care hospitals became increasingly specialized, the role of the nursing home has changed. It was affected by the deinstitutionalization movement in the 1950s and 1960s that saw large numbers of elderly discharged from mental hospitals. Nursing homes began to assume the role of providing specialized care for the elderly. By the 1960s this role was well established, but the nursing home industry was subjected to constant reports of substandard and negligent care and, in some instances, charges of absolute abuse of patients and misuse or embezzlement of their funds. This resulted in even greater scrutiny and regulation by the government.

The Nursing Home Today

Although the nursing home of today suffers from the negative image of the past, it offers a far different environment than it did even 10 years ago. Recent years have witnessed the development of retirement communities that can take one of several forms: they may be self-contained towns, retirement villages, retirement subdivisions, retirement residences, and continuing-care communities (Matteson and McConnell, 1988). These communities provide a variety of levels of care to the residents based on the resident's need. In an "assisted living" arrangement, the resident can maintain maximum independence, seeking help as it is needed. Most of the facilities also maintain a convalescent center, and services such as occupational therapy, physical therapy, and dental care may also be available. The one limiting factor may be the cost of access.

ORGANIZATION AND ADMINISTRATION OF HEALTH CARE INSTITUTIONS

The organizational functioning of health care institutions is not always as clear cut as that of business and industry. Lines of authority and responsibility may vary considerably depending on the size of the facility and the services it renders. The discussion that follows outlines the most common structures.

The Governing Board

Typically health care institutions are governed by a board of directors, a board of trustees, or commissioners. Members of the governing boards may be elected or appointed but usually are influential members of the community who have been successful in their other endeavors. Recently there has been a tendency to have boards composed of individuals with specific management skills, such as business executives, bankers, attorneys, and similar professionals. The governing board sets policy and deals with matters of finance and long-range planning. Recently they have also been accountable for the monitoring of quality control, although this is delegated to the medical staff. They hire an administrator and other key personnel who have responsibility for operating the hospital. Medical and patient care matters are usually deferred to the medical staff.

The Administrator

The administrator has the responsibility for the day-to-day management and supervision of the organization and for implementing the policy established by the board. The administrator has the overall responsibility for managing finances, hiring and supervising personnel, and coordinating organizational activities. In large facilities, assistant administrators may assist with these duties. Although some administrators have had no formal preparation for these responsibilities, today many hospital administrators have been educated for that role with a master's degree in hospital or health administration. Some smaller hospitals may have a nurse as the administrator, especially in Catholic hospitals run by one of the various nursing orders. The administrator of a nursing home must usually possess a credential approved by the state. The administrative position may be assigned one of a number of titles, including president, chief executive officer, executive director, or even superintendent.

The Medical Staff

A physician wishing to bring his or her patients to a particular hospital must apply for *staff privileges*. The bylaws of the organization describe how this process is managed, but it usually involves making application to the medical board and verifying qualifications in terms of education and medical expertise.

Staff privileges may fall into a number of different categories, including active staff, associate staff, courtesy staff, consulting staff, and honorary staff. Usually each hospital has a *chief of staff*, an elected position held by one of the members of the medical staff for a given period of time. Physicians are responsible for monitoring the quality of care provided within the hospital and operate through a number of medical committees. In large hospitals there may be a "chief" for each of the specialty services such as medicine, surgery, obstetrics, and psychiatry.

A nursing home will typically have a medical director who is responsible for medical policy and procedure. In very large institutions this may be a full-time position, but in many it is a part-time responsibility. Each resident must have a personal physician who provides medical supervision and reviews medical care at least monthly. The medical director may serve as the personal physician for some of the residents in the nursing home.

The Nursing Director or Administrator

The top nursing position within any health care institution is that of the nursing director or administrator. Because of the responsibilities associated with this position, its importance within the organization, and the number of employees under this person's supervision (nursing is the largest department in any hospital), there has been a trend in the past few years to use the title nursing service administrator or assistant administrator for nursing services. The title for this position might also be vice-president for nursing. In nursing homes the most common title is director of nursing. In most of these instances the nursing administrator occupies a position on the organizational chart similar to other assistant administrators.

The administrator for nursing services is ultimately responsible for the nursing care provided within the institution. This person generally controls the budget for nursing services and is responsible for organization and staffing of the nursing units. There has been a strong push in recent years to require that nursing service administrators have a master's degree in nursing. Many masters programs in nursing offer a nursing service administration pathway, and an increasing number are offering a combined nursing and business masters program. In some instances, persons filling this role have master's degrees in business administration in addition to their basic preparation in nursing at a baccalaureate level.

To assist with the responsibilities of administering nursing services, the nursing director or administrator may have an assistant for each shift within the hospital. In addition, depending on the size of the facility, there may be clinical specialists in areas such as maternity, pediatrics, oncology, and critical care. Each clinical unit will have a nurse manager who is responsible for supervising the activities of that unit. There has been a growing trend to give this individual greater responsibilities for the management of the unit, including developing and managing the budget, interviewing and hiring employees, and similar activities. In some hospitals these positions may carry the title head nurse, which is a carryover from the earlier days in nursing.

ORGANIZATION OF HEALTH CARE INSTITUTIONS

Hospitals are bureaucratic organizations. By that we mean that they operate and are administered through a number of departments and subdivisions with appointed individuals having responsibility for carrying out various defined functions. This structure determines command and strengthens authority. Often the routines established and the communication paths to be followed are rather inflexible but are established to provide order and structure to the organization. Bureaucracy in hospitals is also a product of their history with its strong military and religious influence.

It is useful for any students entering into this environment to have some understanding of its structure. The following section outlines some of the more commanding aspects of the hospital organization. Students are encouraged to gain greater depth in this area in books devoted entirely to the topic.

The Organizational Chart

Characteristically, hospitals are organized into departments that are generally established based on the function or purpose they serve within the organization. Each will have a described set of tasks to be accomplished by the persons employed in that area. Thus in a typical hospital, you see admitting departments, maintenance and housekeeping departments, medical records departments, outpatient departments, nursing departments, and so on. Which departments are present, the size of these departments, and the specific domain under which they are situated within the organization will depend on the purpose and size of the institution.

The relationship of one department to another is defined in terms of organization structure and is usually depicted in an organizational chart. The number of levels on any chart is determined by the need within the organization to assign authority and responsibility. The greatest authority exists at the top of a pyramid-shaped chart and decreases as you move toward the base. Persons having jobs within the organization that are located at the top of the organizational chart are considered administrators, executives, or "the management," and those closer to the base are considered employees or staff. Often located between these two levels is an area known as "middle management" composed of a group of individuals who coordinate and control activities of specified groups of workers to accomplish the directives established by the executives.

The organizational chart may take one of several forms, reflecting the type of administration operating within that organization. If the organization has chosen to have a *narrow span of control*, that is, has placed the responsibility for overseeing the activities of the organization in the hands of a few individuals, it is said to have a *centralized* or *tall* organizational structure. If, however, the organization has chosen to have a *broad span of control*, then it places responsibility in the hands of a larger number of individuals and is said to have a *decentralized* or *flat* organizational structure.

Of course, many organizations develop variations of these basic structural patterns. In some instances a local institution may have a what appears to be a simple structure but it is complicated by its relationship to a large corporation that manages many health care institutions. You will want to investigate the structure of any organization in which you seek employment.

Channels of Communication

The structure of the organization also spells out the *channel of communications*. Channels of communication run up and down the organizational chart, moving from one level of responsibility and authority to the next. Thus the nursing administrator communicates instructions to the assistant administrator, who will communicate the message to the nursing manager, who communicates with the nursing staff. In return, the staff communicate messages to their nursing manager who communicates with the assistant administrator and so forth. It is generally considered improper and inappropriate to skip or bypass any of the levels in this communication process. It is not appropriate for the staff nurse to communicate a concern to the assistant administrator without first sharing it with the nursing manager.

Chain of Command

Paralleling the channel of communication is the *chain of command*. The chain of command describes the path of authority and accountability from the individuals at the top of the organization to those at the base of the organization. It is also referred to as the *organizational hierarchy*. Typically the nursing administrator gives instructions to and evaluates the performance of the assistant administrator, who in turn gives direction to and evaluates the performance of the nursing manager, and so forth throughout the organization. Working from the base of the or-

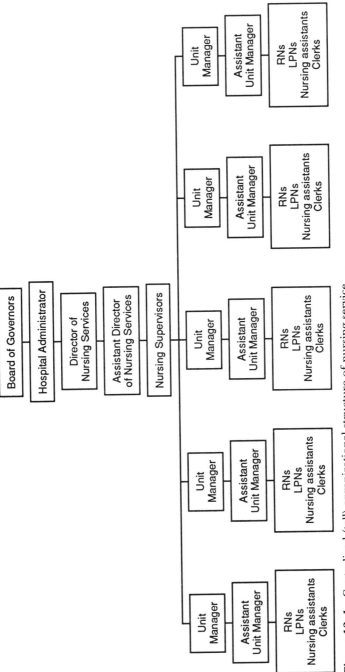

Figure 12-1. Centralized (tall) organizational structure of nursing service.

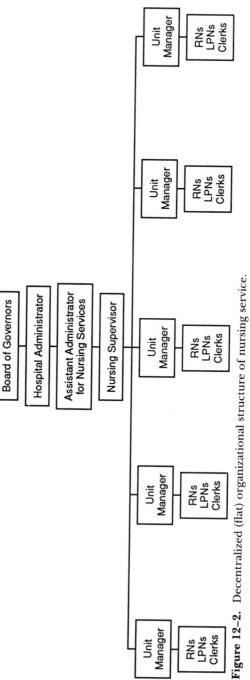

Figure 12–2. Decentralized (flat) organizational structure of nursing service.

ganization to the top, we frequently use the language "reports to." Thus, the staff nurse reports to the nursing manager and the nursing manager reports to the assistance administrator, who reports to the nursing administrator. Again, the length of the "chain of command" and the number of different "reports to" will depend on the size of the organization, being fewer in small organizations and greater in large facilities.

One problem in some complex organizations is that individuals may find that they are responsible to more than one supervisor. As long as these two supervisors share goals and priorities this may pose few problems. If, however, these supervisors have differing priorities, the employee may feel stressed by the conflicting expectations.

Job Descriptions

The responsibilities of all jobs or positions within the organization are spelled out in *job descriptions.* Job descriptions are written statements, usually found in hospital policy manuals, that describe the responsibilities to be assumed by individuals hired into any of the jobs or positions within the hospital. Thus the job description of the staff nurse explains what that individual will do, the job description of the nurse manager outlines that person's responsibilities, and the job description of the admitting clerk will describe the role that person plays within the organization. These job descriptions should form the foundation for the evaluation of the individual working in that role.

ESTABLISHING AND IMPLEMENTING ORGANIZATIONAL GOALS

All organizations must have methods and provisions for establishing their goals and objectives and for implementing them. These often begin with the establishment of broad policies for operation and continue through the development of a mission statement, philosophy of care, and goals and objectives.

The Mission Statement

Health care institutions, like other major organizations, usually have developed *mission statements.* Mission statements are broad declarations of the purpose of the organization. A typical mission statement for a community hospital might read as follows: "Cleaver Community Hospital exists to provide high level health care and services to the citizens of Cleaver County." Mission statements will vary depending on the nature, purpose, and setting of the institution. The mission statement of a university hospital heavily involved in education and research will reflect those commitments. A small community hospital that refers many of its critical patients to a nearby metropolitan hospital will probably not have statements in its mission about research and, in fact, may not be involved in research activities.

The mission statement is implemented through the philosophy of care and goals of the organization. The *philosophy of care* outlines what the organization believes about the care to be delivered to consumers. In other words, the philosophy is a statement of belief. Philosophies of care might include such statements as "Cleaver Community Hospital believes that each individual, regardless of race, religion, economic status, or chosen life style is entitled to personalized, quality care provided with respect for the dignity of the individual."

The philosophy of care, in turn, is implemented through *goals and objectives*. There may be broad goals and objectives to outline and describe the activities of the organization as a whole. There are usually goals and objectives that address in a more specific manner the endeavors of a particular care unit. If the hospital has a hospice unit, the goals and objectives of that department will likely be quite different than the goals and objectives outlined for the birth center for the same hospital.

Policies and Procedures

As mentioned earlier in this chapter, the responsibility and authority for developing policies for the hospital rests with the governing board. The governing board delegates to the hospital administrator the responsibility for determining that these policies are implemented and adhered to. Policies are written and copies are maintained in a policy manual. Usually there is a policy manual in each major department or unit within a hospital. Depending on the area in which you are employed, you will find varying needs for referring to the policy manual in your role as a recently graduated registered nurse. As you might anticipate, the need for special policies related to occurrences in an emergency department, delivery room, or a critical care unit will be greater than those of a general medical or surgical unit. Special unit policies are sometimes termed *protocols*.

Procedure manuals are also found in each unit or department. Procedure manuals spell out how a particular activity or nursing activity is to be completed and is often related in a number of steps. For example, you may find a procedure for managing a patient's epidural analgesia, for administering oncological agents, and for doing a host of basic care procedures such as catheterizations.

Nurses have been given increasing responsibility for affecting and developing institutional policies and procedures. They are serving as representatives to various committees responsible for developing and monitoring policies and procedures. Policies for an individual unit that are within the guidelines of general policy may be developed and adopted by the personnel on that unit. This might include a policy of how scheduling requests are handled. Policies or protocols that relate to specific patient care needs may be reviewed by an appropriate committee of the medical staff before final acceptance. Newly developed policies that are broad in scope must move up the chain of command and be approved by the governing board, but nurses' input at the grassroots level is becoming more commonplace.

Quality Improvement

Quality Improvement (QI), or total quality management (TQM) as it is sometimes called, is a structured program being introduced into many health care organizations as a mechanism to assess and improve care. This is seen by many as the next step after quality assurance programs have been established. Quality assurance often has involved assuring that basic standards for care have been met. Quality improvement helps an organization move beyond these basic standards to an ever-expanding view of quality care.

The first step in quality improvement is defining what the individual organization means by quality of care. This involves consulting consumers as well as providers of health care. Consumers may describe difficult-to-measure qualities such as attitudes toward consumers by employees in the institution. There may also be very practical concerns expressed by consumers such as timeliness in meeting appointments and accessibility of care providers when consumers have questions. Professionals often have other attributes in mind when they speak of quality care. These attributes may include addressing concerns of the whole family as well as those of the individual patient.

Whatever the concerns, quality improvement identifies goals and objectives that represent higher standards of care. After these higher goals and objectives are identified, the next step is developing plans to move toward them. Through quality improvement, health care providers are striving to create a care delivery system that is responsive and caring

Figure 12–3. The first step in quality improvement is to define what the organization means by quality of care.

and that demonstrates the highest standards possible in light of today's health care system.

PATTERNS OF CARE DELIVERY

The nursing department of any health care institution carries major responsibility for the quality of nursing care delivered. Throughout the years, the structure of the delivery of that care has taken a number of different formats. Among the factors influencing the delivery pattern selected are the type of patients served, the type of care provided, the cost of the care, and the number and education of potential employees.

In the following section we describe the typical implementation of various patterns of care delivery. It is important for you to know and remember as you read through these descriptions that there are variations and adaptations made within different facilities of any pattern of care. We have outlined what each pattern typically looks like, but you might find it practiced just a little differently where you are employed.

The Case Method

The case method was the first system used for the delivery of nursing care in the United States. A nurse worked with only one patient and was expected to meet all of that patient's nursing needs. Often the nurse lived in the patient's home or might "special" that patient in the hospital. If working in the patient's home, the nurse often had other household-type duties associated with carrying out nursing care, such as cooking for the patient. This one-to-one relationship had many advantages as far as care was concerned, but the nurses worked long hours and were poorly paid. Advancing technology and changes in cost made this type of care delivery impractical in the hospital.

A variation of the case method is used in most home care agencies. In these situations, the nurse is assigned the "case" and follows that individual through the entire time care is provided by the agency. Although this is not 24-hour-a-day care, it does encompass the totality of the patient's care needs.

The Functional Method

The functional method of care delivery emerged during the Depression of the 1930s. This method allowed for the care of increased numbers of patients in hospitals and for the advancing technology. The division of nursing responsibilities varied from hospital to hospital depending on the number of nurses, nursing students, orderlies, and nurse's aides available. Typically, with the functional method specific tasks were assigned by the head nurse to the various persons employed on the unit according to the level of skill required for performance. A "temperature nurse" took temperatures; a "treatment nurse" cared for wounds, dressing changes, and other treatments to be administered; while a "medicine nurse" would give all of the medications, chart them, and provide a list of replacement needs to the head nurse. A nurse may have more than one of these responsibilities if there were fewer patients or fewer nurses. The head nurse gave "report" to the next shift of nurses who would care for the patients.

The system was economical and efficient, but it had the disadvantage of fragmenting care. No one person was responsible for planning the patient's care. Each staff member charted the aspect of care for which they were responsible. Communication among the different persons who cared for the patient was lacking, and often the patients had no idea who was in charge of their care.

Functional nursing is used in many nursing homes because of its economy and efficiency. The registered nurse may be in charge. The licensed practical nurse may be assigned to give all medications, and the nursing assistants may do all direct personal care. In the long-term care setting, where both staff and residents are there over a long period of time, some of the disadvantages of functional care may be overcome. A specific registered nurse may be assigned to assess each resident and plan appropriate care. That same nurse may be responsible for updating nursing care plans monthly and for assigning and supervising the nursing assistants. The staff may be stable enough to know the residents well and communicate with each other effectively. The resident and family may know all of the staff well enough to be aware of who is in charge. Unfortunately, not all long-term care settings have the resources for this kind of planning and communication.

Team Nursing

The concept of team nursing was introduced in the early 1950s. This approach to patient care is based on having a group of people of different levels of skill assigned to a group of patients. Typically the rooms in a hospital unit are divided between or among nursing teams each led by a registered nurse, who is basically responsible for overseeing the care delivery to her group of patients by the "team."

The team is composed of other registered nurses, nursing students, practical nurses, and nursing assistants, to whom the "team leader" delegates or assigns responsibilities as appropriate. The team works together, with members performing those tasks for which they are best prepared. Often the team leader gives all medications and delegates responsibilities to other members of the team. The team leader gives report to the team that follows on the next shift. A central aspect of its function is the team conference in which the team members plan patient care together with the team leader responsible for seeing that this occurs.

The potential for high-quality care is present in team nursing, but the time required for team conferences and the necessity for constant communication can interfere with achieving the ideal. There remains the concern that patients may not be able to identify the persons responsible for their care. Nurses may also feel some frustration at the lack of autonomy. Without team planning and communication, team nursing may become in reality just a variation of functional nursing.

Figure 12–4. Team conferences, planning, and communication are critical elements of team nursing.

Total Patient Care

Many hospitals have returned to a total patient care type of assignment, in which a registered nurse or licensed practical (vocational) nurse is assigned for all care needs. The assignment is based on the needs of the patient. This nurse cares for a group of four to six patients, depending on how acutely ill each patient is. This returns a greater sense of control to the nurses, giving them a greater sense of autonomy and fostering a greater sense of involvement in patients' outcomes. This type of care focuses on the total person rather than on a collection of tasks or procedures. By maintaining a broad range of skills, the nurse can enjoy the satisfaction that comes from seeing and being involved in the whole spectrum of care.

Primary Nursing

In a pattern of primary care, which came into popular use in the 1980s, one nurse is assigned by the head nurse or nursing coordinator the responsibility for the care of each patient from the time the patient is admitted to the hospital through that patient's discharge planning and discharge. The primary nurse is responsible for initiating and updating the nursing care plan. An associate nurse works with this same patient on other shifts and on the primary nurse's "days off." The associate nurse carries out the plan established by the primary nurse. The obvious benefit for the patient is continuity of care, and patients often express satisfaction in knowing who is responsible for their care. Nurses often find greater job satisfaction because they have more autonomy and control of the care given. More nurses are required for this method of care delivery, and it is more expensive than other methods.

One of the problems associated with primary nursing is the role of the primary nurse. In most facilities every nurse serves as the primary nurse for a few patients and as the associate nurse for the patients of primary nurses on other shifts. Sometimes the nurse finds it difficult to follow plans made by another if there is disagreement. The patient's condition may also change, requiring the plan to be changed without consulting the primary nurse. Another concern is the level of expertise and commitment required of all nurses. Because there is no team leader to help pull things together, patient care will suffer if a nurse is not fully competent to perform all the required tasks. Some hospitals have required that all primary nurses have baccalaureate degrees in nursing, a stipulation hard to assure in any period of nursing shortage. Nursing service administrators in hospitals that have used the primary nurse pattern of care delivery have also expressed concern that nurses have forgotten how to delegate responsibilities. In a work environment in which the nurse provided all care, there was no opportunity to decide who might best carry out various patient care activities if more than one individual was involved in giving that care.

Case Management

Case management is a process of monitoring an individual patient's health care for the purpose of maximizing positive outcomes and containing costs. A key to case management is the identification of a critical pathway for care and treatment that includes specific timelines and standard protocols.

The case manager is an individual assigned responsibility for this process. The case manager may follow the patient from the diagnostic

Figure 12–5. The case manager may follow the patient from the diagnostic phase through hospitalization, rehabilitation, and back to home care.

phase through hospitalization, rehabilitation, and back to home care. The case manager ensures that plans are made in advance for the next needed step. Through this longitudinal relationship, the case manager assists with decision making and helps to assure that the patient receives care that will achieve the most positive outcomes in the most efficient manner. This process helps to eliminate costly delays in progress. For example, one case manager for cardiac surgery patients identified a common problem that was creating lengthened hospital stays. By consulting with the surgeons, a preventive approach to this problem was identified and the average length of stay for these cardiac patients was decreased. This resulted in a significant cost saving to the hospital and a significant increase in well-being for the patients.

Registered nurses are the most common professional group to act as case managers. Case management goes beyond primary nursing to responsibility for managing the patient's interaction with the entire health care system and may not include the provision of any direct care. In some settings social workers also act as case managers. Case managers may be employed by third-party payers (such as insurance companies) or by health care providers.

In some instances case management means including a third party into the patient–physician decision-making process. The case manager from an insurance company may be consulted at the start of the diagnostic process for approval for high-cost diagnostic studies. This case manager must be familiar with the indications for the use of these technologies and when lower cost alternatives would provide adequate information. It is within the responsibility of the case manager to suggest a second opinion or further diagnostic studies.

Preadmission certification may also be performed by the insurance company's case manager. The physician contacts the case manager to obtain prior approval for hospitalization and surgery. In these instances the case manager has the authority to suggest nonhospital treatment if that would achieve the same outcome for the patient. When hospitalization is approved, the case manager begins planning for discharge needs.

During hospitalization, the case manager follows the patient's progress, helps to coordinate various services needed, and supports discharge planning that shortens hospitalization. After discharge, the case manager continues to follow the patient's progress to assure that desired outcomes are being attained.

Case managers who are employed by hospitals typically follow a patient from the time admission is planned through the time of discharge. This case manager might plan the admitting process to ensure that all preadmission workups are completed and that the patient is being admitted at the appropriate time to facilitate follow-through on problems. For example, the hospital case manager might ensure that a patient having a certain series of diagnostic tests be admitted on Monday because the tests can be performed within 5 days only if no weekend intervenes.

Case managers are also helping employers to establish wellness programs that seek to contain health care costs by decreasing the need for services. Blood pressure management, stress management, stopping smoking, and exercise classes may significantly decrease costs of health care for a large corporation. By setting up programs for identification and treatment of those who have substance abuse, there are ultimate savings in major medical costs.

Case managers in private practice may focus on a particular group of clients; for example, the geriatric case manager focuses on managing care for the older client. The private case manager is paid by the client or family, usually based on the hours of service provided. The case manager may help the family to identify all of the options for care and treatment, ask questions to obtain greater understanding of the overall problem, and work with the family in the decision-making process. Private geriatric case managers have been particularly helpful to midlife children trying to plan care for elderly parents who live in a distant city.

Problems for case managers include opposition from physicians who see the role as an infringement on their historical rights of autonomy in decision making. Providers may also believe that the case manager is more concerned with the "bottom line" of cost than with what is best for the individual. In the same vein, accusations are sometimes made that quality is sacrificed to cost containment through case management. Some companies have challenged the theory that case management always results in cost savings. When nurses are carefully overseeing patient care, they may identify additional health care needs as well as facilitating care for known needs. These newly identified needs may then require additional services.

Nurses dramatically change their roles when they assume responsibility for case management. They have increased autonomy and power. They relate more effectively to the business community, and as they do this they are becoming more familiar with health care financing and the many constraints on the system. Case management is a growing arena in which nurses are making significant contributions to health care.

Clinical Ladders

Clinical ladders are mechanisms developed to recognize and reward nurses who remain in direct patient care. Historically, the nurse who looked for advancement was required to move away from the patient into administrative positions. As nursing has developed an increasingly responsible and autonomous profile in health care institutions, nurses have sought ways of recognizing the expertise of those in direct care.

Most clinical ladders establish a pathway with titles and higher levels of pay for those who have demonstrated proficiency in patient care. Sometimes the clinical ladder requires a certain amount of continuing education in a specialty field or certification in a specialty. Peer evaluations, supervisor evaluations, and self-evaluations may be part of the process of obtaining advancement on a clinical ladder. Through this process the nurse is encouraged and supported in developing greater expertise.

CONCLUSION

As a new graduate you will have choices to make in regard to the setting in which you choose to practice. The overview provided in this chapter was designed to assist you in understanding and evaluating organizations you are considering. The focus has deliberately addressed the institutional environment because that is where most new graduates work. In no way is this meant to detract from the opportunities that exist for employment in doctor's offices, clinics, and home health care.

As you move toward the role of an employee in a health care institution, you will find it valuable to understand that organization and how it functions. This chapter has provided a specific focus on patterns of delivery of nursing services to enable you to ask appropriate questions and understand the answers you may receive.

There is no "best" or "perfect" type of organization. Each one will adapt any general pattern to its own situation and needs. In addition, the formal organization is always affected by the way individuals in positions of authority act out the official policy. The challenge for you is to find the organization or setting that provides the optimum "match" with your personal philosophy of nursing and approach to care.

REFERENCES

Collopy B, Boyle P, Jennings B: New Directions in nursing home ethics (A Hastings Center Report Special Supplement, pp 1-16, March-April) Hastings Center Report 21(2), 1991

Donahue MP: Nursing: The Finest Art. St. Louis, CV Mosby, 1985

Haglund CL, Dowling WL: The hospital. *In* Williams SJ, Torrens PR: Introduction to Health Services, 3rd ed, pp 160–211. New York, John Wiley & Sons, 1984

Kalisch PA, Kalisch BJ: The Advance of American Nursing. Boston, Little, Brown & Co, 1986

Matteson MA, McConnell ES: Gerontological Nursing: Concepts and Practice. Philadelphia, Harcourt-Brace-Jovanovich, 1988

Raffel MW, Raffel NK: The U. S. Health System: Origins and Functions, 3rd ed. New York: John Wiley & Sons, 1989

FURTHER READINGS

Aiken LH: Charting the future of hospital nursing. Image 22(2):72–78, 1990

Chaska NL: The Nursing Profession: Turning Points. St. Louis, CV Mosby, 1990

Flood SD, Diers D: Nurse staffing, patient outcomes and cost. Nurs Manage 19: 34–43, 1988

Kane RA, Kane RL: Long-term Care: Principles, Programs and Policies. New York: Springer, 1987

Krieger G, Sullivan J: The case for case management. J Occup Health Safety 1: 92, 1988

Moccia P: 1989: Shaping a human agenda for the nineties: Trends that demand our attention as managed care prevails. Nurs Health Care 10(1):14–17, 1989

Moxley D, Buzas L: Perceptions of case management services for elderly people. Health Soc Work 8:196–203, 1989

Parker M, Secord LJ: Case managers: Guiding the elderly through the health care maze. In Lindeman CA, McAthie M: Readings: Nursing Trends and Issues, pp 271–274. Springhouse, PA, Springhouse Corporation, 1990

Parker M, Secord LJ: Private geriatric care management: Providers, services and fees. Nurs Econ 6(4):165–168, 1988

Smith J: Changing traditional nursing home roles to nursing care management. J Gerontol Nurs 17(5):32–39, 1991

13

Organizations for and About Nursing

Objectives

After completing this chapter, you should be able to

1. *Discuss reasons for the existence of the large number of nursing organizations.*

2. *Identify the purposes of the major structural units of the American Nurses' Association (ANA).*

3. *Discuss the activities and programs of the ANA.*

4. *List some of the activities of the National Student Nurses' Association.*

5. *Identify the major structural units of the National League for Nursing (NLN).*

6. *Discuss the activities and programs of the NLN.*

7. *Discuss the major programs and services of the NLN.*

8. *Identify those criteria for membership in the NLN and the ANA.*

9. *Identify the purposes of accreditation.*

10. *Discuss the major thrust of the specialty organizations.*

11. *Identify the purposes of honorary organizations in nursing.*

12. *List five different groups of nursing organizations and discuss their purposes.*

A student once said that it seems that every time nurses identify a problem, their first action is to form a new organization. This is an exaggeration but has some remnants of truth. To the person initially introduced to the great number of nursing and nursing-related organizations, it may all seem confusing.

A serious concern in the field of nursing is the overlapping of function and interrelationships between some of the various organizations. Unfortunately there has been a spirit of competition rather than one of cooperation in some situations in the past. Because nurses traditionally have not had high incomes, the decision of whether to join none, one, or several organizations has often been an economic as well as a philosophical issue.

Nursing organizations have recently put forth a concerted effort to promote cooperation. Nurses, as a whole, seem to be better informed about the various organizations, and they generally receive better salaries

Figure 13–1. The large number of nursing organizations may seem overwhelming.

than in the past. Unfortunately this has not resulted in significantly greater participation by professional nurses in their organizations. Some people specifically do not join because of philosophical differences, but many nurses seem to be apathetic and do not recognize the importance to the profession of nurses acting together. In an address to the 1978 American Nurses Association (ANA) convention, Senator Daniel Inouye of Hawaii remarked that nurses are the single largest group of health care providers, and that as a result they have potential for power in affecting change if they work together.

AMERICAN NURSES ASSOCIATION

The ANA, the professional association for registered nurses, had its origins in a meeting of nursing leaders at the World's Fair in Chicago in 1890. Through their suggestions and efforts, in 1896 the alumnae organizations of 10 schools of nursing sent delegates to form a committee to organize a professional association. The resulting organization was called the National Associated Alumnae of the United States and Canada. The name was changed in 1899 to the Nurses' Associated Alumnae of the United States and Canada. In 1911 the organization split into Canadian and American groups because the state laws of New York (where the organization was incorporated) did not allow for representatives from two countries. The name American Nurses Association was adopted in the United States.

Membership

In 1982 the ANA adopted a different organizational format, moving from a direct, individual membership to a modified federation structure. The ANA membership is composed of state nurses' associations. The individual nurse belongs to the constituent state organization. Each state is free to establish its own membership plans; however, membership is limited to registered nurses. The only exception to this is the admission to membership of some new graduates who have not yet passed state board examinations. In addition to this change in membership, the ANA has made significant changes in how the functions of the organization are to be carried out.

In 1984 there were more than 1.8 million registered nurses in the United States (RN ranks. . ., 1986). Of these, approximately 185,000 belong to the ANA. From this you can readily see that most nurses do not participate in this organization. The figures are somewhat misleading, however, because it is safe to assume that many of the registered nurses who do not join the organization are not practicing, whereas those who are leaders in the profession usually are members. Nevertheless, although the association is the official voice for the profession, fewer than half of the registered nurses participate in the organization.

One reason for the low level of membership is its high cost. Dues to the national association and the state and district associations are paid together, and in most areas of the country they are more than $250.00 per year. Another reason given for not joining is lack of time to participate in activities. Many nurses have dual responsibilities of job and home and feel they have no time for a professional organization. Other nurses do not see how the benefits available through the association are personally valuable. Some explain that they are just not interested in the issues and concerns in which the organization is involved. Lastly, there are those who do not join because they do not agree with the position of the ANA on major issues.

Figure 13–2. Deciding which organizations to join is an economic as well as a philosophical decision.

Those who are active in the ANA believe that its work is severely hampered by the low level of membership. The organization is limited in funds because of the small number of members. Because some specific programs, such as those involved with collective bargaining, are costly to the state association, there has been a strong move to require nurses to belong to the association if it serves as a bargaining agent. In some states the state association has set a specific percentage of staff that must be members before they will become the bargaining agent.

A current controversy involves differing views over what the purpose of the professional organization should be. Many people believe that the major concern should be what the organization can do for the individual nurse. Others believe that a truly professional view looks at what the individual may contribute to the profession through the organization. Some think that the organization should not be an advocate in the realm of economic security, whereas others see this as essential. Another point of controversy is the organization's stand on political issues.

Policy Making

Every 2 years at the ANA convention, members of the House of Delegates, who have been selected to represent each state nurses' association, meet. The power to set policy and direction for the organization rests with the House of Delegates. This body often takes an official stand on a controversial issue. In the time between conventions, it is the duty of the organization to carry out the directions of the House of Delegates.

The members of the House of Delegates also vote for candidates for all elective offices in the organization. A board of directors is elected to oversee the functioning of the association. The board makes policy decisions during the time between conventions, although it must stay within the framework of the decisions made by the House of Delegates. The officers of ANA (president, vice-president, secretary, and treasurer) are also elected and sit on the board.

The ANA has a large, professionally staffed office in Kansas City. (Plans are currently underway to move the office to Washington, D.C.) Although the volunteers in the organization are essential, the many and varied tasks could not be accomplished without the full-time staff. Business staff are needed for the many purposes of the organization, but some positions are filled by nurses with special expertise. This is especially true of those positions that require the individual to represent the organization and the interests of nurses to other organizations and individuals. The executive director is the chief administrator of the organization and is hired by the board. Throughout the history of the organization the executive director has always been a nurse with administrative expertise. The executive director works cooperatively and supportively with the president and the board.

The ANA supports committees that work on such policies as the ANA Social Policy Statement (American Nurses Association, 1980). These activities are ongoing efforts to support the advancement of nursing as a profession.

The ANA also supports research on topics related to the profession itself, such as the historical patterns of licensure (Snyder and La-Bar, 1984).

ORGANIZATIONAL STRUCTURE

There are many components of the ANA. The policy-making bodies have already been discussed. Other organizational units were developed to enable the organization to address particular needs.

The basic structure is a *federated* model. That means that the ANA is an organization whose members are other organizations. Figure 13-2 provides an overview of the ANA structure. Activities of the organization are focused into the two broad areas represented by the Congress on Nursing Practice and the Congress on Nursing Economics.

Standing committees deal with business and organizational functions of the ANA. These committees are determined by the bylaws and are permanent. The bylaws, finance, and membership promotion committees are examples of standing committees. Special committees and task forces are set up to deal with a particular problem at a particular time. For example, a special task force of the ANA was appointed to develop a statement on scope of practice. This task force reported back to the House of Delegates at the 1987 ANA convention.

The Constituent Assembly includes the presidents and executive directors of the state nurses' associations. This group meets to discuss concerns of common interest, to study issues, and to present a unified voice from the state nurses' associations on topics of national interest. For example, in 1986 it recommended that future membership in the ANA include both professional and technical nurses. This recommendation was presented to the Board of Directors of ANA (Forum. . ., 1987).

Activities

The ANA has been referred to many times throughout this book. As a professional association it has been involved in all the issues that

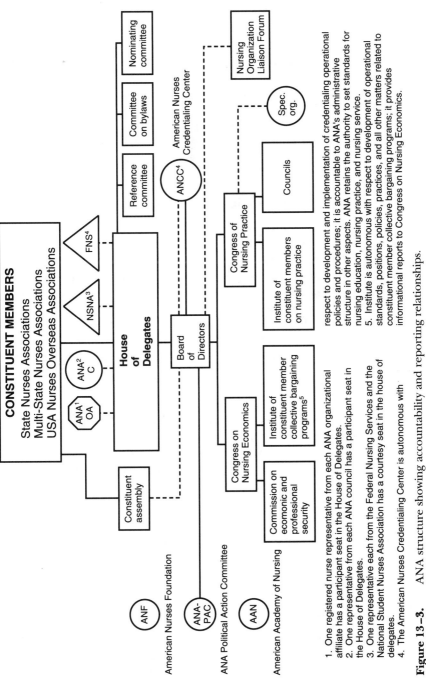

Figure 13–3. ANA structure showing accountability and reporting relationships.

nursing has confronted. The activities of the ANA are carried out by committees, commissions, congresses, and other parts of the organization. There has not been universal support within the nursing community for all the activities that the ANA has championed or for the stands that it has taken. With any group as large as nursing, it is perhaps inevitable that there should be a wide range of viewpoints.

In addition to its activities, the ANA provides direct services to members. These include access to a group professional liability insurance plan and group insurance for health, disability, and accident coverage. From time to time the ANA also provides access to group travel arrangements and purchasing discounts.

Publications and Educational Materials

Through its educational services the ANA produces and distributes a wide variety of educational materials, such as films for nursing, as well as a biennial report entitled *Facts About Nursing*. This report provides basic statistical information used by many organizations and individuals. Reports of committees and commissions and special studies supported by the ANA are also published.

The *American Nurse* is the official organ of the association; official announcements of ANA business are published in this paper. The paper also contains current news of relevance to nursing and health care, editorials, letters, and classified advertisements. The *American Journal of Nursing* is the official journal of the organization. It is published monthly and contains some current news, but its major focus is professional articles. It is published by the American Journal of Nursing Company in New York City and retains autonomy over its own content. The American Journal of Nursing Company is wholly owned by the ANA.

The organization also publishes many pamphlets and informational resources that are of value to nurses. A complete list of publications is available from the organization.

ORGANIZATIONS RELATED TO THE ANA

As the official professional association, the ANA is related to three other organizations in a special way.

National Student Nurses' Association

The National Student Nurses' Association (NSNA) is the professional organization for students in schools of nursing and was started in 1952. Although it works with the ANA and the National League for Nursing (NLN) it is a fully independent organization.

Although the NSNA is an autonomous organization, it has close ties with the ANA. Members of the NSNA serve on selected committees within the ANA, speak to the House of Delegates at the ANA convention to provide a student viewpoint, and work together with the ANA in regard to current issues.

Each state has a state student nurses' association that operates in the same relationship to the state professional organization as the NSNA does to the national organization. State conventions and workshops are held in many states. State issues are addressed by the state association in the same way that national issues are addressed by the NSNA. Local student nurses' organizations may or may not exist in individual schools of nursing. These local organizations may be closely tied to the state and national groups, or they may be independent. It is possible for an individual student to join the state and national student nurses' organizations even if no local counterpart exists.

A major project of the NSNA is "Breakthrough into Nursing," which is designed to recruit and maintain the enrollment of minorities in schools of nursing. The project has enlisted nursing students to speak to minority teenagers to interest them in nursing early in their scholastic careers and to act as preceptors and tutors to increase the retention of minority students when they enroll in schools of nursing.

The NSNA is frequently asked to testify before congressional committees when issues relevant to nursing education are being considered. In this role the organization becomes the public voice for all student nurses.

In 1975 the NSNA developed a Student Bill of Rights. This document carefully balances the rights of students with the responsibilities of students. It supports the view of students as competent adults who are engaged in an educational program. The rights outlined relate to the educational program itself, to the rules and policies of the institution, and to freedom in personal life and decision making.

In the past it was not uncommon for schools of nursing to require membership in the student nurse organization at local, state, and national levels. With increasing emphasis on student rights and freedom of choice, this practice is no longer followed and has led to recruitment problems for many of the student nurse organizations. Students are very busy, with full lives and limited funds. Some do not understand that the efforts of the organization benefit them in larger ways that are not immediately visible. The activities of the student organization cannot occur without a wide membership base for funding and for credibility. Certainly the profession of nursing as a whole and the situation of the individual nursing student would be adversely affected if the NSNA did not remain a viable and active force.

N.S.N.A. STUDENT BILL OF RIGHTS

The following Student Bill of Rights and Responsibilities was adopted by the NSNA House of Delegates in April 1975.

1. Students should be encouraged to develop the capacity for critical judgment and engage in a sustained and independent search for truth.

2. The freedom to teach and the freedom to learn are inseparable facets of academic freedom: students should exercise their freedom with responsibility.

3. Each institution has a duty to develop policies and procedures which provide and safeguard the students' freedom to learn.

4. Under no circumstances should a student be barred from admission to a particular institution on the basis of race, creed, sex, or marital status.

5. Students should be free to take reasoned exception to the data or views offered in any course of study and to reserve judgment about matters of opinion, but they are responsible for learning the content of any course of study for which they are enrolled.

6. Students should have protection through orderly procedures against prejudices or capricious academic evaluation, but they are responsible for maintaining standards of academic performance established for each course in which they are enrolled.

7. Information about student views, beliefs, and political associations which instructors acquire in the course of their work should be considered confidential and not released without the knowledge or consent of the student.

8. The student should have the right to have a responsible voice in the determination of his/her curriculum.

9. Institutions should have a carefully considered policy as to the information which should be a part of a student's permanent educational record and as to the conditions of its disclosure.

10. Students and student organizations should be free to examine and discuss all questions of interest to them, and to express opinions publicly and privately.

11. Students should be allowed to invite and to hear any person of their own choosing, thereby taking the responsibility of furthering their education.

12. The student body should have clearly defined means to participate in the formulation and application of institutional policy affecting academic and student affairs.

13. The institution has an obligation to clarify those standards of behavior which it considers essential to its educational mission and community life.

14. Disciplinary proceedings should be instituted only for violations of standards of conduct formulated with significant student participation and published in advance through such means as a student handbook or a generally available body of institutional regulations. It is the responsibility of the student to know these regulations. Grievance procedures should be available for every student.

15. As citizens and members of an academic community, students are subject to the obligations which accrue them by virtue of this membership and should enjoy the same freedom of citizenship.

Figure 13–4. NSNA Student Bill of Rights.

16. Students have the right to belong or refuse to belong to any organization of their choice.
17. Students have the right to personal privacy in their living space to the extent that the welfare of others is respected.
18. Adequate safety precautions should be provided by schools of nursing, for example, to and from student dorms, adequate street lighting, locks, etc.
19. Dress code, if present in school, should be established by student government in conjunction with the school director and faculty, so the highest professional standards possible are maintained, but also taking into consideration points of comfort and practicality for the student.
20. Grading systems should be carefully reviewed periodically with students and faculty for clarification and better student–faculty understanding.

(Reprinted by permission of the National Student Nurses' Association, Inc © 1978)

Figure 13–4. *(Continued)*

International Council of Nurses

The International Council of Nurses (ICN) is the international organization for professional nursing, with membership composed of national nursing organizations. The ANA, as a constituent member of the ICN, sends delegates to its convention and participates in its activities. The ICN is interested in health care in general and nursing care in particular throughout the world. It works with the United Nations when appropriate and with other international health-related groups, such as the International Red Cross.

The ICN concerns itself with such issues as the social and economic welfare of nurses, the role of the nurse in health care, and the roles of the various national nursing organizations throughout the world and their relationships to their governing bodies. The primary governing body of the organization is the Council of National Representatives, which meets biennially.

The ICN has representatives of 98 national nurses' organizations. Every 4 years a quadrennial congress is held. This meeting is open to all nurses and to delegates from the national organizations. Activities of the organization are carried out by the officers, volunteer nurse members of constituent organizations, and employed staff. The ICN maintains headquarters in Geneva, Switzerland.

American Nurses' Foundation

The ANA established the American Nurses' Foundation (ANF) as a tax-exempt, nonprofit corporation for the purpose of supporting research related to nursing. It is autonomous in financing and governance. The Board of Trustees is composed of members of the Board of Directors of the ANA, other nurse members, and nonnurse members from other health-related fields and from the public.

The ANF maintains a three-pronged approach to supporting research. The first objective is conducting policy analyses to provide nursing leaders and public policymakers with the information they will need for decision making. The second objective is related to developing a group of "nurse scholars" who engage in study in such areas as journalism and public policy. Support is directed toward independent study, research, and doctoral and postdoctoral work for these nurse scholars. The third objective is facilitating the research and educational activities of ANA. This includes providing consultation and funding for those groups within the ANA that wish to initiate projects.

To accomplish its varied objectives, the ANF solicits gifts and contributions from individuals and organizations. These gifts are tax deductible. The $62,000 in research grants awarded in 1986 brought the total that the ANF has contributed to nursing research since 1955 to $1.5 million (Foundation. . ., 1986).

American Academy of Nursing

The American Academy of Nursing (AAN) was established by the ANA as an honorary association within the ANA. The original members were chosen by the Board of Directors of the ANA. The AAN is now an independent organization, and new members are selected by those currently in the AAN. Those elected to the AAN are called fellows and may use the title Fellow of the American Academy of Nursing (FAAN). The purpose of this organization is to recognize those nurses who have made significant contributions to the profession of nursing in general.

THE NATIONAL LEAGUE FOR NURSING

Another major nursing organization is the National League for Nursing (NLN), which was established in 1952 and is often referred to simply as "The League." This organization fused seven organizations or committees into one. The groups were the National League of Nursing Education (1893), the National Organization for Public Health Nursing (1912), the Association of Collegiate Schools of Nursing (1933), the

Joint Committee on Practical Nurses and Auxiliary Workers in Nursing Services (1945), the Joint Committee on Careers in Nursing (1948), the National Committee for the Improvement of Nursing Services (1949), and the National Nursing Accrediting Service (1949).

Originally the National League of Nursing Education was organized under the title of the American Society of Superintendents of Training Schools for Nurses of the United States and Canada. Established in 1893, it was the first nursing organization in the United States. The name was changed to the National League of Nursing Education in 1912.

In 1989, after several years of planning the NLN again changed its structure. The changes were prompted by financial pressures, increased competition, and the need to diversify. In 1982 the NLN lost its bid for development of the state licensing examination for registered and practical nursing, which provided a major part of the operating budget for the organization. Other avenues had to be developed to maintain fiscal stability. Business operations needed to be separated from internal membership discussions and conflicts.

As part of the change the National League for Nursing, Incorporated became a subsidiary of the larger National League for Health Care, Incorporated (NLHC). The president of the NLN serves as a member of the Board of Trustees of the NLHC. Essentially this moved the NLN into a corporate structure, allowing it to be involved in both for-profit and not-for-profit ventures. Monies from the for-profit areas, such as publishing, can be returned to the NLN to provide assistance to support its activities.

Organizational Structure and Membership

The new National League for Nursing, Incorporated retained many of its previous activities and responsibilities. Its stated mission is to advance "the promotion of health and the provision of quality health care within a changing environment by promoting and monitoring effective nursing education and practice through collaborative efforts of nursing leaders, representatives of relevant agencies, and the general public" (Convention '89, 1989, p 387). It continues to offer membership to individuals and agencies and is unique among nursing organizations in its consumer participation. The NLN extends membership to members of the health care team, interested laypersons, institutions concerned with nursing service and nursing education, as well as to registered nurses.

The NLN is governed by a seven-member Board of Governors, three of whom are elected officers; president, president-elect and treasurer. The other members are elected as governors at large, and the final seat is that of secretary, which is filled by the chief executive officer of the NLN. The elected chairman of each of the councils of the NLN are also members of the Board of Governors. At present there are eleven councils:

The Council of Associate Degree Programs
The Council of Baccalaureate and Higher Degree Programs
The Council of Diploma Programs
The Council of Practical Nursing Programs
The Council of Community Health Services
The Council for Nursing Practice
The Council for Nursing Informatics
The Council for Society for Research in Nursing Education
The Council for Nursing Centers
The Council for Nurse Executives
The Council of Constituent Leagues

As you can easily determine by reviewing these titles, they provide representation from the various groups comprising the organization. Four of the councils represent different types of educational programs. Agencies may join any of the various councils, and individual members may maintain membership in more than one council should they so desire.

The final council listed, the Council of Constituent Leagues, represents the various organizations at the state level, although a few heavily populated states have more than one organization and in other less populated areas two states may be combined into one constituent league.

The NLN works in a complementary, rather than competitive, manner with the ANA. Whereas the ANA speaks as the official voice of nurses, the NLN seeks to unite the interests of nursing with those of the community. These two major nursing organizations along with the American Association of Colleges of Nursing (AACN) and the American Organization of Nurse Executives (AONE) form the membership of another group known as the Tri-Council. The Tri-Council is active in uniting and speaking for all nursing on issues and causes that will benefit the public and the profession.

Services Provided by the League

The NLN provides a number of vital services: accreditation, consultation services, continuing education, evaluation and testing, research, and publishing. In addition, the NLN assumes an active role in assuring that nursing has input into health policymaking. It provides information to the US House of Representatives, the US Senate, the Administration, and other policymakers and keeps the membership alert to key legislative issues. Of current interest is a national health care plan that has been developed by the NLN that was presented to Congress in the spring of 1991.

Accreditation

Most students are aware of the accreditation services, especially if they are attending an NLN-accredited school. Accreditation, which is voluntary, is one of the oldest services provided. Initially this was done by the National Nursing Accrediting Service, which, as mentioned earlier, was merged with other groups to form the NLN. It is currently carried out by the Division of Education and Accreditation Service of the NLN. The goals of accreditation include providing the public with well-prepared nurses, guiding students in the selection of a program, assuring the public of the quality of the school and its faculty, and stimulating the continued improvement in schools. Recently there has been a significant push toward evaluating the "outcomes" of the various educational programs rather than focusing more heavily on the process of education and its structure. The criteria for accreditation developed by each educational council reflected outcome-oriented criteria after June 1991.

Designated by the US Department of Education and by the Council on Postsecondary Accreditation as the accrediting body for all nursing programs the NLN currently accredits more than 1500 educational programs. The NLN also provides accreditation to home care and community health programs, which assures consumers that an agency meets national standards for care.

The schools and agencies seeking accreditation request this service and pay for it. Working with published criteria and guidelines, each school or agency prepares a rather involved self-study. After completing the self-study the school or agency is visited by representatives of the NLN. These visitors are either educators from other NLN-accredited schools or community health experts from accredited agencies, whichever is appropriate to the group seeking accreditation. These representatives have been specially selected and prepared to serve as voluntary visitors for the NLN. Their purpose in visiting the school or agency is to assess and evaluate the program and make recommendations about accreditation status. If the program is seeking continuation of ongoing accreditation and the recommendation of the visitors is to renew the accreditation status, the Board of Review does a limited review of the materials before voting on accreditation status. If the program is seeking initial accreditation or if the recommendation of the visitors is to deny

Figure 13-5. Accreditation is designed to help ensure that the desired outcomes of education are achieved.

or defer accreditation or impose other conditions, the program is then reviewed in full by the Board of Review.

The Board of Review is composed of eight nurse educators, one nursing service representative, and one public member, all of whom have been elected by schools that carry accreditation status. The Boards of Review meet twice each year for the purpose of reviewing programs. More and more schools and agencies are recognizing the value of NLN accreditation and are participating in the program.

A list of NLN-accredited programs is published each year in *Nursing and Health Care* and is available in pamphlets listing accredited schools and agencies.

Consultation

The NLN also offers consultation to schools that are seeking to improve their programs or that are initiating new programs and to health agencies that are seeking to improve services. This consultation usually takes the form of personal visits to the school by paid staff and appointed members, but consultations at NLN headquarters or by telephone are also offered.

Continuing Education

The NLN sponsors continuing education workshops and conferences throughout the country, often repeating a workshop in different locations to spare nurses and others the expense of travel. Subjects are determined in consultation with the councils and are geared to current needs and interest. Curriculum, research, accreditation, testing and evaluation, student recruitment and retention, political awareness and health care legislation, and a nurse executive series are regular subjects for continuing education. The NLN has developed and conducted workshops designed to assist the new graduate with the state licensing examination.

The constituent leagues, which are grouped by regional assemblies, offer workshops designed to meet the interests of particular areas of the country.

Evaluation and Testing

Students may also be aware of the testing and evaluation services of the NLN because it is the only testing service exclusive for nursing and health-related disciplines. The testing service provides pre-entrance testing to programs preparing practical and registered nurses as well as to graduate nursing programs. It also prepares achievement tests that can be administered to students who are enrolled in practical and professional programs while in school and proficiency examinations for nursing service personnel. The NLN working with the American Nursing Review also prepares materials and conducts workshops to assist new graduates to prepare for the licensure examination.

Research

When the US government needs figures on nursing education, it cites data gathered by NLN's Division of Research. The division is a primary provider of statistics on nursing education, each year surveying all schools of nursing and of practical nursing for enrollments, admissions, and graduations. It also conducts a yearly survey of newly registered nurses for characteristics of employment. Every 2 years the nurse–faculty census is taken; every 3 years data are gathered on men and minorities in schools of nursing. These data are published in the annual *Nursing Data Book*. The division also publishes the yearly "blue books," which contain essential information on state-approved schools of nursing and of practical nursing.

Other Services

The career information service answers the thousands of inquiries that come in every year about nursing education by mail and telephone. The NLN publishes annual lists of accredited schools of associate degree, baccalaureate, master's, diploma, and practical nursing programs, plus a list of doctoral programs and information on scholarships and loans. (Each of these booklets carries a nominal price.)

The Division of Public Policy and Research monitors the vital signs in Washington, D.C., and communicates its findings on legislation affecting nursing and nursing education through a monthly column in *Nursing & Health Care* and a quarterly newsletter, *Public Policy Bulletin.* Sometimes NLN spokespersons offer testimony on legislation or rulings significant to the organization.

Throughout this book, and especially in Chapter 2, we have referred to the NLN publications. As a nursing student you are already aware of the monthly magazine *Nursing & Health Care,* the official organ of the NLN. This journal focuses on administrative and educational concepts, better methods of care delivery, expanding roles and practice, and material of nursing theory and research. It does not carry articles on direct patient care or specific clinical material. The NLN also has a publications unit, which brings out papers and monographs of selected workshops or topics, the various research and recruitment materials, and nursing studies.

As a nursing student you may also have had the opportunity to watch one of many videotapes prepared by the NLN. *Nursing in America: A History of Social Reform* is widely used in nursing programs to celebrate and share with students the extraordinary achievements of nurses as social activists. Videotapes have also been developed that focus on basic skills, such as patient transfer and personal care, and on topics of interest to nursing educators and administrators.

The NLN consistently has pushed for better services for the consumer through improved education of nurses and improved delivery of services. They have continued a push begun in 1982 to improve the public image of the nurse. Students who wish to learn more about the NLN and its functions are encouraged to obtain the pamphlet *This Is the National League for Nursing* (publication No. 41-1532), available from the NLN in New York (see Appendix B for address).

NATIONAL FEDERATION OF LICENSED PRACTICAL NURSES

The National Federation of Licensed Practical Nurses (NFLPN) is one of the professional organizations for practical nurses. The NFLPN has worked with the ANA in regard to some of its activities and actively supports the need for the practical nurse in health care. State and local groups of the NFLPN are active in regard to educational issues for the licensed practical nurse and have supported the associate degree as an appropriate educational preparation for the responsibilities of the licensed practical nurse in the current health care system.

SPECIALIZED NURSING ORGANIZATIONS

In addition to the two major nursing organizations described, there are many other nursing organizations that have a special focus. These groups may have local organizations only in larger population centers; however, nurses may often join the national organization, regardless of whether there is a local chapter.

Clinically Related Organizations

Some of the earliest specialty organizations were related to specific clinical fields of nursing. A major focus of these organizations is continuing education related to the nursing specialty. One of the earliest specialty organizations was the American Association of Nurse Anesthetists, a group of approximately 24,000 members of whom 40% are male. Most of these groups also have some mechanisms, such as certification, for recognizing achievement in the field. Among them are groups that began as auxiliaries to specialty physicians' organizations such as the NAACOG: The Organization for Obstetric, Gynecological and Neonatal Nurses. This organization was started for nurses affiliated with physicians who were members of the American College of Obstetricians and Gynecologists. As more members joined and nurses became more active, these groups became autonomous. (See Appendix B for a listing of the major specialty groups.)

One concern has been the overlapping of purpose and action between the Councils on Practice of the ANA and the corresponding specialty organizations. One attempt to promote more cooperative effort was the creation of the Nursing Organization Liaison Forum (NOLF).

Groups Related to Ethnic Origin

As the movement for self-determination and preservation of identity arose within ethnic groups in the United States, nurses within ethnic groups began to unite for a greater voice in health care. Some groups are nationally organized. Other ethnic groups may be organized on a more local level.

Honorary Organizations

Sigma Theta Tau is an international organization established in collegiate schools of nursing to recognize those with superior ability, leadership potential, and contribution to nursing. Candidates may be asked to join during the senior year of a baccalaureate program or any time thereafter. Members are required to have a baccalaureate degree in nursing. Sigma Theta Tau has established a nursing library at its headquarters in Indianapolis that has reference abilities to support advanced scholarship. Local organizations may maintain funds to support individual research projects, hold research conferences, and recognize those who have made significant contributions to nursing.

Alpha Tau Delta is a professional nursing fraternity. Students who are enrolled in baccalaureate nursing programs and demonstrate scholarship and personality characteristics in line with the organization's professional goals are eligible for membership.

Religiously Oriented Organizations

The National Council of Catholic Nurses and the Nurses' Christian Fellowship (primarily a nondenominational Protestant group) were organized to assist nurses to share concerns and integrate their work and their religious beliefs. These two organizations place special emphasis on meeting the patient's spiritual needs and on dealing with ethical issues.

Educationally Oriented Organizations

There has been a great deal of change and development since the 1960s as nursing education has moved from the hospital into the educational setting. During this time there has been an increasing emphasis on educational methods, curriculum development, and research.

Regional Organizations

Within several major geographical regions of the United States, organizations open to schools of nursing, members of the state boards of nursing, and interested individuals were developed to promote interstate and interinstitutional cooperation in seeking pathways to improved nursing education and scholarship. These organizations are the Western Institute of Nursing (WIN), the Council on Collegiate Education for Nursing of the Southern Regional Education Board (CCEN/SREB), the New England Board of Higher Education (NEBHE), the Midwest Alliance in Nursing (MAIN), and the Mid-Atlantic Regional Nursing Association (MARNA).

National Organization for the Advancement of Associate Degree Nursing

One of the newest national organizations is the National Organization for the Advancement of Associate Degree Nursing (NOAADN). Organized in 1986, this group was the outgrowth of the development of several state organizations that were originated to focus attention on the value of associate degree education in nursing. The first state to initiate an organization was Texas, where the first chapter was started in 1984.

The NOAADN has four purposes: (1) to speak for associate degree nursing education and practice, (2) to reinforce the value of associate degree nursing education and practice, (3) to maintain endorsement of registered nurse licensure from state to state for the associate degree nurse, and (4) to retain the registered nurse licensure examination for graduates of associate degree nursing programs. To fulfill these goals, seven objectives have been incorporated into the bylaws of the organization that relate to activities soliciting support for associate degree nursing, including legislative activity.

Membership is open to individuals, states, agencies, and organizations, with varying dues assessed each group. In 1987 *AD Nurse* became the official publication for this organization. The title of this publication was later changed to *Advancing Clinical Care.*

American Association of Colleges of Nursing

The American Association of Colleges of Nursing (AACN) was formed to assist collegiate schools of nursing to work cooperatively to improve higher education for professional nursing. Membership is restricted to deans and directors of programs that offer a baccalaureate degree in nursing with an upper-division nursing major and that are part of a regionally accredited college or university. Likewise, hospital schools of nursing have formed the National Association of Hospital Schools of Nursing, the aim of which is to support quality education in diploma programs.

National Council of State Boards of Nursing

The National Council of State Boards of Nursing, Inc. (NCSBN), was organized in 1978 to replace the Council of State Boards that had been part of the ANA. The purpose of this organization is to provide a forum for the state boards to act together regarding matters of common concern, especially the development of the licensing examination. There is one delegate from each state board to this council. One reason given for establishing this independent organization rather than remaining within the ANA was to avoid any potential conflict of interest between the legal licensing authority and the professional organization. Although delegates to the 1978 ANA convention expressed dismay over this change, the ANA did vote to develop a liaison with the new council. The actions of this council are particularly important because its membership represents the legal authority for control of nursing education and nursing practice. Although each state board must operate within its own laws, it does have authority to establish many specific rules and regulations. Working together, the state boards hope to promote uniform standards for the nursing profession.

National Association for Practical Nurse Education and Service

The National Association for Practical Nurse Education and Service (NAPNES) informs the public about the role of the licensed practical nurse, promotes quality education for the practical nurse, develops guidelines and criteria for continuing education for practical nurses, and works with other groups that have similar or related interests. This organization has both institutional and individual memberships available. Institutional memberships are held by schools, practical nurse associations, health agencies, and others with concern for practical nursing education. Individual memberships are open. Many registered nurses who are employed in practical nursing education are members.

North American Nursing Diagnosis Association

The North American Nursing Diagnosis Association (NANDA) is open to individuals as well as to group members. The purpose of this group is to work toward a uniform terminology for nursing diagnosis and to share ideas and information regarding this topic. Individuals identify and research problems nurses manage, prepare documentation, and submit these to NANDA to be included in the consideration process. The individual problems are then reviewed by committees. Those that meet the basic criteria for nursing diagnoses are then submitted to the membership. A national convention held every two years serves as the final forum for debate and discussion of proposed new nursing diagnoses.

The general outline of the taxonomy (classification system) was established by a group of nursing theorists and then accepted by the organization.

Political Action Organizations

There are specific rules and regulations governing the conduct of individuals and groups in the political realm. A nonprofit professional organization may provide expert testimony in regard to an issue but is prohibited from actively lobbying on the behalf of either legislation or a candidate. As nurses have become more politically active, one of the routes they have chosen has been for the formation of specific political groups. The financing of these groups must not be related to any nonprofit organization, and membership must be voluntary. Political action groups are free to undertake lobbying efforts as well as to work on behalf of candidates. Many individual states have political action organizations for nurses. The ANA-CAP is the ANA's political action group (see Chapter 10).

Miscellaneous Organizations

The Gay Nurses' Alliance was an outgrowth of the movement of homosexuals to be accepted without having to disguise their sexual orientation. This group has primarily focused on the issue of gay rights. They also provide a forum for individuals to address the difficulties they may face in the nursing profession.

The American Assembly for Men in Nursing was formed for men who believe that, as a minority in the profession, they need to speak on issues with a united voice. The organization has addressed the issue of discrimination toward men in nursing and seeks to present a view of nursing as a profession in which both men and women can contribute and excel.

Nurses House Inc. provides assistance for nurses in need. It originated from a bequest in 1922 from Emily Bourne, who donated $300,000 to establish a country place where nurses might find needed rest. As the need for a specific residence decreased, those who had become supporters of this endeavor sold the estate and invested the proceeds. Income from the investment and other funds donated by nurses and friends of nurses are used to provide guidance and counseling for nurses with emotional and chemical dependency problems, encouragement to homebound nurses, and temporary financial assistance to nurses who are ill, convalescing, or unemployed. Nurses House seeks members to continue these activities and donations to support them.

OTHER HEALTH-RELATED ORGANIZATIONS

There are a great many of other health-related organizations in the United States. Some are open to nurses as members, and others have more restricted membership. Often the activities of these organizations affect the health care climate in which the nurse works. Knowledge of these organizations may help you to respond more effectively to their actions.

Health Problem-Related Groups

Many organizations focus on a particular illness or group of illnesses, such as the American Heart Association. Public information and education are usually a major part of their efforts. In addition, many of these groups actively support research, professional education, and patient care. Nurses may join these groups as much as any member of the public might because of an interest in supporting the work. In addition, nurses may join such groups because they also make available special educational opportunities regarding patient care. Nurses may actively participate in these organizations, serving on committees and running for office. Some of these organizations hire nurses to serve various educational roles.

Organizations of Other Health Care Professionals

Most health care professionals have a professional association. It is rare, however, to find as large a number of organizations as there are for nurses. One exception is the number of professional organizations for physicians. In addition to the American Medical Association, there are many clinical specialty organizations. These groups focus on the recognition of competence and continuing medical education within their specialty area.

Other professional groups, such as occupational therapists, physical therapists, medical record administrators, and dietitians have their own professional organizations. The American Hospital Association (AHA) is an organization of accredited hospitals throughout the country. The AHA focuses on concerns common to institutional health care providers. The American Nursing Home Association serves the same function for nursing homes.

Accrediting Organizations

Many organizations are important to nurses because they exert their influence through the process of accrediting institutions. The state legally may license an institution or allow it to function within regulations (a process variously called approval, accreditation, or licensing) based on meeting minimum standards for safety and effectiveness. Nongovernmental accrediting bodies also review health care institutions and schools of nursing based on criteria that reflect higher standards. Thus, among hospitals, some are allowed to function by the state, although they do not meet the more rigid criteria set by the Joint Commission on the Accreditation of Healthcare Organizations (JCAHO), formerly the Joint Commission on the Accreditation of Hospitals (JCAH). In the same way, schools of nursing may be approved by the state but may not be nationally accredited by the NLN.

Often a great deal of power is wielded through the criteria set by the accrediting body. One way that nurses have worked to alter conditions for delivering nursing care is by persuading the accrediting body to alter their criteria.

Those nursing programs that are part of colleges and universities are also reviewed by the regional accrediting organization for postsecondary institutions that accredit the college as a whole. Thus a nursing program may seek approval by the state board of nursing, by the NLN, and by the regional collegiate accrediting agency. This system may help to maintain quality in nursing education, but it may also create difficulties if the requirements of the various groups differ.

CONCLUSION

Any discussion of all the organizations related to nursing may seem confusing. It cannot be the most stimulating topic you have encountered; however, these organizations have far-reaching effects on the field of nursing and therefore will have a personal impact on you. We hope the information presented here will help you to be somewhat familiar with the many organizations and perhaps feel more secure when others begin to sprinkle their conversations with the "alphabet soup" of nursing acronyms. A more comprehensive listing of nursing-related organizations is included in Appendix B. We wish you good fortune as you make your personal decisions about membership.

REFERENCES

American Nurses' Association: Nursing: A Social Policy Statement. Kansas City, MO, American Nurses' Association, 1980

American Nurses' Association: The Nursing Practice Act: Suggested State Legislation. Kansas City, MO, American Nurses' Association, 1981

RN ranks grow. AM J Nurs 86(5):603–604, 1986

Snyder ME, LaBar C: Issues in Professional Practice: I. Nursing: Legal Authority for Practice. Kansas City, MO, American Nurses' Association, 1984

FURTHER READINGS

ADN educators organize new group to fight for RN license. Am J Nurs 86(7): 862, 1986

ANA honors nursing leaders. Am J Nurs 82(8):1142, 1982

Allen A: Tri-Council for Nursing issues statement on assistive personnel for the registered nurse. J Post Anesth Nurs 5(4):295–296, 1990

Christy T: The first fifty years. Am J Nurs 71(9):1778–1784, 1971

Convention 1982: ANA votes federation. Am J Nurs 82(8):1246, 1982

Convention '89. Nurse and Health Care 10(7):364–387, 1989

Curtin LL: Creating a culture of competence. Nurs Manage 21(9):l, 7–8, 1990

Facts About Nursing. Publication No. D-92. Kansas City, MO, American Nurses' Association, 1987

Forum considers nursing scope statement. Am Nurse 19:1, 1987

Foundation awards $62,000 in research grants. Am Nurse 18:18, Nov-Dec, 1986

Gilliland K et al: Specialty nursing council: A peer support group for nurses in independent roles. Clin Nurs Spec 4(1):38–42, 1990

Gunning CS et al: Identifying nursing's future leaders. Nurs Outlook 38(2):78–80, 1990

NSNA turns thirty. Am J Nurs 82(7):1024, 1982

Puetz BE: A federation of equals: National Federation of Specialty Organizations. Rehabil Nurs 14(6):316, 1989

Quinn S: ICN: Past and present. Int Nurs Rev 36(6):174–175, 1989

Schmidt MS: Why a separate organization for state boards? Am J Nurs 80(4): 725–726, 1980

Sigma Theta Tau International's "Actions for the 1990s." Reflections 16(1):1–2, 1990

Appendix A:
State Boards of Nursing

APPENDIX A: STATE BOARDS OF NURSING

For specific information regarding licensure requirements, regulations, and fees, write or telephone the specific board.

Alabama
State Board of Nursing
RSA Plaza, Suite 250
770 Washington Avenue
Montgomery, AL 36130
(205) 242-4060

Alaska
Board of Nursing
Division of Occupational
  Licensing
Frontier Building, Suite 722
3601 C Street
Anchorage, AK 99503
(907) 561-2878

Arizona
State Board of Nursing
Suite 350
2001 W. Camelback
Phoenix, AZ 85015
(602) 255-5092

Arkansas
State Board of Nursing
University Tower Building,
  Suite 800
1123 S. University Avenue
Little Rock, AR 72204
(501) 371-2751

California
Board of Registered Nursing
P.O. Box 944210
Sacramento, CA 94244-2100
(916) 322-3350

Board of Vocational Nurse and
  Psychiatric Technician
  Examiners
1414 K Street, Suite 103
Sacramento, CA 95814
(916) 445-0793

Colorado
State Board of Nursing
1560 Broadway, Suite 670
Denver, CO 80202
(206) 894-2430

Connecticut
Connecticut Board of Examiners
  for Nursing
150 Washington Street
Hartford, CT 6106
(203) 566-1032

Delaware
Board of Nursing
Margaret O'Neill Building,
  Box 1401
Dover, DE 19901
(302) 736-4522

District of Columbia
Board of Nursing
614 H Street, N.W., Room 923
Washington, DC 20001
(202) 727-7468

Florida
Board of Nursing
111 Coast Line Drive East,
  Suite 504
Jacksonville, FL 32202
(904) 359-6331

Georgia
Board of Nursing
166 Pryor Street, S.W.
Atlanta, GA 30303
RN (404) 656-3943
PN (404) 656-3921

Hawaii
Board of Nursing
Box 3469
Honolulu, HI 96801
(808) 548-4100

Idaho
State Board of Nursing
280 North 8th Street, Suite 210
Boise, ID 83720
(208) 334-3110

Illinois
Department of Professional
  Regulation
320 W. Washington Street,
  3rd Floor
Springfield, IL 62786
(217) 785-0820

Indiana
State Board of Nursing
Health Professions Bureau
402 West Washington Street,
  Room 041
Box 82067
Indianapolis, IN 46204
(317) 232-2960

Iowa
Iowa Board of Nursing
State Capitol Complex
1223 E. Court Avenue
Des Moines, IA 50319
(519) 281-3255

Kansas
State Board of Nursing
Landon State Office Building
900 SW. Jackson Street,
  Suite 551-S
Topeka, KS 66612-1256
(913) 296-4929

Kentucky
Board of Nursing
4010 Dupont Circle, Suite 430
Louisville, KY 40207
(502) 897-5143

Louisiana
Board of Nursing
150 Baronne Street, Room 907
New Orleans, LA 70112
(504) 568-5464

Board of Practical Nurse
  Examiners
Tidewater Place
1440 Canal Street, Suite 1722
New Orleans, LA 70112
(504) 568-6480

Maine
State Board of Nursing
State House Station #158
Augusta, ME 04330
(207) 624-5275

Maryland
Board of Nursing
4201 Patterson Avenue
Baltimore, MD 21215
(301) 764-4747

Massachusetts
Board of Registration in Nursing
100 Cambridge Street,
  Room 1519
Boston, MA 02202
(617) 727-9961

Michigan
Board of Nursing
Department of Licensing
and Regulation
Ottawa Towers North
611 W. Ottawa, Box 30018
Lansing, MI 48909
(517) 373-1600

Minnesota
Board of Nursing
2700 University Avenue W.,
#108
St. Paul, MN 55114
(612) 642-0567

Mississippi
Board of Nursing
239 North Lamar Street,
Suite 401
Jackson, MS 39201
(601) 359-6170

Missouri
State Board of Nursing
P.O. Box 656
Jefferson City, MO 65102
(314) 751-0681

Montana
Board of Nursing
Division of Professional and
Occupational Licensing
Arcade Building, Lower Level
111 N. Jackson
Helena, MT 59620-0407
(406) 444-4279

Nebraska
Board of Nursing
Department of Health, Bureau of
Examining Boards
P.O. Box 95007
Lincoln, NE 68509
(402) 471-2115

Nevada
Board of Nursing
1281 Terminal Way, Suite 116
Reno, NV 89502
(702) 786- 2778

New Hampshire
Board of Nursing
Division of Public Health Services
Health and Welfare Building
6 Hazen Drive
Concord, NH 03301-6527
(603) 271-2323

New Jersey
Board of Nursing
P.O. Box 45010
Newark, NJ 07101
(201) 648-2570

New Mexico
Board of Nursing
4253 Montgomery N.E.,
Suite 130
Albuquerque, NM 87109
(505) 841-8340

New York
State Education Department
Division of Professional Licensing
Services
Cultural Education Center,
Room 9B30
Albany, NY 12230
(518) 474-3843

North Carolina
Board of Nursing
P.O Box 2129
Raleigh, NC 27602
(919) 782-3211

North Dakota
Board of Nursing
919 S. 7th Street, Suite 504
Bismarck, ND 58504
(701) 224-2974

Ohio
Board of Nursing
77 S. High Street, 7th Floor
Columbus, OH 43266-0316
(614) 466-3947

Oklahoma
Board of Nurse Registration and
  Nursing Education
2915 Classen Blvd., Suite 524
Oklahoma City, OK 73106
(405) 525-2076

Oregon
State Board of Nursing
10445 SW. Canyon Road,
  Suite 200
Beaverton, OR 97005
(503) 644-2767

Pennsylvania
State Board of Nursing
Department of State
Box 2649
Harrisburg, PA 17105-2649
(717) 783-7142

Rhode Island
Board of Nurse Education and
  Registration
Cannon Health Building,
  Room 104
3 Capitol Hill
Providence, RI 02908
(401) 277-2827

South Carolina
State Board of Nursing
220 Executive Center Drive,
  Suite 220
Columbia, SC 29210
(803) 731-1648

South Dakota
Board of Nursing
3307 South Lincoln Avenue
Sioux Falls, SD
57105-5224
(605) 335-4973

Tennessee
Board of Nursing
283 Plus Park Blvd.
Nashville, TN 37247-1010
(615) 367-6232

Texas
Board of Nurse Examiners—RN
Box 140466
Austin, TX 78714
(512) 835-4880

Texas Board of Vocational Nurse
  Examiners
9101 Burnet Road, Suite 105
Austin, TX 78758

Utah
Division of Occupational and
  Professional Licensing
Board of Nursing
160 E. 300 South
P.O. Box 45802
Salt Lake City, UT 84145-0802
(801) 530-6628

Vermont
Board of Nursing
Redstone Building
26 Terrace Street
Montpelier, VT 05602
(802) 828-2396

Virginia
Board of Nursing
Department of Health
  Professions
1601 Rolling Hills Drive
Richmond, VA 23229-5005
(804) 662-9909

Washington
Board of Nursing—RN
Department of Health
P.O. Box 1099
Olympia, WA 98507-1099
(206) 753-2206

Board of Practical Nursing
1300 SE Quince Street, EY-28
Olympia, WA 98504
(206) 753-2807

West Virginia
Board of Examiners for
  Registered Nurses
Embleton Building
922 Quarrier Street, Suite 309
Charleston, WV 25301
(304) 348-3572

Board of Examiners for Practical
  Nurses
Embleton Building
922 Quarrier Street, Suite 506
Charleston, WV 25301
(304) 348-3572

Wisconsin
Bureau of Health Service
  Professions
Box 8935
Madison, WI 53708
(608) 266-3735

Wyoming
Board of Nursing
Barrett Building, 2nd Floor
2301 Central Avenue
Cheyenne, WY 82002
(307) 777-7601

U.S. TERRITORIES

American Samoa
American Samoa Health Service
  Regulatory Board
LBJ Tropical Medical Center
Pago Pago, American Samoa
(684) 633-1222 ext. 206

Guam
Board of Nurse Examiners
P.O. Box 2816
Agana, Guam 96910

Northern Mariana Islands
Board of Nurse Examiners
Public Health Center
P.O. Box 1458
Saipan, Northern Mariana Islands
  96950
(011-670) 234-8950

Puerto Rico
Office of Regulations and
  Certification of Health
  Professionals
Attn: Board of Nurse Examiners
Call Box 10200
San Juan, PR 00908
(809) 725-8161

Virgin Islands
Board of Nursing
Medical Arts Complex, Suite 13
P.O. Box 4247, Charlotte Amalie
St. Thomas, VI 00803

Appendix B:
Nursing-Related
Organizations

APPENDIX B: NURSING-RELATED ORGANIZATIONS

Nursing-Related Organizations

Overall Professional Organizations

	Year Established	Membership Eligibility	Publications (monthly unless otherwise noted)
American Nurses' Association (ANA) 2420 Pershing Road Kansas City, MO 64108	1896	RNs only	*American Journal of Nursing, The Amercan Nurse* (for others, write for list)
International Council of Nurses (ICN) Box 42 1121 Geneva 20, Switzerland	1900	National professional nurse organizations	
National Federation of Specialty Nursing Organizations (NFSNO) 22 Euclid St. Woodbury, NJ 08096		Specialty nursing organizations	
National Student Nurse Association (NSNA) 55 West 57th Street New York, NY 10019	1953	Officially enrolled students of RN and RN baccalaureate programs	*Imprint* (5 times/yr)
National League for Nursing (NLN) 350 Hudson Street New York, NY 10014	1952	Individuals and agencies interested in the profession of nursing and delivery of nursing care	*Nursing and Health Care* (for others; write for list)

Organizations Related to Scholarship and Leadership in Nursing

Organization	Year	Membership	Publication
American Academy of Nurses (AAN) c/o American Nurses' Association 2420 Pershing Road Kansas City, MO 64108	1973	Members elected by current members, based on contribution to nursing Use title "Fellow" (FAAN)	*Nursing Outlook* (bimonthly)
Alpha Tau Delta 14631 North 2nd Drive Phoenix, AZ 85023	1921	Students in baccalaureate programs in nursing	*Captions of Alpha Tau delta* (biennial)
Sigma Theta Tau International 550 West North Street Indianapolis, IN 46202-3163	1922	High achievers: senior students in baccalaureate, master's, and doctoral programs; outstanding RNs with baccalaureate or higher degree	*Image, Reflections* (newsletters, both quarterly)

Groups Related to Ethnic/Racial Origin

American Indian Nurses Association (AINA) PO Box 1588 Norman, OK 73071	1972	Student nurses and RNs of American Indian ancestry	*Newsletter of the AINA* (bimonthly)
National Black Nurses Association, Inc, 1012 Tenth Street, NW Washington, DC 20001	1971	African-American RNs	*Journal of National Black Nurses' Association* (twice yearly)

APPENDIX B: NURSING-RELATED ORGANIZATIONS *(continued)*

Nursing-Related Organizations

	Year Established	Membership Eligibility	Publications *(monthly unless otherwise noted)*
National Association of Hispanic Nurses 2300 West Commerce Street San Antonio, TX 78207	1976	Hispanic nurses, associate/all nurses	Newsletter (quarterly)
Phillipine Nurses Association of America, Inc. 459 Joan Street South Painfield, NJ 07080		Filipino nurses and those interested in their issues	
Association of Black Nursing Faculty in Higher Education, Inc. 5823 Queens Cove Lisle, IL 60532		Nursing faculty members of African-American background and those interested in their issues	

Educationally Oriented Associations

	Year Established	Membership Eligibility	Publications *(monthly unless otherwise noted)*
American Association of Colleges of Nursing (AACN) One Dupont Circle NW Suite 530 Washington, DC 20036-1110	1969	Collegiate program with upper-division major in nursing	*Journal of Professional Nursing* (bimonthly) *AACN Newsletter* (10 times/yr) (for others, write for list)
Council on Collegiate Education for Nursing for the Southern Regional Education Board (SREB) 1340 Spring Street NW Atlanta, GA 30309	1963	Colleges and universities in the southern states that have nursing programs	Write for list

496

Organization	Founded	Membership	Publication
Mid-Atlantic Regional Nursing Association (MARNA) 350 Hudson Street New York, NY 10014	1981	Agencies preparing persons in health care and that deliver health care	*Marnagram* (quarterly)
Midwest Alliance in Nursing, Inc. (MAIN) 2511 East 46th Street, Suite E-3 Indianapolis, IN 46205	1979	Agencies engaged in providing direct nursing care or teaching persons to provide direct care	*MAINlines* (bimonthly newsletter)
National Association for Practical Nurse Education and Service, Inc. (NAPNES) 1400 Spring Street, Suite 310 Silver Springs, MD 20910	1941	All persons interested in LPN/LVN education	*Journal of Practical Nursing* (quarterly) *NAPNES Forum*
National Organization for the Advancement of Associate Degree Nursing (NOAADN) Amarillo College PO Box 447 Amarillo, TX 79178	1985	Open	*Advancing Clinical Care*
North American Nursing Diagnosis Association (NANDA) St. Louis University School of Nursing 3525 Caroline Street Room 439 St. Louis, MO 63104	1976	RNs	*Nursing Diagnoses*
New England Organization for Nursing Hewitt Hall, University of New Hampshire Durham, NC 03824	1964	Colleges and universities in the New England states that have nursing programs	Write for list

APPENDIX B: NURSING-RELATED ORGANIZATIONS (continued)

Nursing-Related Organizations

	Year Established	Membership Eligibility	Publications (monthly unless otherwise noted)
Western Institute of Nursing (WIN) PO Drawer P Boulder, CO 80302	1957	Colleges and universities in the western states that have nursing programs	Write for list
Occupational or Specialty-Related Nursing Organizations			
Advocates for Child Psychiatric Nursing 267 Pikley Place San Francisco, CA 94123			
American Academy of Ambulatory Nursing Administration North Woodbury Road, Box 56 Pitman, NJ 08071	1974	RNs in administration of ambulatory nursing	
American Association of Critical Care Nurses (AACN) One Civic Plaza Newport Beach, CA 92660	1969	RNs, LPNs., student nurses	Heart and Lung Journal (bimonthly) Focus on Critical Care (bimonthly)
American Association for the History of Nursing PO Box 90803 Washington, DC 20003	1980	Anyone interested in the history of nursing	The Bulletin (4 times per year)

Organization	Founded	Membership	Publications
American Association of Neuroscience Nurses (AANN) 218 North Jefferson Suite 204 Chicago, IL 60606	1968	RNs	*Journal of Neuroscience Nursing* (bimonthly)
American Association of Nurse Anesthetists (AANA) 216 Higgins Road Park Ridge, IL 60068	1931	RNs who are certified registered nurse anesthetists (CRNAs)	*American Association of Nurse Anesthetists Journal* (bimonthly) *AANA Bulletin* (bimonthly)
The American Association of Nurse Attorneys (TAANA) 720 Light Street Baltimore, MD 21230-3826	1982	Nurses who are attorneys or are in law school and attorneys in nursing schools	*Inside TAANA* (newletter, quarterly)
American Association of Occupational Health Nurses (AAOHN), Inc. 50 Lenox Pointe Atlanta, GA 30324	1942	RNs practicing in an occupational health setting	*AAOHN Journal* *AAOH News*
American Association of Spinal-Cord Injury Nurses 75-20 Astoria Blvd. Jackson Heights, NY 11370-1178			
American Burn Association c/o Dr. Charles E. Hartford Burn Treatment Center Crozier-Chester Medical Center 15th and Upland Avenue Chester, PA 19013		Professionals working with burn patients	

APPENDIX B: NURSING-RELATED ORGANIZATIONS *(continued)*

Nursing-Related Organizations

	Year Established	Membership Eligibility	Publications (monthly unless otherwise noted)
American College of Nurse Midwives (ACNM) 1522 K Street, NW, Suite 1120 Washington, DC 20005	1955	RNs who are certified Nurse Midwives or students in accredited programs	*Journal of Nurse Midwifery* *Quickening* (newsletter)
American Holistic Nurses Association 401 Lake Boon Trail, Suite 201 Raleigh, NC 27607	1981	Active: RN, LPN/LVN Contributing; all others	*Journal of Holistic Nursing* (annual) *Beginnings* (newsletter)
American Nephrology Nurses Association (AANA) North Woodbury Road Box 56 Pitman, NJ 08071	1969	RNs, LVNs employed in the field	*Journal of AANA* (6 times per year) *AANA Update* (newsletter)
American Organization of Nurse Executives 840 North Lake Shore Drive Chicago, IL 60611		RNs in administrative positions	
American Public Health Association (APHA) Public Health Nursing Section 1015 15th Street, NW Washington, DC 20005	1972	All persons interested in Public Health Various categories of membership available	*American Journal of Public Health* *The Nation's Health*

Organization	Year	Membership	Publication
American Radiological Nurses Association 10110 Forum Park Drive Houston, TX 77036	1981	Active: RNs employed in radiologic nursing Associate: other RNs and LPNs in radiologic nursing	*ARNA Images* (4 times/yr)
American Society of Ophthalmic Registered Nurses (ASORN), Inc. PO Box 193030 San Francisco, CA 94119	1976	RNs working in ophthalmology	*Insight* (newsletter)
American Society for Parenteral and Enteral Nutrition—Nurses' Committee 8630 Fenton Street, Suite 412 Silver Springs, MD 20910-3803	1975	Multidisciplinary: professionals working with parenteral and enteral nutrition	
American Society of Plastic and Reconstructive Surgical Nurses, Inc. Box 56, N. Woodbury Road Pitman, NJ 08071	1975	Active: RNs, LPNs working in the field Associate: RNs, LPNs interested in the field	*Journal of Plastic and Reconstructive Surgical Nursing*
American Society of Post-Anesthesia Nurses 11512 Allecingie Parkway Richmond, VA 23235	1980	RNs, LPNs, Anesthesiologists, CRNAs	*Breathline* *Journal of Post Anesthesia Nursing* (quarterly)
American Urological Association Allied 11512 Allecingie Parkway, Suite C Richmond, VA 23235	1972	Active: RNs, LPNs, PAs, technicians Associate: industry, physicians	*AUAA Journal* (quarterly) *Urogram* (newsletter)

APPENDIX B: NURSING-RELATED ORGANIZATIONS (continued)

Nursing-Related Organizations

	Year Established	Membership Eligibility	Publications (monthly unless otherwise noted)
Association for Practitioners in Infection Control 505 E. Hawley Street Mundelein, IL 60060	1972	Active: professionals in infection control Associate: others	AJIC (bimonthly) (others: write)
Association for the Care of Children's Health 3615 Wisconsin Avenue, NW Washington, DC 20016	1965	All individuals interested in children's health	Children's Health Care (for others, write for list)
Association of Operating Room Nurses (AORN) 10170 East Mississippi Avenue Denver, CO 80231	1949	Active: RNs employed in OR or in a related educational program or in research	AORN Journal
Association of Pediatric Oncology Nurses Suite 3A 11512 Allecingie Parkway Richmond, VA 23235	1976	RNs	APON Newsletter (quarterly) (for others, write for list)
Association of Rehabilitation Nurses 5700 Old Orchard Road, 1st Floor Skokie, IL 60077	1974	Regular: RNs Associate: all interested persons	Rehabilitation Nursing (bimonthly journal) Pamphlets
Coalition of Nurse Practitioners, Inc. PO Box 123 East Greenbush, NY	1980	Nurse practitioners and students in nurse practitioner programs	Coalition Communique (quarterly)

Organization	Year	Membership	Publication
Department of School Nurses of the National Education Association (NEA) 1201 Sixteenth Street, NW Washington, DC 20036	1968	School nurse members of the NEA	*The School Nurse*
Dermatology Nurses' Association North Woodbury Road Box 56 Pitman, NJ 08071	1981	Active: RNs, LPNs/LVNs involved in dermatology	*DNA Focus* (bimonthly newsletter)
Drug and Alcohol Nursing Association 113 W. Franklin Street Baltimore, MD 21201	1979	Active: nurses caring for clients with drug- and alcohol-related disorders Associate: all others	*DANA Newsletter* (quarterly)
Emergency Nurses Association (ENA) 230 East Ohio Suite 600 Chicago, IL 60611	1970	RNs	*The Journal of Emergency Nursing Emergency Nursing Core Curriculum*
Flight Nurse Section Aerospace Medical Association Washington National Airport Washington, DC 20001	1964	Designated flight nurses and RNs who are members of Aerospace Medical Association	*Aviation, Space, and Environmental Medicine*
International Association for Enterostomal Therapy (IAET), Inc. 2081 Business Center Drive Suite 290 Irvine, CA 92715	1968	Active: graduate of accredited IAET program	*Journal of Enterostomal Therapy*
Intravenous Nurses' Society, Inc. 2 Brighton Street Belmont, MA 02178	1973	Nurses interested in intravenous therapy	*Journal of Intravenous Therapy*

APPENDIX B: NURSING-RELATED ORGANIZATIONS (continued)

Nursing-Related Organizations

	Year Established	Membership Eligibility	Publications (monthly unless otherwise noted)
NAACOG: The Organization for Obstetric, Gynecologic, and Neonatal Nurses 409 12th Street, SW Washington, DC 20024-2191	1969	RNs and allied health individuals in OGN area	Journal of Obstetric, Gynecologic and Neonatal Nursing (JOGN) (bimonthly) NAACOG Newletter
National Association for Health Care Recruitment PO Box 93851 Cleveland, OH 44101-5851	1975	Active: health care recruiters	Recruitment Directions (10 times/yr)
National Association of Neonatal Nurses 191 Lynch Creek Way Petaluma, CA 94954	1984	Regular: RNs Associate: all others	Neonatal Network: The Journal of Neonatal Nursing (bimonthly)
National Association of Orthopaedic Nurses North Woodbury Road Box 56 Pitman, NJ 08071	1980	RNs, LPNs, LVNs	Orthapaedic Nursing (for others, write for list)
National Association of Pediatric Nurse Associates/Practitioners (NAPNAP) 1101 King's Highway North, Suite 206 Cherry Hill, NJ 08034	1973	RNs with advanced education who are primary care practitioners in pediatrics	The Pediatric Nurse Practitioner (newsletter) The Journal of Pediatric Health Care

Organization	Founded	Membership	Publications
National Association of School Nurses Lamplighter Lane, PO Box 1300 Scarborough, ME 04074	1969	Active: RNs employed by educational institutions Other categories for students, retirees, organizations	*School Nurse Journal* *NAS Newsletter* (quarterly)
National Flight Nurses Association 6900 Grove Road Thorofare, NJ 08086-9447	1981		*Aeromedical Journal* (bimonthly) *Across the Board* (quarterly)
National Nurses Society on Addiction 5700 Old Orchard Road, First Floor Skokie, IL 60077	1983	Regular: RNs Associate: all others	*Annual Review of Nursing and the Addictions* Quarterly newsletter
Nurse Consultants Association, Inc. 414 Plaza Drive, Suite 209 Westmont, IL 60559	1979	RNs with 60% of income from consultant-type sources	Quarterly newsletter Annual membership directory
Nurses Organization of Veteran's Affairs 6728 Old McLean Village Drive McLean, VA 22101			
Society for Peripheral Vascular Nursing (SPVN) 309 Winter Street Norwood, MA 02062	1982	Active: currently licensed nurses	*SPVN Journal* (quarterly)
Society of Gastroenterology Nurses and Associates, Inc. 1070 Sibley Tower Rochester, NY 14604	1974	Individuals employed as gastrointestinal nurses or assistants	*Gastroenterology Nursing* (bimonthly)

APPENDIX B: NURSING-RELATED ORGANIZATIONS (continued)

Nursing-Related Organizations

	Year Established	Membership Eligibility	Publications (monthly unless otherwise noted)
Society of Otorhinolaryngology and Head-Neck Nurses, Inc. 439 N. Causeway New Smyrna Beach, FL 32169	1976	RNs actively working in ORL/head-neck nursing	ORL-Head and Neck Nursing (4 times/year) Update (quarterly newsletter)
Transcultural Nursing Society College of Nursing University of Utah 25 S. Medical Drive Salt Lake City, UT 84112	1979	Nurses and nonnurses	Biannual newsletter
World Federation of Neurosurgical Nurses Avenue Appia 1211 Geneva 27 Switzerland		Professional nurses working in neurosurgery	
Miscellaneous			
American Assembly for Men in Nursing PO Box 31753 Independence, OH 44131	1971	All men in nursing	*Interaction*
National Nurses for Life 1998 Menold Allison Park, PA 15104			

Nurses' Alliance for the Prevention of Nuclear War 225 Lafayette Street Room 207 New York, NY 10012	1981	RNs, students, allied health, general public	*Aegis* (quarterly newsletter)
Nurses Christian Fellowship 6400 Schroeder Road PO Box 7895 Madison, WI 53707	1948	Christian students and RNs	*Journal of Christian Nursing* (quarterly)
Nurses Educational Funds 555 West 57th Street New York, NY 10019	1911	Donors welcome	Semiannual newsletter
Nurses Environmental Health Watch 33 Columbus Avenue Sommerville, MA 02143			
Nurses' House, Inc. 350 Hudson Street New York, NY 10014	1925	Payment of annual contribution	

Appendix C: State Nursing Organizations

APPENDIX C: STATE NURSING ORGANIZATIONS

Alabama State Nurses' Association
360 North Hull Street
Montgomery, AL 36197
(205) 262-8321

Alaska Nurses' Association
237 East Third Avenue
Anchorage, AK 99501
(907) 274-0827

Arizona Nurses' Association
1850 E. Southern Avenue, Suite 1
Tempe, AZ 85282
(602) 831-0404

Arkansas State Nurses' Association
117 South Cedar Street
Little Rock, AR 72205
(501) 664-5853

California Nurses' Association
1855 Folsom Street, Room 670
San Francisco, CA 94103
(415) 864-4141

Colorado Nurses' Association
5453 East Evans Place
Denver, CO 80222
(303) 757-7484

Connecticut Nurses' Association
Meritech Business Park
377 Research Parkway, Suite 2D
Meriden, CT 06450
(203) 238-1207

Delaware Nurses' Association
2634 Capitol Trail, Suite C
Newark, DE 19711
(302) 368-2333

District of Columbia Nurses' Association, Inc.
5100 Wisconsin Avenue, NW, Suite 306
Washington, DC 20016
(202) 244-2705

Florida Nurses' Association
PO Box 536985
Orlando, FL 32853-6985
(305) 896-3261

Georgia Nurses' Association, Inc.
1362 West Peachtree Street, NW
Atlanta, GA 30309
(404) 876-4624

Guam Nurses' Association
Post Office Box 3134
Agana, GU 96910
(671) 646-5801

Hawaii Nurses' Association
677 Ala Moana Blvd., Suite 301
Honolulu, HI 96813
(808) 531-1628

Idaho Nurses' Association
200 North 4th Street, Suite 20
Boise, ID 83702-6001
(208) 345-0500

Illinois Nurses' Association
20 North Wacker Drive, Suite 2520
Chicago, IL 60606
(312) 236-9708

Indiana State Nurses' Association
2915 North High School Road
Indianapolis, IN 46224
(317) 299-4575/4576

Iowa Nurses' Association
100 Court Avenue, 9LL
Des Moines, IA 50309
(515) 282-9169

Kansas State Nurses' Association
700 S.W. Jackson, Suite 601
Topeka, KS 66603
(913) 233-8638

Kentucky Nurses' Association
1400 South First Street
PO Box 2616
Louisville, KY 40201
(502) 637-2546/2547

Louisiana State Nurses' Association
712 Transcontinental Drive
Metairie, LA 70001
(504) 889-1030

Maine State Nurses' Association
PO Box 2240
Augusta, ME 04330
(207) 622-1057

Maryland Nurses' Association, Inc.
5820 Southwestern Boulevard
Baltimore, MD 21227
(301) 242-7300

Massachusetts Nurses' Association
340 Turnpike Street
Canton, MA 02021
(617) 821-4625

Michigan Nurses' Association
2310 Jolly Oak Road
Okemos, MI 48864
(517) 349-5640

Minnesota Nurses' Association
1295 Bandana Blvd. N, Suite 140
St. Paul, MN 55108-5115
(612) 646-4807

Mississippi Nurses' Association
135 Bounds Street, Suite 100
Jackson, MS 39206
(601) 982-9182

Missouri Nurses' Association
206 East Dunklin Street, Box 325
Jefferson City, MO 65101
(314) 636-4623

Montana Nurses' Association
104 Broadway, Suite G-2
PO Box 5718
Helena, MT 59604
(406) 442-6710

Nebraska Nurses' Association
941 O Street, Suite 707-711
Lincoln, NE 68508
(402) 475-3859

Nevada Nurses' Association
3660 Baker Lane, Suite 104
Reno, NV 89509
(702) 825-3555

New Hampshire Nurses' Association
48 West Street
Concord, NH 03301
(603) 225-3783

New Jersey State Nurses' Association
320 West State Street
Trenton, NJ 08618
(609) 392-4884

New Mexico Nurses' Association
909 Virginia NE, Suite 101
Albuquerque, NM 87108
(505) 268-7744

**New York State Nurses'
Association**
2113 Western Avenue
Guilderland, NY 12084
(518) 456-5371

**North Carolina Nurses'
Association**
Box 12025
103 Enterprise Street
Raleigh, NC 27605
(919) 821-4250

**North Dakota Nurses'
Association**
Green Tree Square
212 North Fourth Street
Bismarck, ND 58501
(701) 223-1385

Ohio Nurses' Association
4000 East Main Street
Columbus, OH 43213-2950
(614) 237-5414

Oklahoma Nurses' Association
6414 North Santa Fe, Suite A
Oklahoma City, OK 73116
(405) 840-3476

**Oregon Nurses'
Association, Inc.**
9600 SW Oak Street,
  Suite 550
Portland, OR 97223
(503) 293-0011

**Pennsylvania Nurses'
Association**
2578 Interstate Drive
PO Box 8525
Harrisburg, PA 17105-8525
(717) 657-1222

**Rhode Island State Nurses'
Association**
Hall Building South
345 Blackstone Boulevard
Providence, RI 02906
(401) 421-9703

**South Carolina Nurses'
Association**
1821 Gadsden Street
Columbia, SC 29201
(803) 252-4781

**South Dakota Nurses'
Association, Inc.**
1505 South Minnesota, Suite 6
Sioux Falls, SD 57105
(605) 338-1401

Tennessee Nurses' Association
545 Mainstream Drive, Suite 405
Nashville, TN 37228-1207
(615) 329-2511

Texas Nurses' Association
Community Bank Building
300 Highland Mall Blvd.,
  Suite 300
Austin, TX 78752-3718
(512) 452-0648

Utah Nurses' Association
1058A East 900 South
Salt Lake City, UT 84105
(801) 322-3439/3430

**Vermont State Nurses'
Association, Inc.**
500 Dorset Street
South Burlington, VT 05403
(802) 864-9390

**Virgin Islands Nurses'
Association**
PO Box 583
Christiansted
St. Croix, VI 00820
(809) 773-2323, ext. 116/118

Virginia Nurses' Association
1311 High Point Avenue
Richmond, VA 23230
(804) 353-7311

**Washington State Nurses'
Association**
2505 2nd Avenue, Suite 500
Seattle, WA 98121
(206) 443-9762

**West Virginia Nurses'
Association, Inc.**
2 Players Club Drive, Bldg. #3
PO Box 1946
Charleston, WV 25327
(304) 342-1169

**Wisconsin Nurses'
Association, Inc.**
6117 Monona Drive
Madison, WI 53716
(608) 221-0383

Wyoming Nurses' Association
Majestic Building, Room 305
1603 Capitol Avenue
Cheyenne, WY 82001
(307) 635-3955

Index